Reflexology

Susan Cressy

Heinemann

Heinemann Educational Publishers,

Halley Court, Jordan Hill, Oxford OX2 8EJ

Part of Harcourt Education

Heinemann is the registered trademark of Harcourt Education Limited

First published 2002

2006 2005 2004

10 9 8 7 6 5 4 3 2

A catalogue record for this book is available from the British Library on request.

ISBN 0 435 45104 9

Designed, typeset and illustrated by Hardlines, Charlbury, Oxon

Printed and bound in Italy by Printer Trento S.r.l.

Tel: 01865 888058 www.heinemann.co.uk

CONTENTS

Acknowledgements

I would like to thank all my former and present students who provided me with the inspiration to continue writing.

My close friend and colleague Terri Melnyk, for contributing her time and energy in helping with the photographs and for her critical analysis of the text and foot maps.

Jennifer Zucker, Kathy Fitzgerald, David Morris, Faye Ramjaun, Judith Provan, Bryn Williams, Jayne Salt, Helen Stewart, and all the staff at David Lloyd Health and Beauty, Manchester for their contributions to the photographic sessions.

Sue Zachariassen and Jennifer Zucker for proof reading.

Pen Gresford, commissioning editor at Heinemann, whose persuasive powers convinced me to write this book, Rachel Gear, senior editor, and all at Heinemann who have been involved in its production.

Janine Corciulo of Lido's, Altrincham, Cheshire (www.lidos-spa.co.uk) for kindly supplying illustrations and photos.

Sumita Lynch at Tulsi Health and Beauty Spa for kindly supplying photos.

Finally I would like to thank my family for their constant support and encouragement, and for enduring neglect over the last twelve months and, in particular, my son Thomas for giving up his precious holiday and allowing me to use his feet in the photographs.

Photo acknowledgments

The author and publishers would like to thank Sally Smith (photo research and photoshoot direction), Gareth Boden (photography) and Tony Poole (photographic assistance).

Gareth Boden, p.11, 12, 17, 37, 65, 66, 67, 68, 69, 70, 71, 72, 73, 74, 75, 76, 77
Lido's p. 173 (bottom), 176, 192, 201, 203 (bottom)
Medipics p. 45, 46, (top), 126 (malignant melanoma)
Science Photo Library p. 44 (top). 98
Science Photo Library/Biophoto Associates p.44 (bottom), 46 (middle)
Science Photo Library/Dr. P. Marazzi p.46 (bottom), 47, 126 (eczema, psoriasis and rosacea)
Science Photo Library/Gaillard Jerrican p. 28
Science Photo Library/Michael Donne p. 83
Science Photo Library/Oscar Burriel p. 84 (top)
Science Photo Library/St Bartholomew's Hospital p.126 (top)
Science Photo Library/Steve Horrell p. 84 (bottom)
Tulsi Health and Beauty Spa p. 173 (top), 203

Preface and

Introduction

Preface

Reflexology is a natural holistic therapy using special techniques on the feet and hands to stimulate specific points and initiate a beneficial response in another area of the body. As people are becoming more and more aware of the benefits of holistic therapies in general, there is an increasing demand from students for comprehensive, professional courses of study. There are, therefore, different methods and techniques taught by practitioners of reflexology and whichever technique is employed, they all achieve the same results when performed correctly by a professional and competent reflexologist.

To become a fully competent and professional reflexologist it is essential to acquire the required knowledge to support the development of practical skills. The purpose of this book is to provide a comprehensive source of reference for the student, teacher and qualified reflexologist to include the practice of reflexology, the importance of consultation, client care and the provision of aftercare advice. I have included the essential anatomy and physiology of the foot and all the body systems with their corresponding reflex points, thus providing an understanding of the body and how it works. I have also devoted a complete chapter to stress and the effects it has on the body, as this is an important factor for the reflexologist when providing treatment.

I have worked with students in beauty and holistic therapy for seventeen years and the one area that I am consistently asked to provide information for is the setting up of a business. I have devoted several chapters to all stages of business planning to include market research, finding premises and equipment, obtaining professional advice, raising finance, the legal requirements and formulating a business plan for a new or existing business. I have continued with an operational plan which provides essential information concerning the practical aspects of running a business and increasing profits.

This book covers all the requirements of the VTCT Diploma and other awarding bodies, and will be helpful to all teachers and students of reflexology whichever course is undertaken. In response to many requests I have written the text in a form which is easily accessible to all. The book provides the information in easy-to-read sections with assessment and application of knowledge to reinforce what has been learnt, as well as case studies and a professional code of ethics. I only hope that you enjoy reading this book as much as I have enjoyed researching and writing it.

Susan Cressy

2002

Introduction

What is reflexology?

Reflexology is a non-invasive therapy performed on the feet and using special manipulations with varying degrees of pressure to provide benefits to the client that are both physical and emotional. It is based on the principle that there are reflex zones in the feet which are linked by energy pathways to corresponding parts of the body and, when pressure is applied, it stimulates the movement of energy along these pathways.

The body is programmed to heal itself and this is happening all the time whether it is a cut or a bruise in the tissues, a broken bone or a torn muscle. The systems and organs in the body are constantly working together to heal and repair, from the brain which is the control centre to the circulatory system which transports necessary nutrients to the tissues, to the nervous system which stimulates responses from other systems and organs. Energy is essential to keep everything working and this is provided by the food we digest.

The body is like a complex machine in which all the parts need to be working together to maintain the balance required for maximum effect. If this balance is disrupted for any reason then the component parts will function less effectively. When a blockage occurs, caused by stress, injury or disease in one part, the rest of the body compensates and works harder to try and achieve balance. This may eventually cause further problems.

Reflexology is a **holistic** treatment, as the aim of the reflexologist is to treat the whole person, body, mind and spirit, to induce a state of balance and harmony, stimulating the body's own potential to heal both physically and emotionally.

The pressure for stimulating movement of energy along the pathways is applied using specific finger and thumb massage techniques and is quite different from general body or foot massage that provides a manipulation of the soft tissues in the body. A good reflexologist not only needs sensitive hands to perform the specialised massage techniques but also intuition and an understanding of human nature, as the relationship between the client and practitioner plays an important part of the healing process.

Reflexology is a beneficial treatment that may be used on any person, old or young, male or female. There is an increasing interest in this natural form of therapy consistent with the increased demand for complementary therapies in general.

People are far more aware through the media of the options available to us in maintaining our own health in a much more natural way. We are also beginning to question the validity of some of the more traditional methods used to cope with illness and stress. The success of complementary therapies in dealing with stress and related conditions is the best form of advertising available and many people are more inclined to try other therapies when they have achieved benefits from another.

History of reflexology

The practice of reflexology is evident throughout history and has appeared in different ages and cultures from East to West. The earliest records and the oldest documentation have been found in Egypt in picture form on the walls of tombs. There is a scene depicting the possible practice of reflexology on the wall of a tomb at

Saqqara. This tomb belonged to Ankhmahor, a highly respected physician and influential official, second only to the king. It is also depicted on papyrus showing medical practitioners treating patients' hands and feet in 2500 BC. Egyptian medical practitioners were renowned throughout the world for their expertise and their work was well documented by the artists of the day.

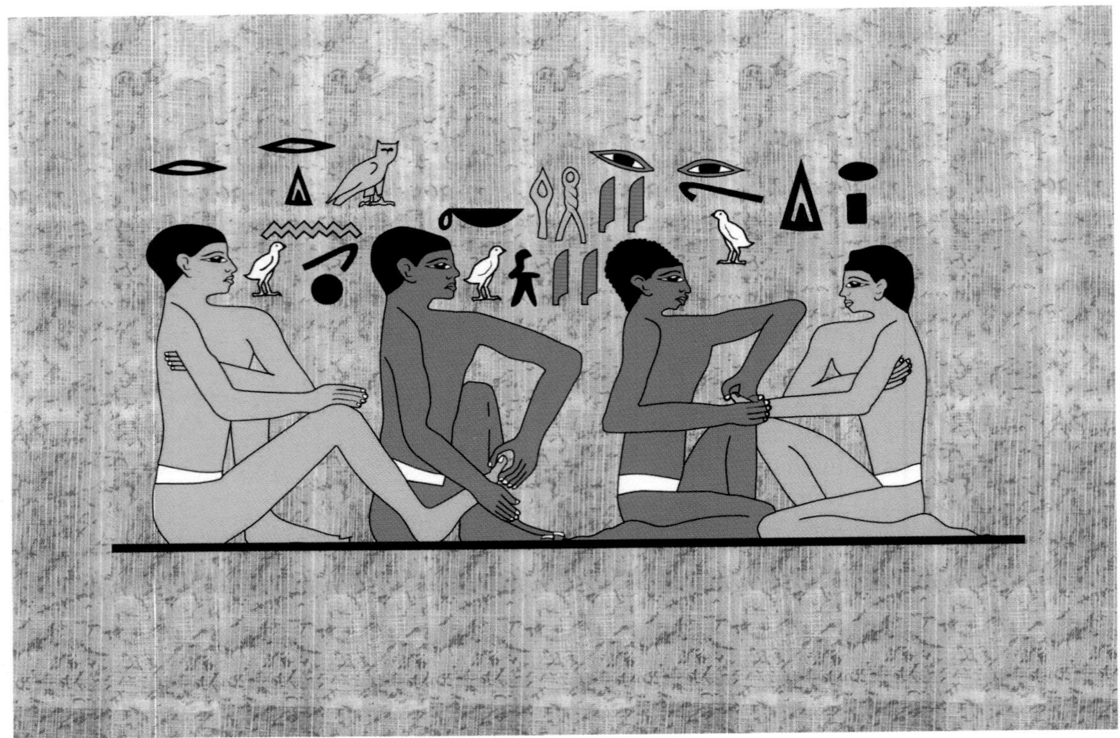

Figure 1 *Ancient Egyptian reflexology treatment*

Reflexology was also practised in ancient India and it is said that Buddhist monks who travelled to China took with them the techniques and practice of reflexology; some time later they travelled to Japan, spreading their teaching.

Before this the Chinese had been using acupuncture for healing and by 2500 BC had divided the body into longitudinal meridians, which they said constituted the body's energy system. Those practising acupuncture believed that pain or illness was caused when one or more of these meridians were blocked, disrupting the body's natural flow of energy and creating an imbalance. The acupuncturist used needles to unblock this energy flow. The Japanese used a form of pressure massage called shiatsu to achieve the same effects. Instead of using needles they applied pressure, using fingers or thumbs, to the acupuncture meridian points and this helped to unblock the energy flow in the same way.

Although there is no evidence to support it, there is a theory that a form of reflexology was passed down to the native Americans by the Incas. The Cherokee Indians have practised for centuries a form of reflex pressure on the feet to heal and balance the body systems.

Reflexology was practised in the United States in the early 20th century by Dr William Fitzgerald, who practised medicine in Boston, London and Vienna before becoming head of the Nose and Throat Department of St Francis Hospital in Connecticut.

It was during this time that he claims to have discovered **zone therapy**. While working with patients he discovered that applying pressure to certain points in the nose, mouth, throat and on the tongue deadened the sensation in certain areas of the body. He also found that exerting pressure on the hands and feet produced pain relief. These discoveries led him to map out areas of the body and their connections, as well as noting the conditions affected by the pressure points, and call it zone therapy. He divided the body into ten equal longitudinal zones, which ran from the top of the head to the tips of the toes, and used these for their anaesthetic effect. His findings show that those parts of the body that are in each zone are linked by a flow of energy and that the parts of the body in each zone can have an effect on each other.

Zone therapy

The longitudinal zones

There are five zones at either side of the midline of the body, and all the organs and structures that lie within the same zone are related to each other. When one reflex point is stimulated then the entire zone will be affected. The zones on the right side of the body are represented in the right foot and the zones in the left side of the body are represented in the left foot. The ten zones terminate on the soles of the feet and the palms of the hands.

- **Zone 1** runs from the big toe, up the body to the brain and then down to the thumb
- **Zone 2** runs from the second toe up to the brain and down to the index finger.
- **Zone 3** runs from the third toe up to the brain and down to the middle finger
- **Zone 4** runs from the fourth toe up to the brain and down to the ring finger
- **Zone 5** runs from the little toe up to the brain and down to the little finger.

Eunice Ingham, who became known as the 'mother of modern reflexology', developed zone therapy much further by mapping the entire body on the feet and developing the reflex points. She also discovered that an alternating pressure actually stimulated healing rather than just having an anaesthetising effect. She spread the word and taught zone therapy to other professionals such as chiropodists, osteopaths, naturopaths, physiotherapists and massage therapists. Her work continues today through her nephew Dwight Byers, director of The International Institute of Reflexology in St Petersburg, Florida.

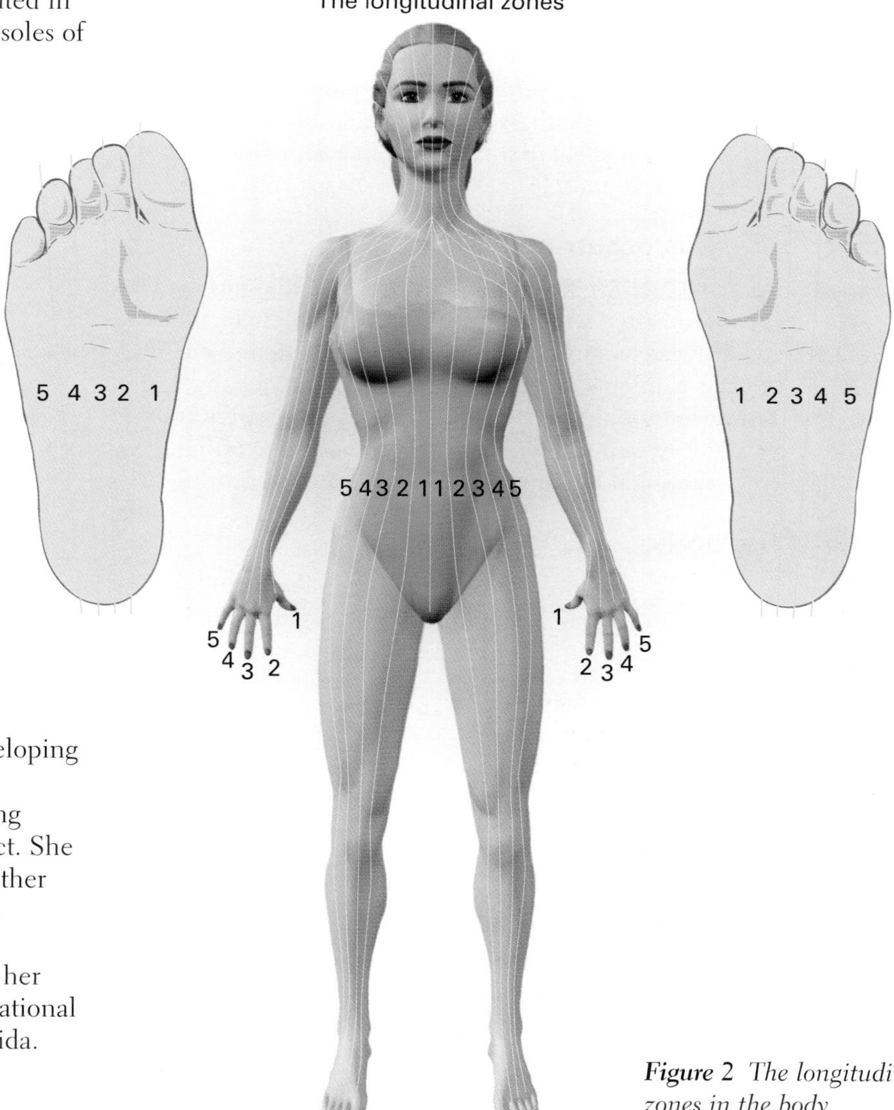

Figure 2 *The longitudinal zones in the body*

The benefits of reflexology

Balances energy

The human body is full of energy, which is known by different names throughout the world. In India it is called '**prana**', in Tibet it is '**lung-gom**', in Japan '**sakia-tundra**', or '**ki**', and in China '**ch'i**'. In the West we refer to it as '**life force**', '**vital energy**' or '**vital force**'.

In physical terms the human body consists of a mass of cells made up of chemical substances that are a collection of atoms. Each atom consists of protons with a positive charge, neutrons with no charge and electrons with a negative charge; this means the body is a mass of energy fields which all influence each other. This energy is circulating around the body influencing the different organs and different areas and helping to maintain homeostasis (a state of balance). When this energy flow is impeded the body does not function efficiently because it is out of balance. It is believed that reflexology helps to unblock the congestion in the energy pathways, returning the body to a balanced state and improving the client's physical and emotional well-being.

Provides pain relief

Reflexology is also known to stimulate the body to produce endorphins, the body's own natural painkiller. When the reflexologist stimulates the pituitary gland reflex during treatment it may increase the amount of endorphins released into the body to suppress pain. The relaxing effect of treatment can also help to reduce the amount of pain as it relieves tension in muscles.

Prevents problems occurring

The environment in which we live is constantly bombarding us with stressors, pollution, food contaminated with chemicals, a hectic lifestyle, poor diet, to name but a few! Together these factors contribute to poor health and encourage disease. Regular reflexology treatments together with the necessary changes in lifestyle and diet can help to prevent problems occurring by alleviating stress and preventing an imbalance in the body systems. It will also help to boost the immune system, making it more effective, enabling it to fight off infection.

Detoxifies the body

Reflexology is believed to improve the function of the lymphatic system, detoxifying and cleansing internally and stimulating the excretory systems to rid the body of waste. It also helps the skin to function more efficiently, removing toxins and the build up of waste.

Aids relaxation

Reflexology helps to balance emotions, is an antidote to stress and induces relaxation, promoting restful sleep. This relaxed state allows the energy to flow more easily, thereby revitalising the body.

Increases circulation

Blood supply to the organs in the body is vital for them to function effectively, as it supplies all the necessary nutrients and oxygen required and removes waste products. Tension in the body restricts blood flow and, as reflexology relaxes the whole body, this allows the blood supply to flow more easily.

Stimulates the nervous system

The nerves convey messages from the central nervous system to all parts of the body and through reflexology the nerve endings are stimulated. This encourages the opening of neural pathways allowing messages to travel unimpeded so that all the organs and systems of the body may be able to to work together effectively.

SNAPSHOTS

Clients who attend for reflexology treatment are diverse. The husband of a regular client of mine had suffered whiplash after a car accident. He found it very painful moving his neck and so avoided having physiotherapy. His wife persuaded him to try reflexology and it wasn't long before he was a devotee when the stress he was suffering, from a heavy workload, seemed to disappear. The mobility in his neck also improved and he was sleeping for eight hours a night after previously having trouble sleeping.

Another regular client is a woman in her early fifties who has suffered pain for many years due to a severe case of rheumatoid arthritis and several slipped discs. She is unable to take medication to ease the pain as she has a condition which causes her to suffer an allergic response to most medication. She has become a firm believer in the benefits of reflexology and attends regularly even when her mobility is poor.

- Treatment requirements
- Consultation
- Assessing the foot
- Contraindications
- Conditions of the feet
- Anatomy and physiology of the foot

Preparing for **Reflexology**

1 Treatment requirements

The treatment room

The nature of the reflexologist's work enables them to work in a wide variety of places and practices. Wherever they work the requirements will always be the same.

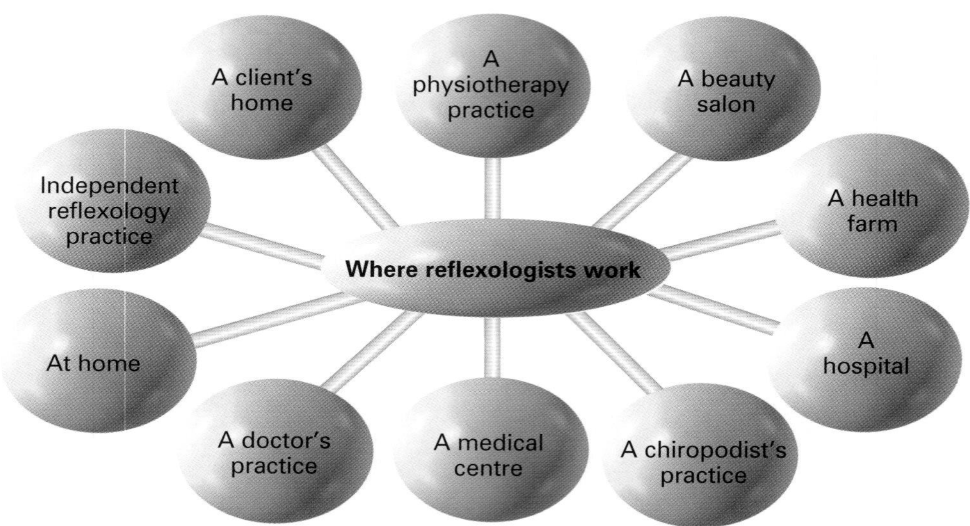
Where reflexologists work
A client's home
A physiotherapy practice
A beauty salon
A health farm
A hospital
A chiropodist's practice
A medical centre
A doctor's practice
At home
Independent reflexology practice

Figure 1.1 Some of the places and practices where reflexologists can work

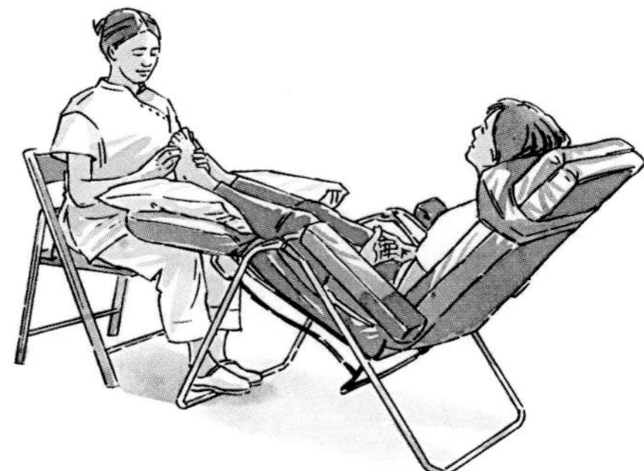

Figure 1.2 A home visiting reflexologist using a portable couch to provide treatment

Whatever the location it is important to create the right atmosphere for a successful treatment. Treatment should be provided in comfortable surroundings that are warm, well ventilated and with adequate light, which could be altered with the use of dimmer switches to provide the right atmosphere for each individual client.

The atmosphere should be quiet, calm, with little distraction. Ideally, the colour scheme should be soothing, but with a professional look which will be calming and reassuring to the client. Privacy is important during the consultation as you may have to discuss personal issues with your client, and during treatment in order to create the right atmosphere for relaxation and self-healing.

Music playing discreetly in the background can help clients to relax. Switch your telephone onto the answer machine when you are with a client, if you do not have the luxury of a receptionist or other members of staff to take your calls. Ask your client to switch off her mobile phone if she has one, so she will have total relaxation and her treatment will not be disturbed.

If possible, separate treatment rooms should be available, but if this is not an option the area should be separated from the rest by using curtains or screens. Dividing doors are available which are soundproof and easy to move backwards and forwards to create large or smaller areas for treatment.

Equipment

Reflexology requires very little equipment. When setting up a reflexology practice think about the amount of working space available and how portable the equipment is for visiting clients at home.

The following items will enable you to provide a thorough and professional treatment:

- A comfortable treatment couch, preferably multi-positioned. This will allow your client to relax totally and gain maximum benefit from the treatment. Full-size massage couches are often used and these should have an adjustable back to allow your client to sit or recline in the most comfortable position for them. Mobile couches are available which can be assembled very quickly and easily transported.
- A stool with back support so there is no strain on your back. It also allows you to sit in an appropriate position to your client, so that you can see your client's body language and physical reactions, which often provide valuable feedback during treatment.
- A comfortable chair for your client during consultation (room permitting). In a small room or work area the client may have to sit on the treatment couch for the consultation as well as for treatment.
- Pillows or cushions for support, placed behind the head and neck and under the knees to reduce pressure on the lower back and to ensure the client is not physically tense during treatment due to discomfort or pain.
- Blankets and sheets to provide a cover for the couch and to ensure the client is warm throughout treatment. Some clients do begin to feel cold if lying for any length of time, immobile.
- Paper towel roll to cover the sheets and blankets on which the client is lying, for hygiene reasons.
- Towels to roll up for support under the ankles, to dry the hands or feet and to cover the feet when necessary.
- Tissues, cotton wool, foot cleanser or wet wipes for feet and hands.
- A small covered waste receptacle with a waterproof lining in which to store waste.
- Cream or oil. This is not used by all reflexologists when providing reflexology treatment but is pleasant for the client when providing relaxation massage or as aftercare to keep the skin soft and supple.
- A small trolley or table to place consumable items and paperwork.

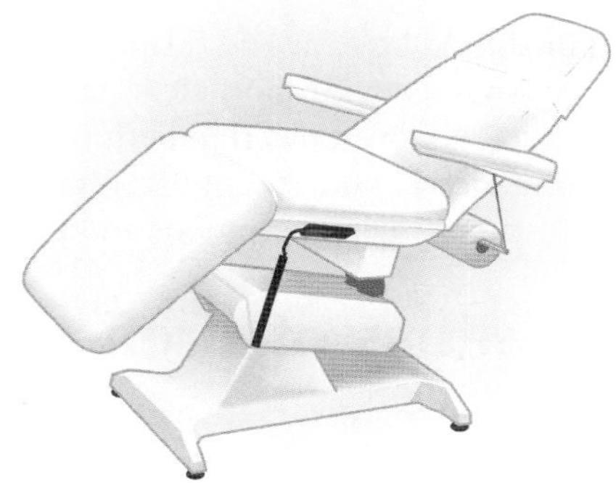

Figure 1.3 *A multi-position treatment couch*

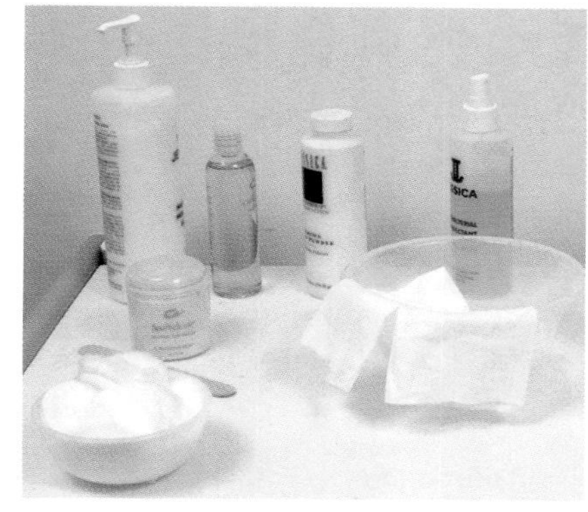

A selection of products should be prepared before you begin the treatment

Hygiene

For hygienic purposes, it is important that you wash your hands before and after each client. Ideally, there should be a wash basin, pump soap dispenser and towels available in or close to the treatment room or area. If this is out of the question because of the location then anti-bacterial wet wipes should be used.

Your appearance

The first impression a client has of you must be a positive one, therefore your appearance should be professional, whatever you wear. Choose your clothes for comfort and ease of movement. There is no particular code of dress that is required in general; however what you wear may depend on where you work. Here are a few examples.

- A hospital or medical environment may require you to wear their standard uniform.

- In a therapeutic practice you may wear the uniform relevant to your current position.
- When working from home, or visiting a client's home, it is often preferable to be more informally dressed; however this is a personal choice. The clothes you wear should be clean, neat and tidy, reflecting a positive professional image.
- When treating children or the elderly, a more informal approach to appearance may be adopted as it may be less intimidating to the client.

Hair should be neat and tidy and tied back if it is long. The hands and nails should be well groomed with short clean nails. Jewellery should be kept to a minimum and be discreet. No overpowering perfumes or aftershave should be worn. You will inspire confidence in your client if you create the right atmosphere for treatment, provide the most appropriate equipment and present a professional appearance at all times.

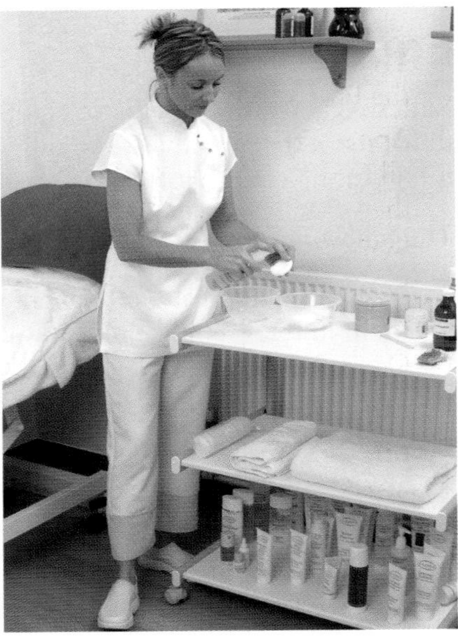

The appearance of the reflexologist is important in giving the right impression to clients

Qualities of a reflexologist

As a reflexologist you are providing the client with the opportunity to take responsibility for their own health and well-being. A partnership will develop when the client has a genuine desire to overcome any problems with your help and support. To achieve this, you need to have certain qualities. They should be:

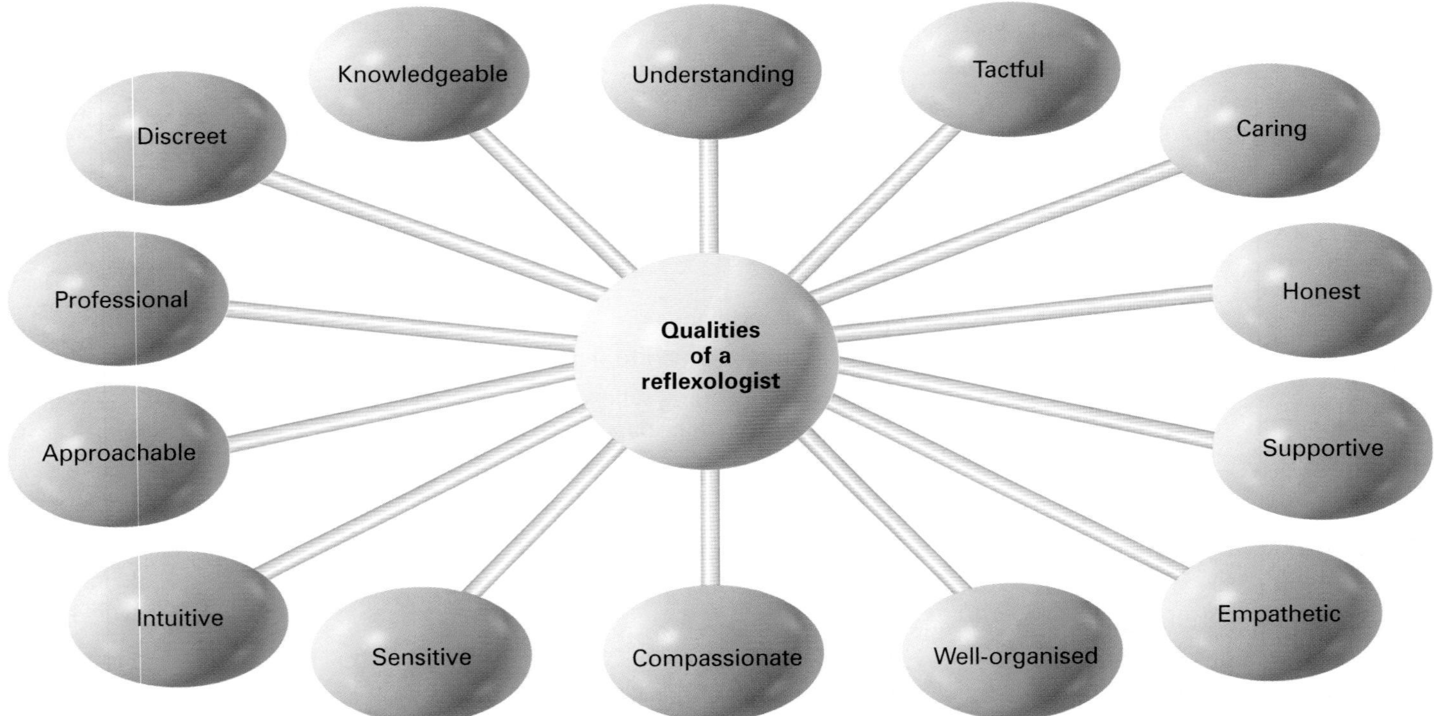
Qualities of a reflexologist
Knowledgeable
Understanding
Tactful
Discreet
Caring
Professional
Honest
Approachable
Supportive
Intuitive
Sensitive
Compassionate
Well-organised
Empathetic

Figure 1.4 *The qualities required by a reflexologist*

- **Professional** in all aspects of the business, following the industry code of practice, complying with the law, maintaining standards and ensuring client confidentiality at all times.
- **Knowledgeable** about reflexology in order to provide an excellent service and be able to answer any questions the clients may ask. To know as much possible about other treatments that will complement reflexology, nutrition and lifestyle advice.

- **Well-organised**, to ensure that time is not wasted on any unnecessary activity and the time you spend with each client is used effectively.
- **Approachable**, so that clients will find it easy to talk to you and provide you with all the relevant information you need. The response they receive should make them feel comfortable. This is particularly important when you first encounter a new client as it sets the tone for your future client/therapist relationship.
- **Sensitive** to the client's feelings and moods, knowing instinctively how to respond, when to listen and when to offer advice.
- **Compassionate** and sympathetic when the client has suffered in any way.
- **Empathetic**, in order to be able to understand your client's feelings.
- **Intuitive** (having an immediate insight, or knowing something instinctively), which is a skill that you will develop with time.
- **Understanding** will allow you to be tolerant of different personalities and problems you may encounter.
- **Caring** is important in any therapeutic treatment. Caring about the client and the outcome of treatment allows you to provide the best treatment you can and develop a good relationship with your clients.
- **Honesty**, in not making false claims to your client about the treatment you are providing, being clear about your charges and not misleading the client in any way.
- **Tactful** in your approach, not offending anyone, avoiding controversial subjects and never making assumptions that may cause embarrassment.
- **Discreet**, as you may have several clients who are related to each other, are friends or neighbours. Never discuss your clients with others or divulge any information which should remain confidential.
- **Supportive**, as many of your clients may have family problems, be worried about exams or their job. They may be trying very hard to lose weight or conquer an addiction. Provide advice and information if it is requested and always listen as this often helps considerably.

These qualities will engender an atmosphere of trust, allowing the client to communicate their requirements without feeling self-conscious and knowing that anything that is said or recorded remains confidential. It gives the client confidence in the ability of the reflexologist and provides the basis of a successful, professional relationship.

Preparing your client for treatment

The client must be seated or reclining comfortably with sufficient support for the head and neck. The lower legs must be well supported with the knees slightly bent to prevent tension in the lower leg muscles, and the feet should be in a relaxed position. If the client is uncomfortable this may create tension in the body which will impede the natural energy flow. Whatever the position, the client's face should always be visible to the reflexologist as their facial expression can often provide relevant information. You must also ensure that the client will be warm enough during the whole of the treatment time. A large towel may be placed over the client but if the client is very cold a lightweight duvet may be used.

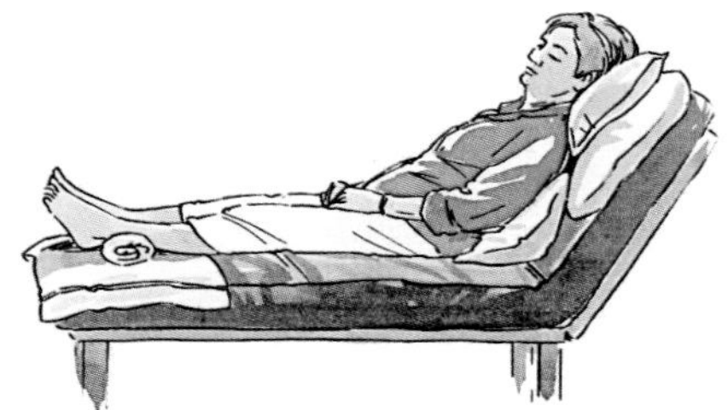

***Figure 1.5** Client in position for treatment, with head back and supported and ankle supported with towel*

PRACTICE IN CONTEXT

1 Consider the different working environments that a reflexologist may encounter when providing treatment. Compare and list the differences there would be in the atmosphere that you would wish to create – in a treatment room at home, in a hospital and when it is part of a beauty salon.

2 Reflexology is a therapy which provides a personal service requiring your client to discuss many personal issues. The first impression you make is therefore important in establishing a relationship with your client, so you must consider your appearance and body language (non-verbal communication) carefully.

Discuss in a group or with a partner what you consider to be 'good' body language and what you consider to be 'bad' body language and the impact that both will have in establishing a professional relationship.

ASSESSMENT OF KNOWLEDGE

1 Why is it important to choose an appropriate colour for the treatment area?

2 Why must the treatment area be private?

3 What are the advantages of using a multi-positioned treatment couch?

4 When choosing a chair for the reflexologist, what is the most important consideration to prevent backache?

5 What must be provided to maintain a high level of hygiene?

2 Consultation

Client consultation

Assessing the client

The initial consultation is an important process as it is the first step in establishing a professional and beneficial working relationship with the client. This initial consultation requires more time, although consultation will occur naturally to a lesser degree before and after treatment at each subsequent session.

The importance of consultation

The therapeutic relationship you will develop with your client is important, and this starts with the initial consultation. The consultation provides the client with the opportunity to talk to the reflexologist and discuss her reasons for having treatment. She can ask any questions concerning reflexology, its effects, how long it takes, how often she will need to attend and what aftercare advice you can give her to reinforce the treatment at home.

Consultation also allows the reflexologist to establish the needs of the client and the outcome she hopes to achieve from the treatment. You can also use this opportunity to explain the benefits of treatment and devise a treatment plan specifically designed to suit the client.

At each subsequent treatment you can obtain feedback from the client, which allows you to monitor the results of treatment. You should ask her how she felt after the last treatment, whether anything changed that needs to be noted in her records, and whether she had any noticeable reaction and has seen any improvements.

Methods of consultation

During the consultation, different methods will be used in assessing the client and providing information. These will be observation; questioning and listening; reference to client records; and use of visual aids.

Observation

As soon as the client enters the room, general observations may be made about the way in which he or she walks, the distribution of weight on their feet, and whether there is any evidence of tension in the body or lack of flexibility. The posture may be noted: is the head held straight, are the shoulders relaxed and level, is there any curvature of the spine, and are the hips and knees level? Any problem you note may help when questioning and assessing the client during the consultation.

Non-verbal communication is often as informative as questions as a client will express themselves through their body language. Are they smiling, or are their lips tightly pursed? Do they have an open posture or are their arms closed or shoulders hunched forwards? Does their breathing pattern appear even or do they seem short of breath? The client's state of relaxation may be noted; if they appear ill at ease and uncomfortable this may indicate a general nervousness, particularly if this is their first visit. However it could indicate that the client is under stress, feeling generally low or suffering from a physical pain or discomfort. With further questioning of the client these initial observations may be reinforced or dismissed, allowing you to formulate an appropriate treatment plan.

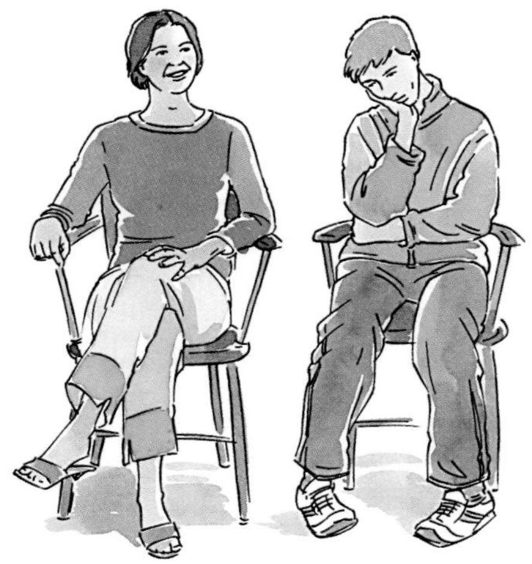

Figure 2.1 *Observing posture and body language provides valuable information during consultation*

A client's physical appearance may also indicate their physical and emotional condition at the time. If they have clear skin with glossy hair and bright eyes, are well groomed and walk with a light step, this will indicate a person in general good health. However, if they have blemished skin with a greyish pallor, lank, lifeless hair and dull eyes, this could be symptomatic of depression, lethargy or other problems.

Observation of the feet

A detailed observation of the feet will be carried out during consultation and any tender or problem areas must be noted on a blank diagram of the feet together with other observations about the:

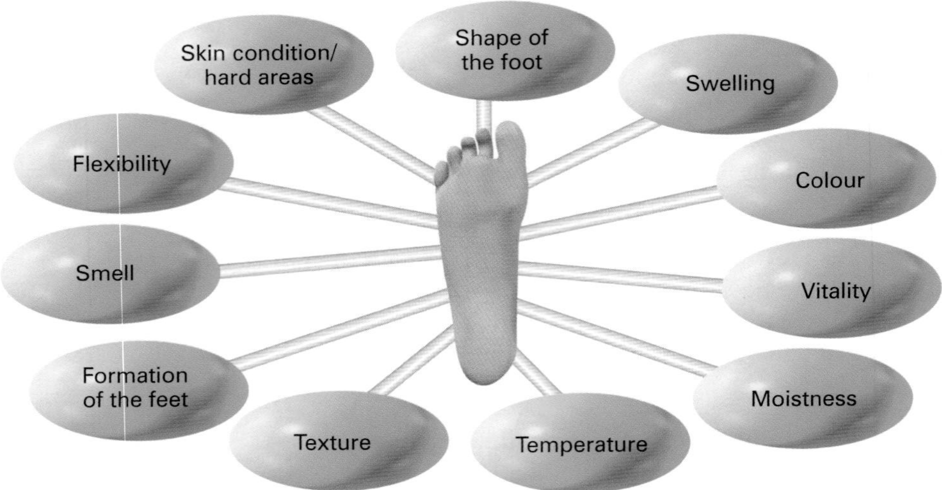

Figure 2.2 In observing feet a reflexologist takes several conditions into account

It is also useful to compare the differences in each foot, as they are not always identical. This may indicate an imbalance on one side of the body; for example one shoulder may be higher than the other, or there may be a difference in the curve of the spine on the medial aspect of the foot, which may indicate an abnormal curvature of the spine.

Questioning and listening

This is an essential part of the consultation process and different types of questions may be used.

Open questions

These allow a free response from the client, giving them the opportunity to express their wishes and provide you with all the information required to formulate an appropriate treatment plan. These questions always start with words such as: How, What, Why, When, Where? You may begin by asking, 'What made you decide to try reflexology?' The answer is often quite revealing. Most recently a client of mine responded by saying:

'I have been suffering with severe mood swings for two years and am now waking at night with hot flushes and I feel that this is the beginning of the menopause although I am still menstruating. I was on the pill for many years from my early twenties to my middle thirties and I do not want to continue taking hormone tablets. I have been recommended to you by a friend who is enthusiastic about the results of reflexology treatment.'

She continued in this vein for some time and seemed relieved to have someone to confide in. From one simple open question I had gained a great deal of information about her medical history.

Occasionally an open question provides a response, which is not related but provides an insight into the client's emotional state. A client recently attended for treatment as she felt it would help with her high blood pressure. The question I asked was, 'When did you last have your blood pressure checked?' Her response was:

'The doctor checked it last week as I was having dizzy spells. It's not surprising really as I have just moved from Bath to Manchester to be near my daughter. She doesn't think I should live so far away and on my own. My husband died ten years ago and I should have been celebrating my 50th wedding anniversary. I don't know a soul up here, I've left the home I had for thirty five years and she's got her own life to lead...'

A question about her medical condition provided me with far more information about her emotional state and this was useful when formulating a treatment plan.

The answers to these sort of questions will provide detail as well as an insight into the client's emotional well-being, his/her confidence and energy levels. Open-ended questions allow an unrestricted response, and to build up goodwill it is a good idea to start the questions with one that will put the client into a relaxed frame of mind. This question does not need to have any relationship to the treatment process; it could concern the weather, their general well-being, how they arrived for their appointment or even where they live.

Closed questions

These call for responses which are strictly limited and are used to elicit specific information from the client, or when a yes/no answer is sufficient. These are valuable when recording essential information such as name, address, telephone number, medical history, etc. This information is required to maintain professional records and ensure a smooth running service.

Probing questions

These are useful when you need to find out a little more information than the client is offering, to clarify a point or to expand on a relevant issue. One of my clients is a nurse and I completed a consultation record card in detail. She said she had no problems with her bones and joints and no gynaecological problems. When I was completing the physical assessment of her feet I felt a clicking sensation in her shoulder reflex and a lumpy feeling was evident in the uterus reflex area. I questioned this client further about these areas and eventually she told me she had a shoulder injury that had been caused by an incorrect lifting technique when she had been moved after an operation. She had also been on and off HRT for short periods of time before stopping altogether. She had recently suffered some spasmodic heavy bleeding with accompanying pain. The probing questions were required in this case to ensure a more detailed and correct medical history was recorded. Because this client was a nurse, she had an informed and detailed knowledge of all things medical and had a tendency to dismiss obvious signs and symptoms until they were pointed out.

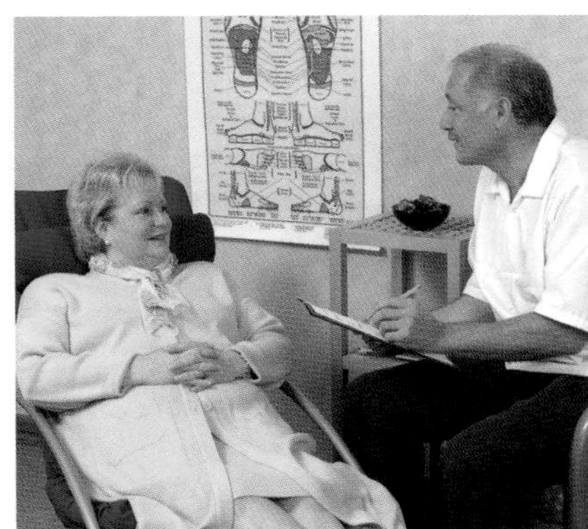

A consultation with a client

It is also very important to listen to your client and summarise what they have said to show you have understood or to clarify a point. Good communication with a client requires active listening, which helps to receive and understand the true message being conveyed. Because we think much more quickly than we speak, it often means that we are formulating our response before the client has delivered the whole message; therefore we may only remember certain parts of the information and may have eliminated something important. To actively listen you must ensure that you:

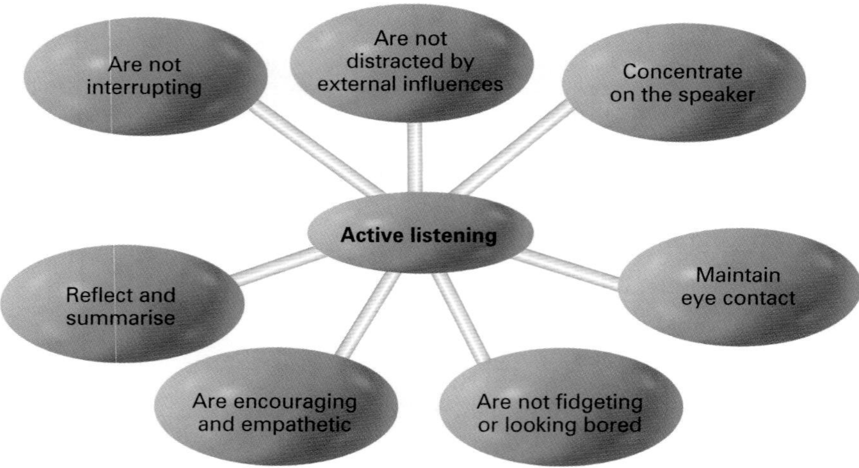

***Figure** 2.3 The requirements of active listening*

Ask a friend or colleague to write a synopsis of a recent event in their lives. They must then speak for approximately five minutes about this event whilst you listen carefully and then repeat the story back to them. Your partner must then make a note of how much of the story you have recounted accurately. This will show if you have the ability to 'actively' listen.

Reference to client records

As a result of the assessment, all relevant information will be recorded in detail on a record card or in a case file. This information provides the foundation of the case history you will compile whilst treating the client and will include:

- personal details
- medical history
- client objectives and expectations
- client's lifestyle
- treatment record (see page 22)

Personal details

The personal details will include name, date of birth, address and telephone number, enabling you to communicate with your client when necessary. For those clients with a busy lifestyle, and to make it easier for you to contact them in this age of increasing technology, it is advisable to record mobile phone numbers, fax numbers and email addresses. In some cases the client's date of birth may be surrendered reluctantly. It may however be significant if their age does not reflect their physical appearance; for example they may appear older and this may indicate a problem, illness or lifestyle factor that should be taken into account.

Medical history

The medical history will include the name, address and telephone number of the client's doctor and any medication the client is taking, their height and weight, any health problems and any complaints for which the client is seeking help.

Past medical history is also important as this may contribute to any current problems. The family medical history may also provide useful information. There are certain general areas which need to be noted.

- General state of health
- Past/present illness
- Emotional trauma
- Operations/after-effects of anaesthetic
- Accidents or injuries sustained
- Muscular/skeletal problems
- Digestive problems
- Circulatory problems
- Gynaecological problems
- Nervous system
- Immune system disorders/problems
- Allergies
- Skin problems
- Medication
- Current medical treatment

This information will also highlight any reason why the treatment may be contraindicated or adapted to suit the client. When you suspect the client has a contraindication to treatment, explain why and how long she will need to wait before having treatment. You must not alarm her, be reassuring in your approach and sensitive to her feelings when discussing possible contraindications. In some cases you may need to refer her to her GP for advice (see Chapter 4).

Aims, objectives and expectations

It is most important for you to know why the client requires a reflexology treatment. It may be as a source of relaxation, stress relief or to ease a physical problem. However the majority of clients are asking for your advice; they may have tried other forms of therapy or have been recommended to you by a friend, colleague or medical practitioner.

Providing as much information as possible will help your client to become aware of how reflexology works and understand that the body is capable of self-healing, and that this is an important aim in treatment. A client will not have unrealistic expectations of treatment if you explain how reflexology works and make it clear that a reflexologist does not diagnose disease, recommend or adjust medication. This treatment must **not** be used to replace orthodox medicine, but is used alongside medical treatment to complement it.

Client's lifestyle

It is important to find out as much as you can about your client's lifestyle, as it will help in understanding any problems they may have. The environment in which the client lives and works may also have a bearing on their general health and well-being.

The time they spend working, relaxing, socialising or running the home will provide an indication of how stressful the client's life is and how much time they have to relax. It will also allow you to plan the client's appointments around her other responsibilities or activities.

Diet and nutrition will also have an effect on the client's health and energy levels, as will their eating patterns. When and how they eat may be affected by their lifestyle, and their food intake may also have a bearing on physical problems that they are having, or if they are feeling low or depressed.

Treatment record

This should include all the dates the client attends for treatment, the end-of-session evaluations of the treatment and any comments you may think useful to record or the client wishes to make. This enables you to adapt or change the treatment plan. A note must also be made of the date of any referral to a medical practitioner, the response and the date it was received.

Use of visual aids

Using visual aids reinforces verbal information given to the client during consultation. Charts of the foot showing reflex points and zones of the body will help the client understand the principles of reflexology. Leaflets providing information about general foot care and samples of products used on the feet, which may be available to buy, are useful for the client to have, allowing them to continue caring for their feet at home.

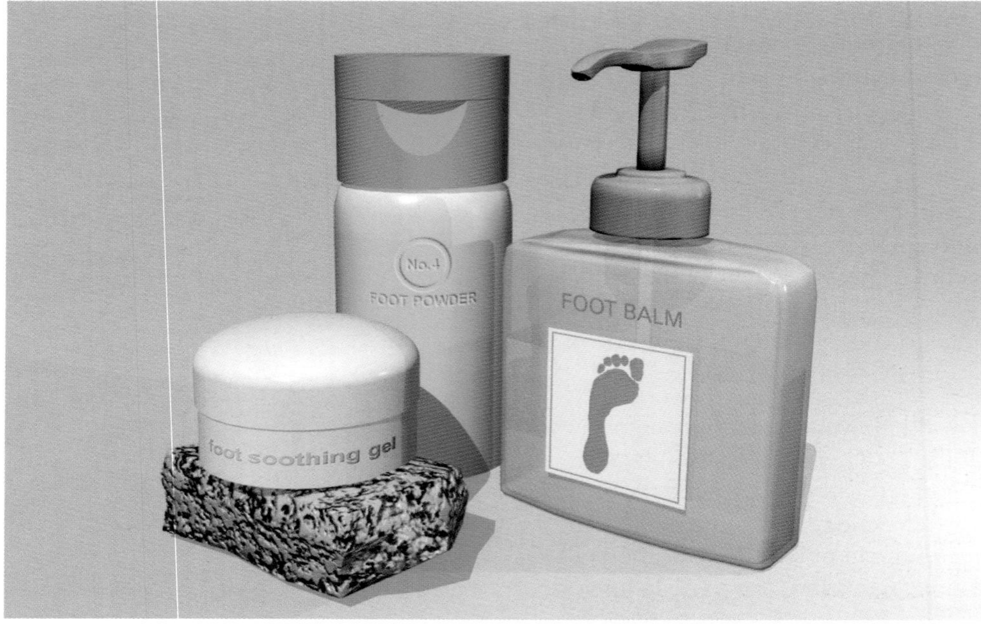

***Figure** 2.5 Using visual aids reinforces information provided during consultation*

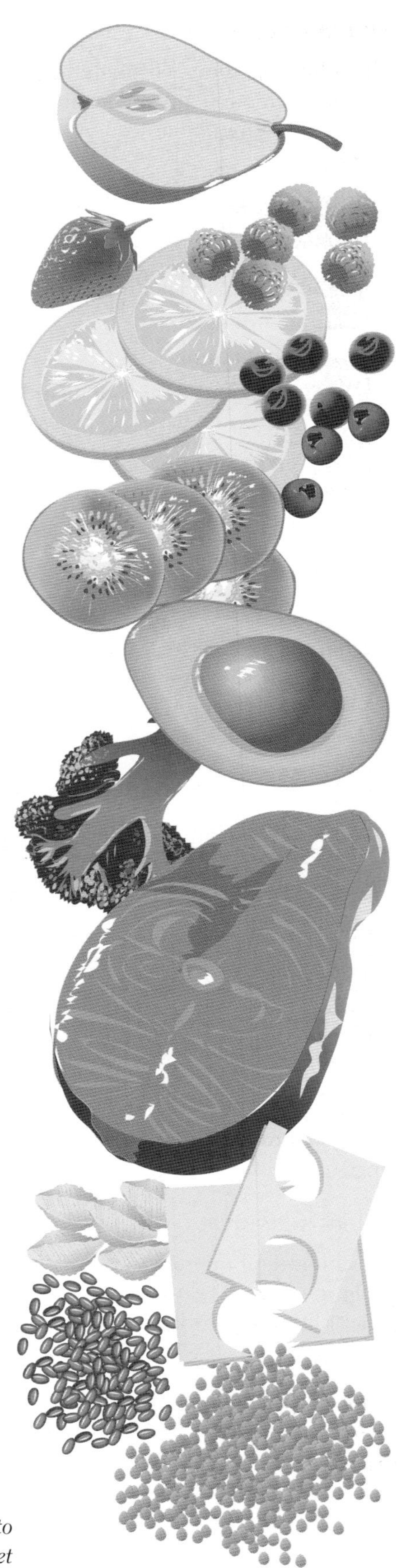

***Figure** 2.4 A selection of foods to provide a healthy diet*

The consultation process

The following chart provides an overview of the steps taken in a consultation with a client.

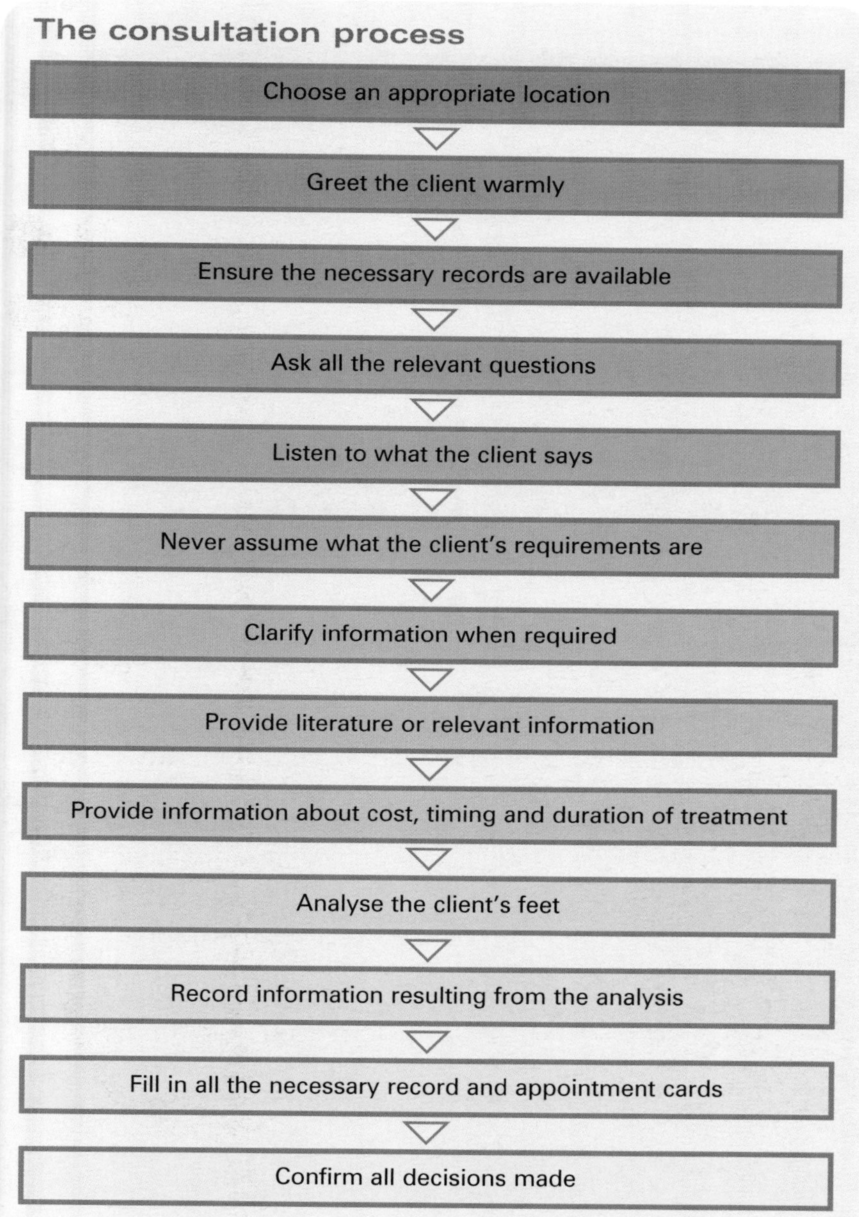

The consultation process
Choose an appropriate location
Greet the client warmly
Ensure the necessary records are available
Ask all the relevant questions
Listen to what the client says
Never assume what the client's requirements are
Clarify information when required
Provide literature or relevant information
Provide information about cost, timing and duration of treatment
Analyse the client's feet
Record information resulting from the analysis
Fill in all the necessary record and appointment cards
Confirm all decisions made

A full treatment will normally accompany the initial consultation, therefore extra time must be allocated when booking the first appointment for each client to accommodate the consultation process. Fifteen to twenty minutes should be sufficient.

A short consultation will occur at each subsequent treatment to provide the feedback required from the last treatment and allow discussion about any new issues which may affect the treatment plan. Treatment may then be adapted if necessary.

Reflexology consultation record

REFLEXOLOGY CONSULTATION RECORD

PERSONAL DETAILS	
Name	
Address	
Tel./ Fax/ e-mail	
Birthdate	
Client objectives	
MEDICAL HISTORY	
Dr. Name	
Address	
Tel. No.	
Height Weight	
General state of health	
Illness past/present	
Operations/anaesthetic	
Accidents/injuries	
Muscular problems	
Skeletal problems	
Digestive/excretory problems	
Circulatory disorders	
Gynaecological problems	
Nervous problems	
Emotional trauma	

Immune problems	
Allergies	
Skin	
Current medical treatment	
Medication	
Family medical history	
LIFESTYLE	
Marital status	
Professional status	
Exercise	
Energy level	
Sleep pattern	
Ability to relax	
Free time	
Diet	
Vitamin supplements	
Food allergies/intolerance	
Eating disorder	
Type & no. drinks daily	
Smoke	
Other comments	
Client signature	
Reflexologist signature	
Date	

REFLEXOLOGY CONSULTATION RECORD

PERSONAL DETAILS	
Name	Susan Rawlinson
Address	10, Menstone Road Bromborough Wirral CN5 R52
Tel./ Fax/ e-mail	0151 443 4291
Birthdate	10-4-52
Client objectives	Relaxation, Relieve pain in joints
MEDICAL HISTORY	
Dr. Name	Dr. Thompson
Address	Roslobie Park Health Centre Withington Staffs
Tel. No.	0161 205 1979
Height Weight	5' 5" 11st 4lbs
General state of health	Good, a little tired + slightly stressed, blocked left ear, tired eyes
Illness past/present	All childhood illnesses
Operations/anaesthetic	None
Accidents/injuries	None
Muscular problems	Dropped arches both feet
Skeletal problems	Short left leg, pain in left hip, knee, ankle and foot
Digestive/excretory problems	Occasional indigestion and IBS
Circulatory disorders	None
Gynaecological problems	Menopause
Nervous problems	None
Emotional trauma	None

Immune problems	None
Allergies	None
Skin	Dry, clear skin
Current medical treatment	HRT
Medication	Prempak – C
Family medical history	Osteoporosis prevalent in maternal family
LIFESTYLE	
Marital status	Married with 3 children aged between 17 and 23
Professional status	Working full time – teaching and research – independent consultant
Exercise	Attends health club twice a week, Aerobic exercise – bike + rower + weights
Energy level	Good
Sleep pattern	6 hours
Ability to relax	Good
Free time	Very little at the moment
Diet	Low carbohydrate
Vitamin supplements	Antioxidant A, C + E selenium and zinc
Food allergies/intolerance	None
Eating disorder	None
Type & no. drinks daily	Tea 6/7 cups daily Wine 4/5 glasses weekly Water 2 glasses
Smoke	No
Other comments	Client appeared tense, limping slightly. Arrived straight from work.
Client signature	Susan Rawlinson
Reflexologist signature	T. Melnyk.
Date	27th August 2001

An example of a completed consultation record

Details of the consultation

The consultation is a two-way process and careful use of questioning together with active listening will provide you with all the information required. Try and be as detailed as possible when completing the client's medical record as this will provide valuable information about your client.

General state of health

Open questions will help to provide you with detailed information. You must determine whether they have any general weakness or specific problems. The client will explain why she is trying reflexology, if it is related to her health, and will provide you with a list of complaints or symptoms which may be worrying her. Occasionally you may find the client has tried a treatment, which may not have been successful, or they require additional help in treating a specific problem. It may be they are suffering from a recurring minor problem such as headache, migraine or period pains, they may be feeling generally unwell but not be able to pinpoint the problem or they may be suffering a more serious chronic illness.

Past/present illness

You may start by asking about any childhood illness or recurring problems that may indicate the immune system is not working effectively; or it may indicate that recovery from illness is not always complete. Ask how present illness is affecting the client. For example, is it restricting them in any way or are they still able to work? Is it affecting their sleep pattern, which in turn may cause other problems?

Operations

Any operations clients have had should be recorded as they may have caused adverse effects, for example, recovery may have been slow or complications may have occurred. The after-effects of an anaesthetic may also cause problems.

Accidents or injuries

Record any major accidents, the length of the recovery period, and if they have been left with any disability. Clients may suffer from small recurring accidents, such as falling over or crashing into things. Find out from questioning why this is happening.

Muscular/skeletal problems

These problems may be noticeable from your physical assessment; however sometimes the client is not aware that they have a problem until questioned. They may have problems caused by previous injury, they may suffer persistent aches and pains, so ask if these are in the muscles or the joints.

Digestive/excretory problems

These may be indicated by infrequent or too frequent bowel movement, diarrhoea, constipation or haemorrhoids. Other indicators are pain or discomfort after eating, indigestion, flatulence, or a sickly feeling after eating certain foods.

Circulatory problems

There may be a family history of high or low blood pressure or a heart condition. The client may have cold hands and feet, chilblains or suffer from fluid retention. Does the client suffer from varicose veins or phlebitis or are they diabetic?

Gynaecological problems

Check if the menstrual cycle is regular, whether the client suffers painful periods and if they are heavy or light, or whether the client suffers with premenstrual syndrome. Are they taking the contraceptive pill? Is there a history of miscarriage or problems conceiving? If they have children, did they suffer problems during pregnancy or in childbirth? Is the client suffering symptoms of the menopause or perimenopause, have they had problems in the past or side-effects from treatment?

Nervous system problems

These may be evident from observing the client; however you may need to ask if they are suffering from a disorder of the nervous system, mood swings, headaches or nervous tension. Have they had problems in the past, accidents or after-effects of operations or illness?

Emotional trauma

This may be caused by many things: bereavement, divorce, shock, illness in the family, losing a job, problems with children or supporting older, infirm relatives. Sensitivity is required when questioning the client – if you have gained their confidence and you use open questions, they will probably confide in you details they feel comfortable with. Emotional stress can give rise to illness, either real or merely perceived by the client.

Immune system problems

Clients may have suffered from glandular fever in the past which may affect the immune system and its responses. They may be taking medication, which has an effect on the immune system or suffer from an illness such as rheumatoid arthritis or lupus. They may have constant recurring problems as a result of an inefficient immune system.

Allergies

The client will be able to provide information about allergies as they are often a visible problem, the most common allergy being contact dermatitis, a skin irritation caused by exposure to a sensitiser. The eyes and nose are often affected causing symptoms such as watery eyes, redness and swelling of the eyes, sinus congestion and sneezing or a constantly runny nose. The sensitisers are many and varied, and questioning the client about diet, work and general lifestyle may expose the culprit. Eczema is visible and often caused by contact with a sensitiser or sometimes by foods ingested. The client may suffer from nut allergy or have an allergic response to bees or wasps or other insect bites. There are also some clients who may feel they have an allergy or intolerance to certain foods.

Skin problems

This may show as excessively dry skin, redness or vascularity, or lots of papular eruptions (spots) on the face. Particular areas of the face correspond with different systems within the body, therefore this may be an indication of sluggishness in one of the other systems. The general colour of the skin and puffiness could also indicate further problems. These could be problems with the digestive system or the endocrine system if there is a hormonal imbalance.

Current medical treatment

You need to find out if a client is having medical treatment, as you may require permission from a general practitioner or specialist before commencing reflexology treatment.

Medication

Any medication the client has been taking is recorded along with the period of time they have been using that medication, what it has been prescribed for, any side-effects, and the dosage given as this may indicate the severity of the problem. Doctor's permission may be required (see page 42) before reflexology commences as the medication may be eliminated from the body more quickly after treatment and this may alter the required effect of the medication.

Family medical history

Knowing your client's family medical history provides you with more detailed information (see pages 18–19).

Lifestyle

Completing the lifestyle section of the record card may be a valuable means of assessing areas of the client's life which may be causing problems, and which, with guidance, she may be able to change for the better.

Home

The home environment may be busy and stressful if it combines looking after children and working; for example sleep patterns may be disrupted with a new baby or an elderly parent. Family discord or other problems may cause emotional stress and this in turn may affect diet and energy levels.

Work

The working environment may be causing stress either through physical problems such as repetitive strain injury, lifting or carrying heavy weights, exposure to hazardous substances or simply pressure from overwork or disputes with colleagues or management. The client may have a job which requires standing for hours at a time or sitting behind a desk speaking on a telephone all day, or sitting in front of a computer screen. Over a period of time, all these jobs and lack of exercise will cause physical problems such as back pain, cramps, varicose veins, haemorrhoids and oedema.

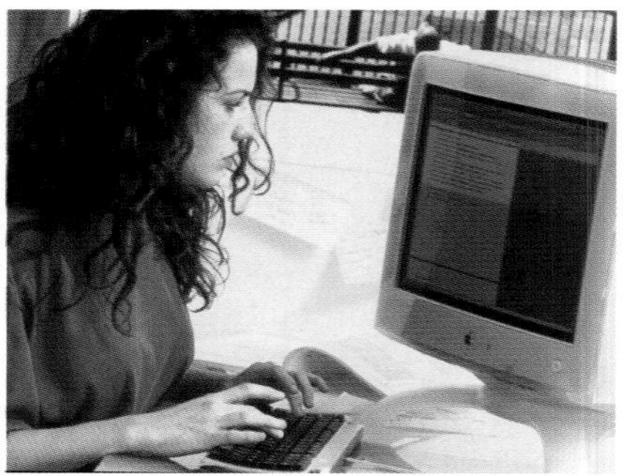

Sitting in the same position for long periods of time at work can lead to physical problems

Leisure

Leisure time is important as it helps people relax and cope with stress. Regular exercise helps in maintaining a healthy body but only if this is not excessive or will not cause injury. Clients may have hobbies and pastimes that are causing problems, or pursue very active or dangerous sports which may cause repetitive strain injury.

Energy levels

Find out if the client's energy levels are high or low, if they are constant or uneven, and if the client recovers quickly with rest or are constantly tired.

Sleep

When the client complains of poor sleeping patterns, it is important to look at the way in which they sleep to see if they lie in a comfortable position to support the spine and reduce tension in muscles. Also do they find it easy to get back to sleep after waking during the night, do they catnap a great deal during the day and do they feel refreshed after a short sleep or do they continually feel tired?

Diet

Note when the client eats, if the diet is balanced, if they eat in a hurry and whether they take vitamin supplements. Food intolerance and allergies should also be recorded and the client may indicate an eating disorder, past or present. A balanced diet contains all the necessary nutrients required for growth maintenance and repair in the right quantity to maintain a healthy body weight. This diet must include a combination of carbohydrate, protein, fat, minerals, vitamins and fibre.

The amount of fluid they take in daily and the types of drinks must also be recorded, as many clients do not drink sufficient water, leading to problems which may be easily rectified. Water comprises about two-thirds of the body weight and the body's need for water is second only to its need for air. The balance of water retained in the body is carefully regulated by the kidneys and under normal circumstances about 1 litre of water and other fluids should be drunk daily. This is necessary to maintain the health of body cells, to aid digestion and the transportation of substances around the body and to dilute waste products, thus aiding elimination. It also contributes to the maintenance of body temperature.

Signing the record card

Always ask your client to sign the record card when you have completed it together, as it provides evidence that the client agrees with the information which has been recorded. Your signature on the record card is useful if any other therapist has to treat the client in future and needs to clarify information. It also shows that you and the client agree that the information is accurate.

The Data Protection Act 1984

If you use a computer to store records and client details, this Act requires you to register with the Data Protection Registrar. Once registered you must comply with the principles of good information handling practice, set out in the Data Protection Act, which states that you must:

- obtain and process data fairly and lawfully
- hold information only for the purposes specified in your register entry
- use information only for those purposes and disclose it only to the people listed in your register entry
- only hold data which is adequate and relevant
- ensure that data is accurate and kept up to date
- hold information for no longer than is necessary
- allow individuals access to information held about them
- take security measures to prevent unauthorised or accidental access to, alteration, disclosure or loss and destruction of information.

An important aspect of the relationship you establish with your client is based on trust. It is important therefore to reassure your client that the information you have on record is stored securely and will remain confidential.

PRACTICE IN CONTEXT

1 Think about your feelings when you have been in a new or unknown situation, when you may have been a little apprehensive, worried or unsure of what is expected of you. Consider how you would like to be treated, what would put you at ease and make a list of things you may provide to make your clients feel comfortable.

2 Try and become more observant as you go about your daily activities, make a mental note of mannerisms that people adopt when they are feeling tired, angry, shy, frightened, antagonistic, happy, sad, sociable or withdrawn. The more observations you make the more practised you will become at understanding your client.

3 Practise completing a consultation record card by filling one in with all your own details, then try and complete a record card for each of your fellow students. The more cards you complete the easier it will become to ask the right questions during consultation.

ASSESSMENT OF KNOWLEDGE

1 How often should consultation with a client occur?

2 Why is it important to record a client's medical history?

3 What is the importance of using probing questions during consultation?

4 What are the requirements of active listening?

5 What are the 13 steps to be followed during the initial consultation process?

6 Why must your signature and that of the client appear on the record card?

3 Assessing the foot

To provide the most effective reflexology treatment you must first assess the foot, looking for all the visual and sensory clues that will provide you with the information you need to carry out treatment. This information will help you to decide which are the main reflexes to treat.

The shape of the foot

The shape of the feet usually corresponds with the size and shape of the person. If the client is tall and slim then the feet are usually long and thin, if the client is small and round then the feet will be small and round. Particular characteristics also show on the feet, for example if the client has broad shoulders then the area of the foot corresponding to the shoulders will be wide; if the client has a long neck then the toes will be long.

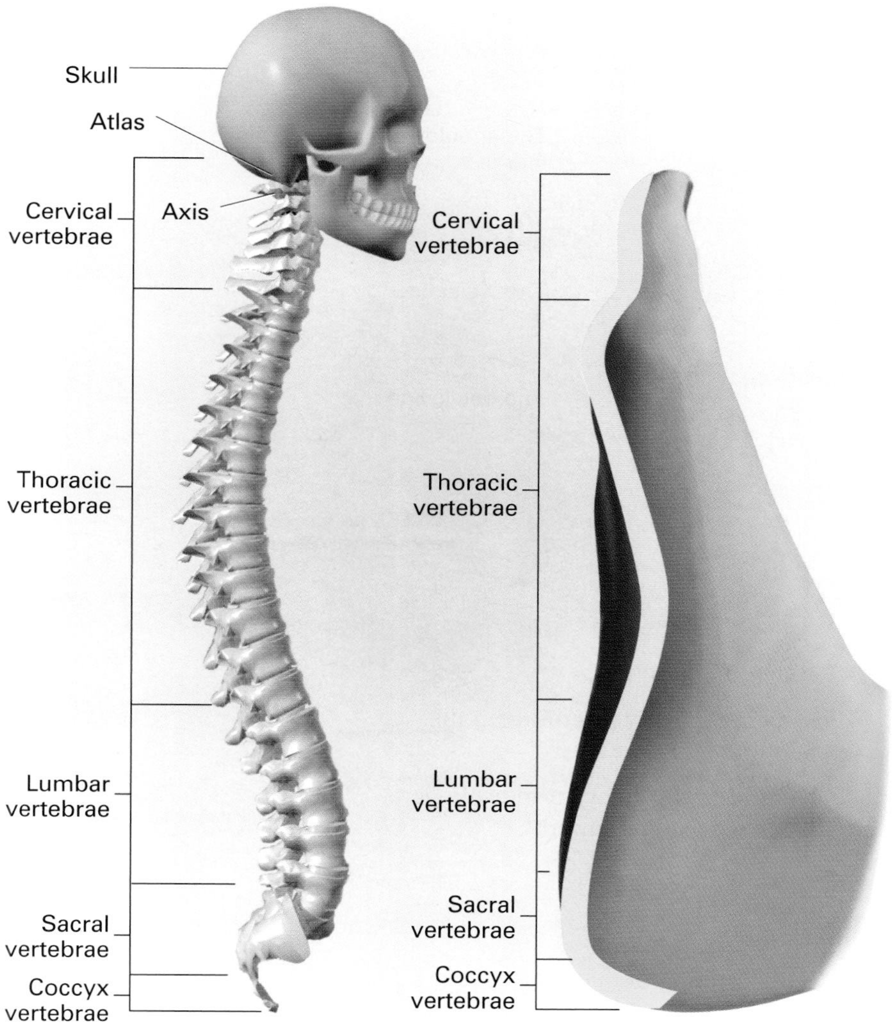

Figure 3.1 The vertebral column represented on the foot

The spine is mirrored in the foot when viewed from the side with the four natural curves of the vertebral column matching the natural curves in the foot when viewed from the side.

Transverse sections of the feet and body

The sole of the foot is divided horizontally into four distinct sections which correspond with four sections of the body, and these are:

1. The head and neck area above the shoulder line on the toes.
2. The thoracic area, the trunk between the neck and diaphragm with the lung, heart, oesophagus and other structures, on the ball of the foot.
3. The abdominal area on the arch of the foot between the ball and the heel.
4. The pelvic area on the heel of the foot.

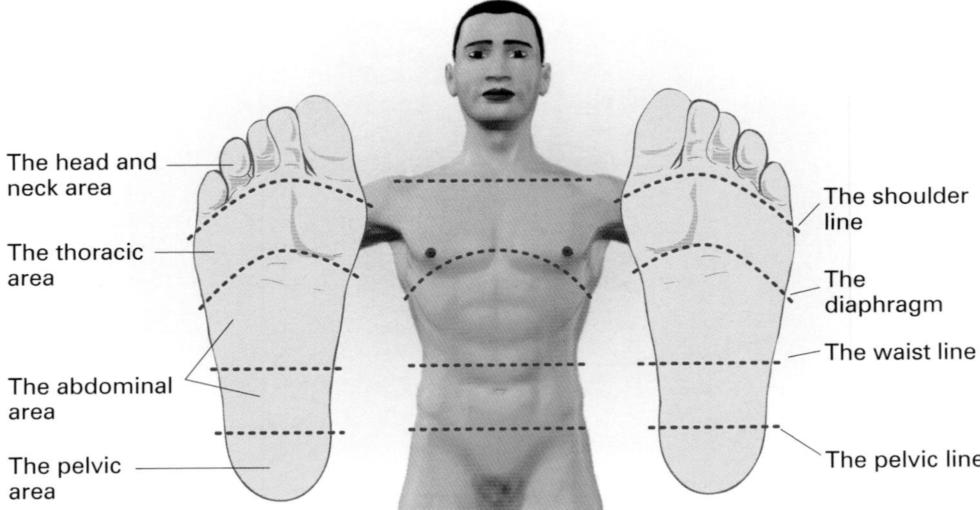

Figure 3.2 *Transverse zones*

These areas are divided by lines which are:

1. The shoulder line located just below the toes.
2. The diaphragm line located just below the metatarsal bones.
3. The waist line located in the middle of the foot from the bony protrusion at the base of the fifth metatarsal on the lateral aspect of the foot.
4. The pelvic line located at the base of the heel, found by putting your index fingers at either side of the foot on the ankle bones and drawing a line inwards.

There are four other distinct areas and these are:

1. The ankle which is the location for the reproductive system.
2. The medial aspect (inside) of the foot which is the location of the spine.
3. The lateral aspect (outside) of the foot is the location of the joints and ligaments.
4. The dorsal surface of the foot is the location for the ribs, breasts, circulation and lymph as well as face, teeth and neck.

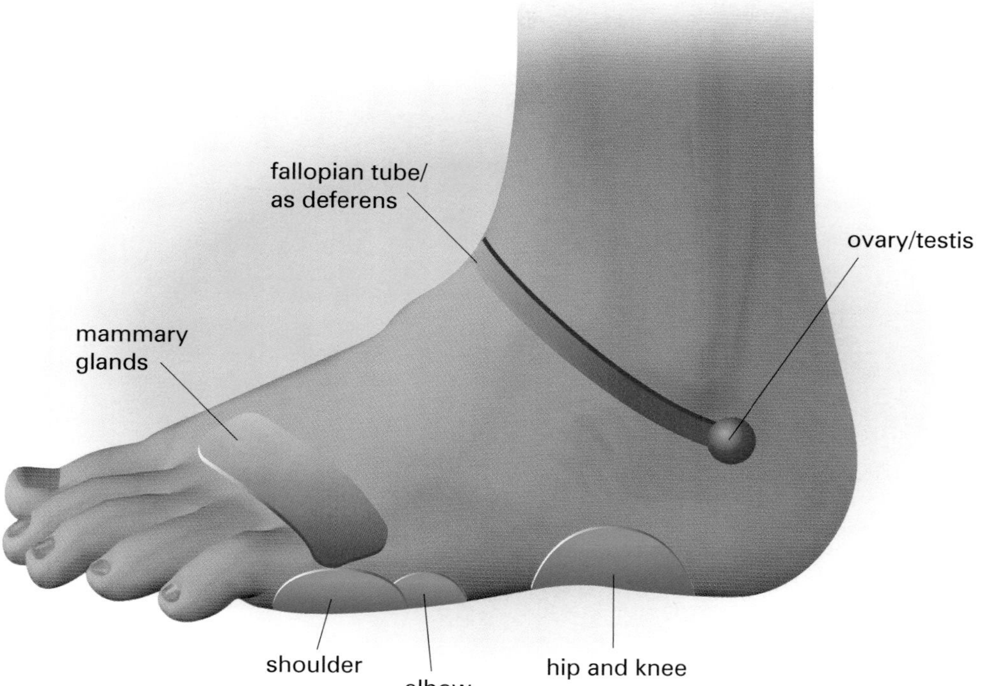

Figure 3.3A Lateral view of the foot to show reproductive area and joints

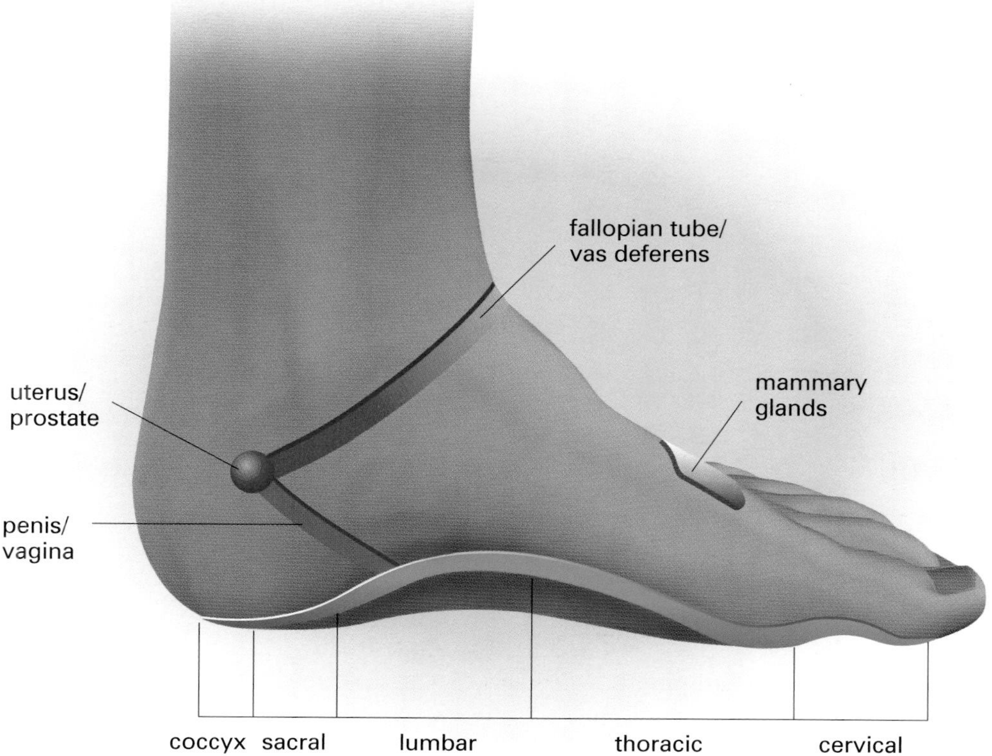

Figure 3.3B Medial view of the foot to show reproductive area and spine

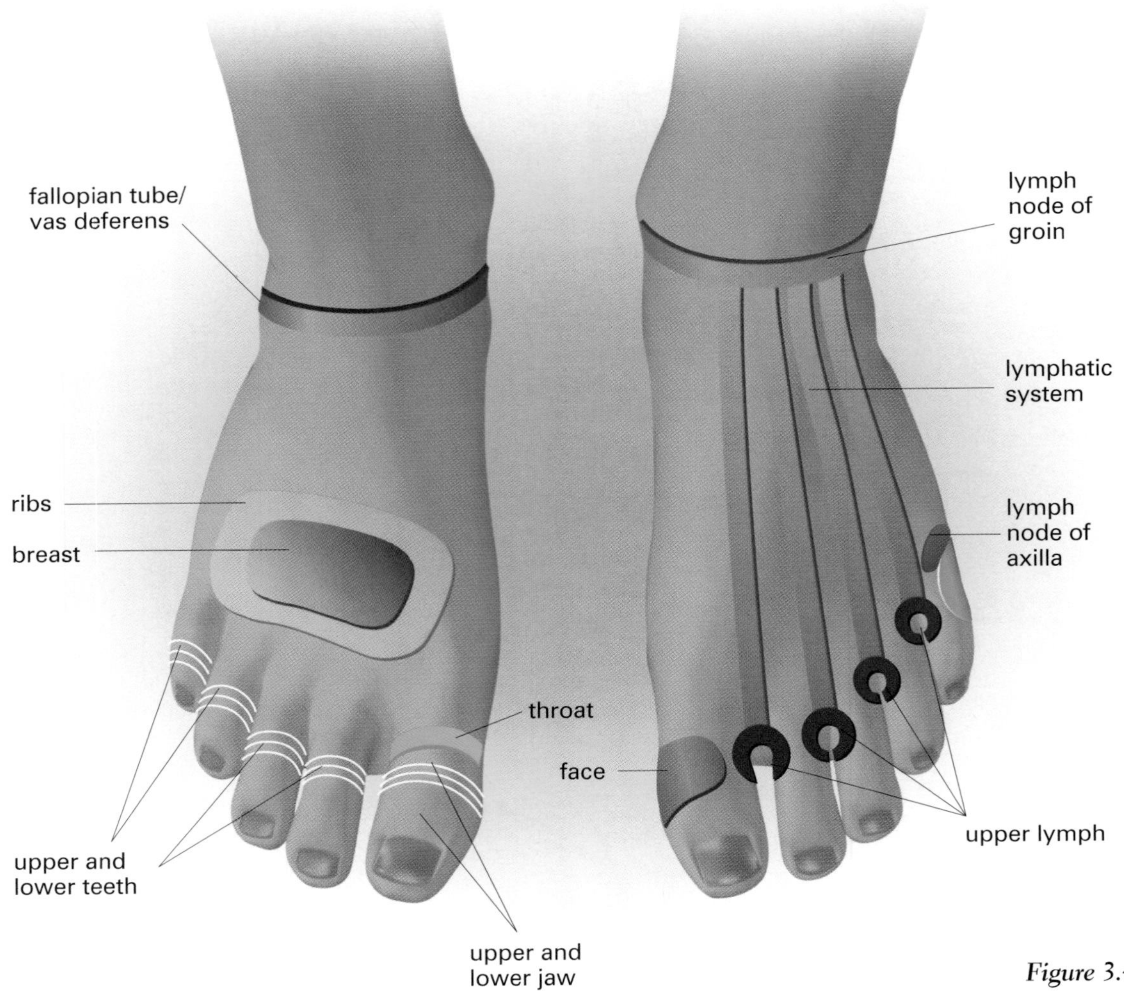

Figure 3.4 *Reflex areas on the feet (dorsal view)*

The following tables show reflex points in each section.

Head and neck	Thoracic	Abdominal	Pelvic
Pineal	Thyroid	Liver	Sciatic nerve
Hypothalamus	Parathyroid	Gall bladder	Sigmoid flexure
Pituitary	Lungs	Stomach	
Sinuses	Heart	Pancreas	
Nose	Thymus	Duodenum	
Mouth	Oesophagus	Spleen	
Eyes	Trachea	Kidneys	
Ears	Bronchii	Adrenal glands	
Upper lymphatic	Solar plexus	Small intestine	
	Diaphragm	Ilio caecal valve	
		Appendix	
		Large intestine	
		Bladder	
		Ureter	

Ankle	Medial aspect	Lateral aspect	Dorsal aspect
Ovaries	Cervical area	Shoulder	Breasts
Testes	Thoracic area	Upper arm	Upper lymph
Fallopian tubes	Lumbar area	Elbow	Ribs
Vas deferens	Sacrum	Forearm	Lungs
Uterus	Coccyx	Wrist	Face
Prostate		Hand	Teeth
Lymph/groin		Hip/Pelvis	Thyroid/Neck
Vagina		Knee	Vas deferens
Penis		Leg	Fallopian tube

NOTE: It is most important to spend time familiarising yourself with these different zones in the body and where the reflex points are situated. Try and focus on one particular area at a time and work with a partner to test each others knowledge.

Assessing the client

The reflexologist does **not** diagnose in the medical sense but does assess the client using a combination of methods to provide a picture that will indicate where any imbalance in the body lies. The methods used are:

- **Questioning** the client during the consultation, which provides specific information and is an excellent foundation on which to work.
- **Listening** to what the client is telling you. Often information will be given during consultation and during or after treatment which may have a bearing on a particular problem. It could be a small thing of no significance to the client but you may recognise it as the cause or part of the cause of a particular problem.
- **Observation** of the feet to recognise physical signs which may indicate a problem in a particular zone or over a reflex point.
- **Palpation** (examining through touch) will provide an indication of weak or sensitive areas showing where imbalance is occurring. The client will respond to painful or sensitive areas and the reflexologist should be able to feel any differences in texture on different parts of the foot. The strength and flexibility of the foot will also be felt and how resistant the tissues are to the touch, which indicates the stamina or vitality of the client. A tense foot will indicate tension in the body and a limp foot may indicate general weakness or lack of muscle tone.

Physical signs

The most common physical signs that will be observed are:

- *Corns*, which are small areas of hard skin that have formed in response to pressure or friction.
- *Calluses*, which are large areas of hardened skin, that build up to protect against pressure, friction, or wear and tear.

The presence of these two conditions may be an indication of an internal problem which has caused the reflex area to become more sensitive to pressure and friction and susceptible to the formation of corns, calluses, etc.

- *Plantar warts or verrucae*, viral infections, which may be located on weak reflex points.
- *Bunions* or lumps could indicate other mechanical problems.
- *Flat feet* may put more pressure on reflex points causing an imbalance in energy flow.
- *Scars* may affect energy flow.
- *Nail abnormalities* may be an indication of disease, vitamin or mineral deficiency.
- *Skin disorders*
- *Odour* may indicate imbalance in some systems.
- *Pigmentation* may indicate that the client has had surgery in a part of the body corresponding with the reflex point. A yellow colour may indicate imbalance in the liver, excess toxins or bile in the system. Very pale feet may indicate poor circulation.
- *Puffiness* or slight swelling will show possible areas or systems affected by fluid imbalance or other internal disorders.
- *Sweaty feet* may be an indication of thyroid imbalance.
- *Cracks* or fissures, particularly around the heel area, may indicate a hormonal imbalance or a lack of fat in the diet.
- *Dry flaky skin* may show dehydration, a skin disorder or poor circulation.
- *Variations in colour* may indicate a build up of toxins in the area, fluid retention or mucus. The extremes in colour may also be caused by circulatory disorders.
- The *temperature of the feet* if they are cold may indicate circulatory problems or if they are hot, illness or imbalance in metabolism.

Location of a tactile/physical sign

The location of a physical sign is important as it provides an indication of where the flow of energy has been disrupted. The most common physical signs which will be felt by the reflexologist are:

- A **change in texture** when the skin may alternate from smooth and moist to rough and dry or it may feel hard or soft to the touch. Sometimes you may feel a resistance or the finger or thumb may press easily into the tissue.
- A **crunchy feeling**, which has often been described as small crystals underneath the skin or gritty-like tiny grains of sand.
- A **bubble under the skin** – when moving slowly over the foot you may feel as though there is a tiny bubble just under the surface of the skin, which moves as you touch it.
- A **popping sensation** similar to the sensation you feel when you press a piece of bubble wrap.

- **A lack of mobility or stiffness** – when massaging the feet a resistance may be felt when there is a lack of mobility or stiffness in the foot.
- **Lethargy** is evident when the foot appears lifeless and is probably leaning to one side away from the midline of the body.
- **Vitality** is evident when the foot is in an upright but comfortable and relaxed position.

During treatment the client may experience different sensations as you work over the reflex points. It is important the client is aware of these and informs you of them. They may include:

- a sensitivity to touch, even the lightest of pressure
- sharp sensations as though a pin or the reflexologist's nail is scratching the skin
- pain or discomfort
- a dull ache.

Supporting the foot

The foot should be held firmly but gently and the pressure you exert should be comfortable for the client and sufficient enough to stimulate the body's healing potential. There are different support holds for the foot when working on different areas. These will be demonstrated by your tutor or instructor and you may choose the most comfortable for you and each individual client.

All the information from the assessment should be recorded and kept as part of the client's case history, as in the case of the following assessment record card.

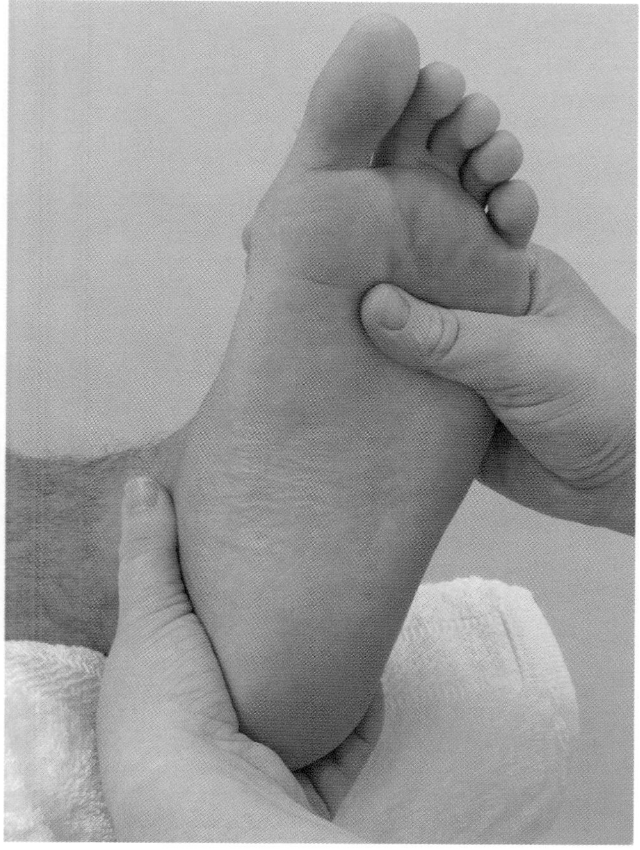

Supporting the foot

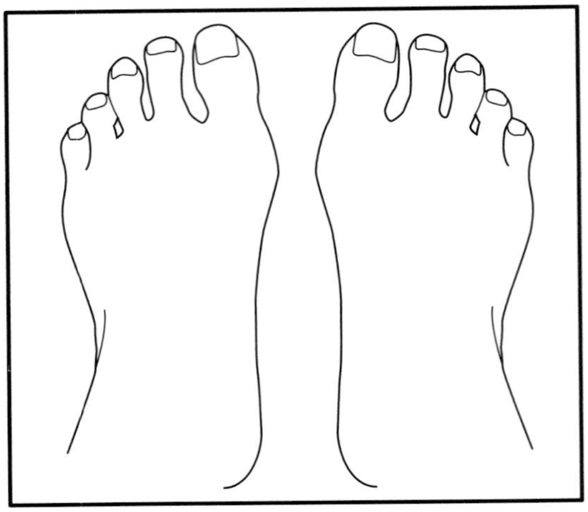

FOOT ASSESSMENT RECORD

NAME ______________________________

DATE ______________________________

REFLEXOLOGIST ______________________________

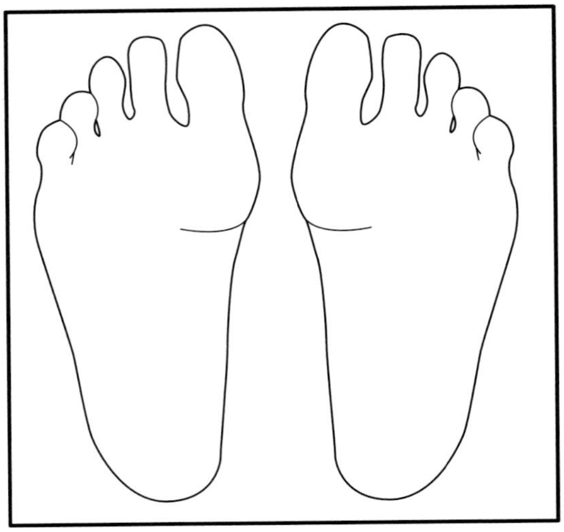

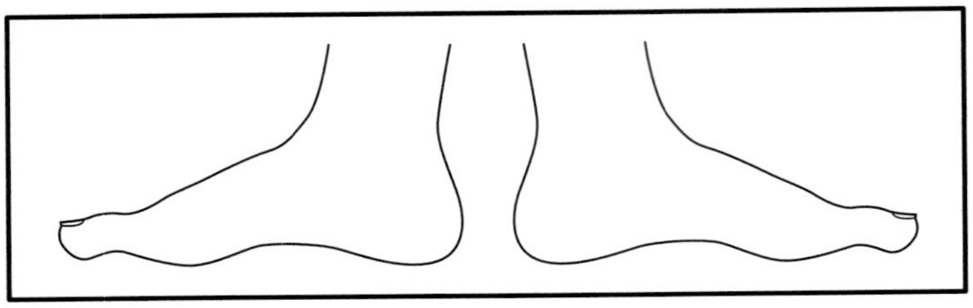

VISUAL ASSESSMENT

RESULT OF PALPATION

CLIENT FEEDBACK

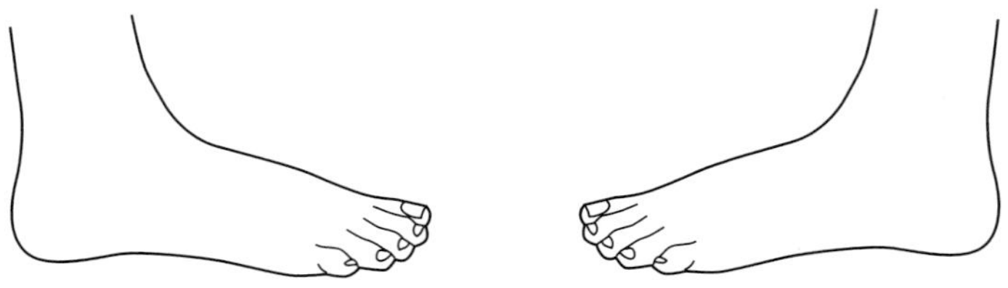

Figure 3.5 Record of foot assessment

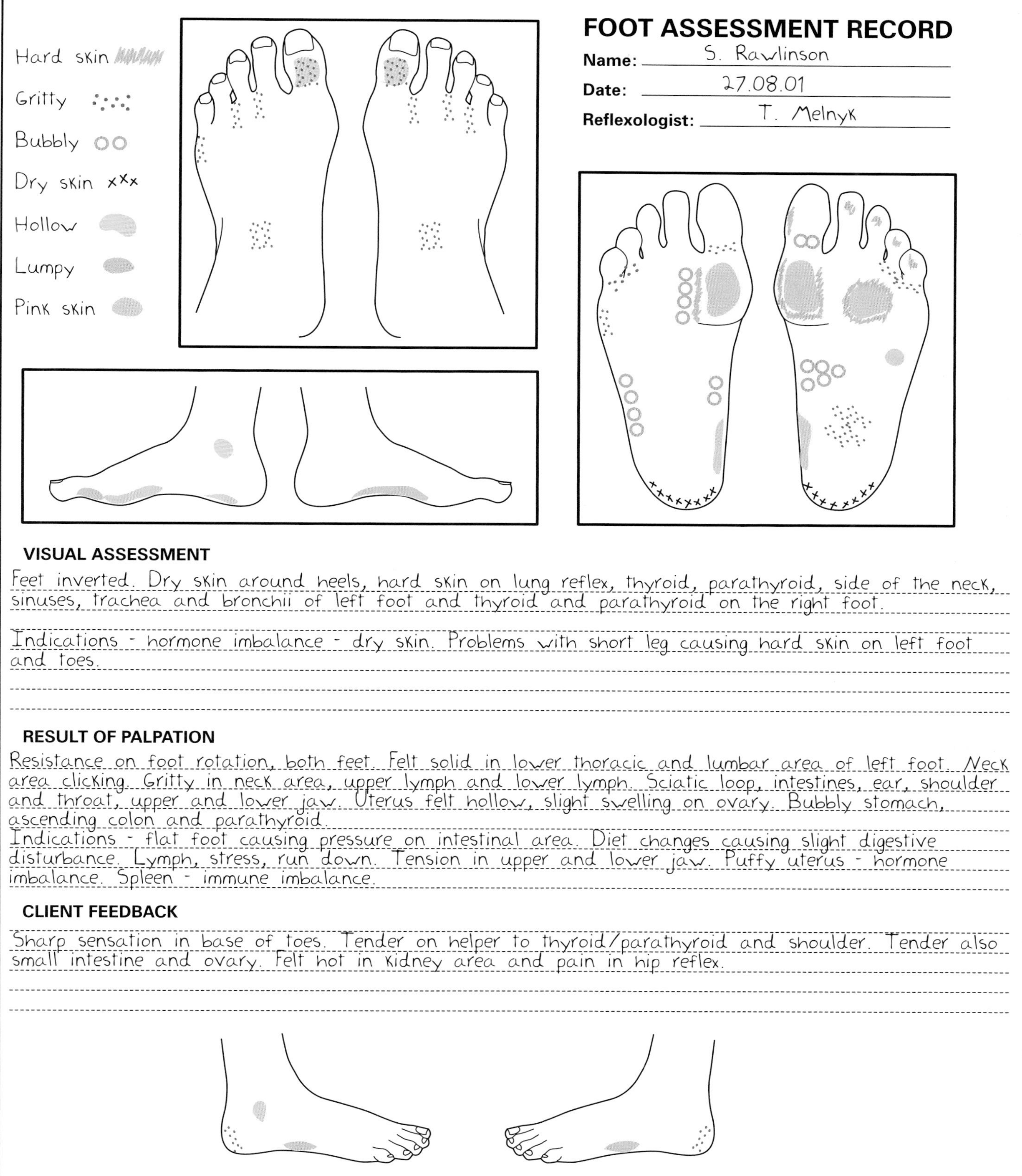

FOOT ASSESSMENT RECORD

Name: S. Rawlinson

Date: 27.08.01

Reflexologist: T. Melnyk

Hard skin
Gritty
Bubbly
Dry skin xxx
Hollow
Lumpy
Pink skin

VISUAL ASSESSMENT

Feet inverted. Dry skin around heels, hard skin on lung reflex, thyroid, parathyroid, side of the neck, sinuses, trachea and bronchii of left foot and thyroid and parathyroid on the right foot.

Indications - hormone imbalance - dry skin. Problems with short leg causing hard skin on left foot and toes.

RESULT OF PALPATION

Resistance on foot rotation, both feet. Felt solid in lower thoracic and lumbar area of left foot. Neck area clicking. Gritty in neck area, upper lymph and lower lymph. Sciatic loop, intestines, ear, shoulder and throat, upper and lower jaw. Uterus felt hollow, slight swelling on ovary. Bubbly stomach, ascending colon and parathyroid.

Indications - flat foot causing pressure on intestinal area. Diet changes causing slight digestive disturbance. Lymph, stress, run down. Tension in upper and lower jaw. Puffy uterus - hormone imbalance. Spleen - immune imbalance.

CLIENT FEEDBACK

Sharp sensation in base of toes. Tender on helper to thyroid/parathyroid and shoulder. Tender also small intestine and ovary. Felt hot in kidney area and pain in hip reflex.

Figure 3.6 *Completed foot assessment record*

PRACTICE IN CONTEXT

1 Starting with family and friends or colleagues, look at the shape of their feet and record the shape of the foot in relation to the shape and size of the body and note how often they correspond. Familiarise yourself with the position of the horizontal dividing lines on different sized feet.

2 Working on two different sets of feet at the same time, concentrate on one aspect of assessment at a time until you are familiar with that method of assessing the foot. Start with the visual aspect by observing the feet and making detailed notes of the outcome.

3 Continue with palpation, close your eyes and concentrate solely on feeling the feet without the visual signs to distract you, again making notes of your findings.

4 Finally look at the physical characteristics that appear on the feet and note their significance.

This exercise will help to provide you with a greater understanding of the differences that are evident in each individual.

ASSESSMENT OF KNOWLEDGE

1 Which reflex points are located on the lateral and medial aspects of the foot?

2 During the physical assessment of the client what indicates the stamina and vitality of the feet?

3 What is a callus?

4 List four sensations the client may feel during treatment.

5 What colour would the feet appear if the client had poor circulation?

4 Contraindications

A contraindication is any reason why the reflexologist cannot give the client a treatment for a specific reason. It is a common belief amongst practitioners that there are no contraindications as it is a gentle, non-invasive holistic treatment that cannot do any harm and any stimulation that does occur is very gentle. There are however some occasions when the permission of a medical doctor or specialist needs to be given before treatment commences or when special care must be taken, or the treatment adapted.

It is always advisable to err on the side of caution when treating any client you feel may be at risk.

Conditions that contraindicate treatment

There are certain conditions that are generally thought to contraindicate reflexology treatment and these are:

- **Heart disease** A client with heart disease may have several different but related problems. They will probably be taking medication and this may, on occasion, have an effect on the working of the heart. The degree of heart disease will vary and if the heart is working inefficiently this may have a negative effect on other systems of the body; in such a case it is inadvisable to carry out a general treatment which releases toxins into the body that overloads already weakened systems.
- **Thrombosis** Thrombosis is the formation of a blood clot and is thought by many practitioners a reason not to give a reflexology treatment. This is because the nature of the treatment increases the circulation and this increases the possibility of a blood clot moving and causing damage.
- **Post-operative treatment** There is an increased risk of thrombosis immediately after an operation.
- **Temperature** If the client has a fever the body is already fighting to heal itself, therefore treatment may release more toxins into the system. It is advisable to wait until the fever subsides before commencing treatment. Body temperature is controlled by the hypothalamus and the normal body temperature is about 37°C.
- **Infectious disease** There is a possibility of cross-infection to yourself and other clients.
- **Conditions requiring surgery**.

If the feet have any of the following problems then treatment cannot be given, unless the problem area is small and can be covered and protected, preventing discomfort for the client and cross-infection.

- cuts or abrasions in the skin
- undiagnosed lumps and bumps
- severe bruising to the area

In these cases the reflexologist could work on the reflex points on the hands or cross reflexes.

Taking special care

Special care must be taken in certain circumstances or medical permission sought to carry out treatment. For example:

- The client is undergoing medical treatment.
- During pregnancy, particularly the first sixteen weeks when there is a history of miscarriage.
- People with diabetes have a slower rate of healing, their skin is thinner and bruises easily, therefore less pressure should be used, particularly over the pancreas. Great care should be taken not to scratch the skin and in some circumstances treatment time should be shortened.
- Epilepsy requires extreme care when working the head and brain areas.
- Arthritic feet require gentle pressure.
- Osteoporosis requires gentle pressure as bones are fragile.
- Broken bones or sprains, gentle pressure or hand reflexes may be treated.
- If a client is on strong medication, which is obviously given in particular doses, reflexology may hasten its elimination from the system thus not allowing the medication to have the desired effect. Therefore medical permission must be sought before starting treatment.

Each client is an individual and must be treated as such. As you become more knowledgeable, more experienced at assessing a client, more skilled in the application of reflexology treatment and more intuitive, you will be able to recognise automatically when to provide treatment and how to adapt treatment for each client.

Permission for treatment

It is important to ensure that your client agrees with your assessment and that a doctor's permission is sought when in doubt about providing treatment. The client must obtain permission for treatment from their medical practitioner and it is always advisable to have a written copy of this permission in your client's case file.

It is not advisable to use words like 'consent' or 'permission' to medical practitioners as this could have an effect on their own insurance.

The following is an example of a form for obtaining permission from a medical practitioner to carry out reflexology on a client who is receiving medical treatment.

The Complementary Therapy Clinic
Hardwicke Crescent
Sheffield SH5 10A

Dear Dr ....

Mrs ......NAME...... has recently attended my clinic for reflexology, a non-invasive complementary holistic treatment. During consultation it was established that she is receiving medical treatment and is currently prescribed the following ..MEDICATION.. I appreciate you have limited time to respond to such queries so I have included a reply slip for you to complete and return, in the envelope provided, confirming if reflexology treatment may be given. Thank you for your assistance in this matter.

Yours sincerely

Joseph Thomas

✂ --

Mrs ....

- ❑ May receive reflexology treatment.
- ❑ May not receive reflexology treatment.
- ❑ Must wait .... months to have reflexology treatment.
- ❑ Please arrange a telephone appointment to discuss this matter further.

Signed .... **Date** ....

Cross reflexes

These are corresponding reflex areas in the body or 'areas of referral'. The cross reflex may be worked (i.e. to treat or manipulate) when you are prevented from working on the corresponding area, due to injury, damage or tenderness. When the foot may not be treated at all, then the corresponding reflex points on the hand may be worked.

Also if there is a particular reflex point on the foot that is tender or sore then the corresponding reflex may be worked on the foot. For example, if you wanted to treat the shoulder reflex because the client had a frozen shoulder but that area on the foot had a cut in the skin, then you could treat the hip reflex lower down, and as they are cross reflexes the shoulder will benefit.

When different organs in the same longitudinal zone are treated, energy blockages may be removed thus benefiting other organs within that zone.

The cross reflexes are shown in Figure 4.1.

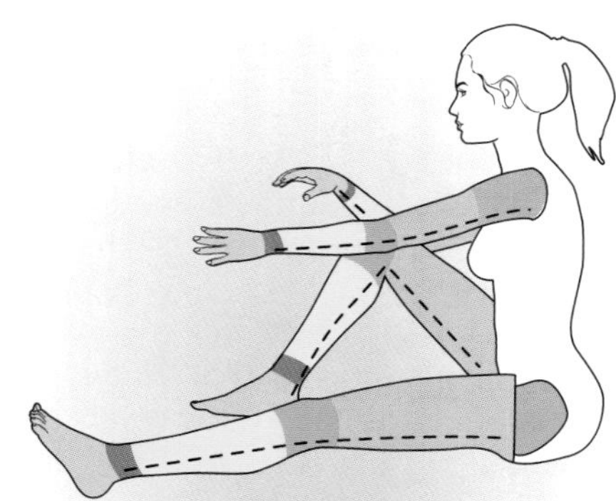

Foot	=	Hand
Sole of foot	=	Palm of the hand
Dorsum	=	Back of the hand
Big toe	=	Thumb
Small toes	=	Fingers
Ankle	=	Wrist
Lower leg	=	Forearm
Knee	=	Elbow
Thigh	=	Upper arm
Hip	=	Shoulder

Figure 4.1 *Cross reflexes or areas of referral in the body*

PRACTICE IN CONTEXT

1 Using a medical dictionary or other source of reference, research some of the conditions which contraindicate treatment.

2 Discuss with your tutor and colleagues the experiences they may have had with a client who has had to obtain GP approval before treatment. Collect examples of letters they may have written to and received from doctors or other health care professionals.

ASSESSMENT OF KNOWLEDGE

1 Define the word contraindication.

2 Why do most reflexologists believe that there are few contraindications to reflexology?

3 Why do some practitioners feel it is inadvisable to treat a client immediately after an operation?

4 How can you adapt treatment for a client who has severe bruising on the foot?

5 Which condition requires extreme care when working reflexes in the head and brain area?

6 Name the cross reflex in the body for (a) the sole of the foot, (b) the hip and (c) the ankle.

5 Conditions of the feet

It is important that you recognise the many conditions which affect the feet, the possible effects that these conditions may have on the body and how they may be responsible for or caused by other problems in the body. In some cases you will be able to advise the client to seek professional advice from a doctor or chiropodist.

Many clients suffer problems such as corns and bunions without ever having treatment for them. You may be able to point out to a client the physical benefits of having professional treatment from a chiropodist and advise her to consult her doctor if she has a condition which is causing pain. I have a client who had dropped arches, a condition she had suffered with all her life, which were particularly severe on her left foot. In her words she said, 'I thought it was something I had to live with.' When I recommended a visit to her doctor to discuss the pain she was suffering in her knee, ankle and hip, she was immediately referred to her local hospital and the podiatrist supplied her with insoles and a lift on the sole of her left shoe. Within weeks the pain in her joints had reduced considerably.

Problems of the feet

Arthritis

This is a condition which attacks the lining of joints and causes swelling, stiffness and pain. **Osteoarthritis** is degenerative, attacking the cartilage around the ends of bones and affecting the weight-bearing joints; it is worse in those who are overweight or have an impaired blood supply. **Rheumatoid arthritis** is a chronic condition mainly affecting the elderly. The origin is unknown, but it is thought to be triggered by a virus or emotional stress.

Athlete's foot (tinea pedis)

This is a fungal infection affecting the foot. It lives in the keratin (the protein in the skin) and produces enzymes which then break the skin down. The moist, warm conditions in which the feet live – tight shoes and socks, toes pressed closely together – make it an ideal environment for the growth of this fungus. The characteristics of this condition are general itching, a peeling and softening of the skin between the toes, and the skin on the top of the foot by the affected area can become red and may also itch. Athlete's foot may also infect the skin on the soles of the feet. This may be in patches or across the entire sole; it is often dry, may crack, be sore and itchy. It is not contagious in all cases; there are some people who are repeatedly exposed to this fungus yet rarely affected.

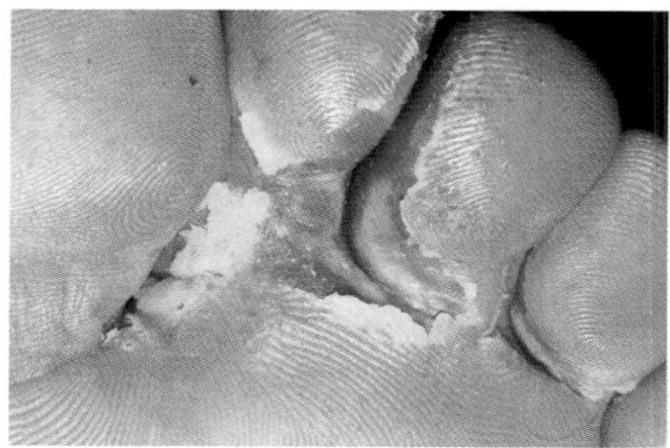

Tinea pedis

Bunion (hallux valgus)

Bunion is a common term used to describe a prominence on the side of the big toe joint. This condition can be caused by wearing ill-fitting shoes and is the result of joint displacement. The big toe may be forced into an unnatural position by pressure over a period of time. Inflammation and swelling of the bursa (the fluid surrounding the joints) occurs. A bunion may develop as a result of a combination of different factors. These may be a strong hereditary factor, abnormal foot function, arthritic conditions, trauma and neuromuscular conditions. It may also be caused by a weakness at the joint between the big toe and the metatarsal. These factors may cause the big toe to deviate inwards and in extreme cases over or under the second toe. A lump may form on the inside of the foot at the base of the big toe and this may become inflamed and painful.

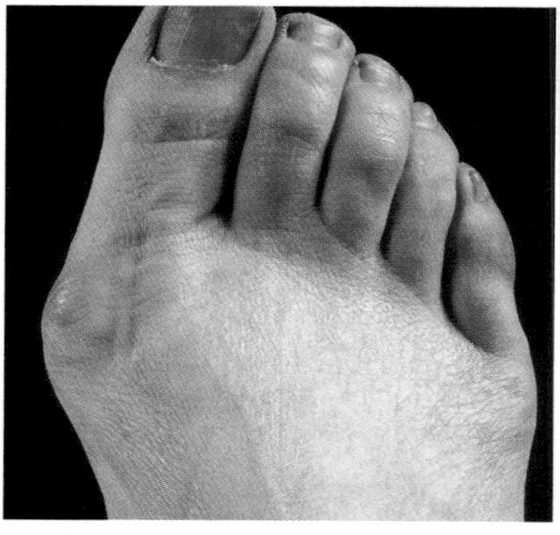

A bunion

Callus

This is a patch of hard, thickened skin which accumulates as a result of pressure on the foot. The most common sites are the weight-bearing heel and the ball of the foot as they take the most impact when walking. Calluses are often intrinsic, associated with uneven weight distribution caused by an abnormality of gait or bone structure and will continue to develop if the problem is not addressed. A burning sensation is often felt in the area because of the irritation of the nerve endings in the skin.

Corn

A corn is a type of callus, a thickened dense area of skin, forming a raised appearance and situated on pressure areas such as the joints of toes, the ball and heel of the foot. They are most commonly caused by ill-fitting shoes and develop as a protection against constant friction. They may also occur on the sole of the foot, when pressure is exerted continuously in one point, creating a hard cone of skin which penetrates deep into the tissue causing pain. This may be caused by an imbalance in posture with weight-bearing heavily in one place. Another common type of corn appears between the toes; this is a soft corn that does not have a hard central mass and it is usually sore when opposing toes move against each other.

Chilblains

These are painful itchy areas on the feet, varying in colour from dull blue to red. The cause is an inadequate blood supply; however the condition is aggravated by cold and damp. Those most susceptible are the elderly and those who work in cold, hot or damp conditions.

Diabetes

This condition has an effect on the feet because of the reduced blood supply and nerve supply to the muscles and skin tissue. The healing properties of the skin on the feet is impaired and there is an increased chance of infection. The feet may appear cold and pale in colour and the skin is usually dry. As the nerve supply is reduced the sensitivity to pain is reduced. This loss of sensation in time can lead to poor muscle control and impaired balance.

Enlarged curvature of the nail (onychogryposis)

This is an enlarged nail caused by an increase in the production of the horny cells of the nail plate. This leads to a curvature of the nail resembling a ram's horn. It is more common in the elderly and the big toe is most frequently affected. The causes are age, persistent friction from a shoe over a period of time, neglect or injury.

Fallen arches (pes planus)

This is a condition due to partial or total collapse of one or both arches of the feet. There are several causes and these include weak muscles, injury, being overweight, ill-fitting shoes or it may be hereditary. This condition causes the ankle to lean inwards causing a weak joint. It produces pain and tiredness in the foot and in some cases in the lower leg up to the knee. The foot acts as a natural shock absorber for the body and without sufficient support this is lost creating problems in the spine and lower back pain. Clients may complain of a 'burning' sensation in the foot when the ligaments and arches are no longer providing sufficient support.

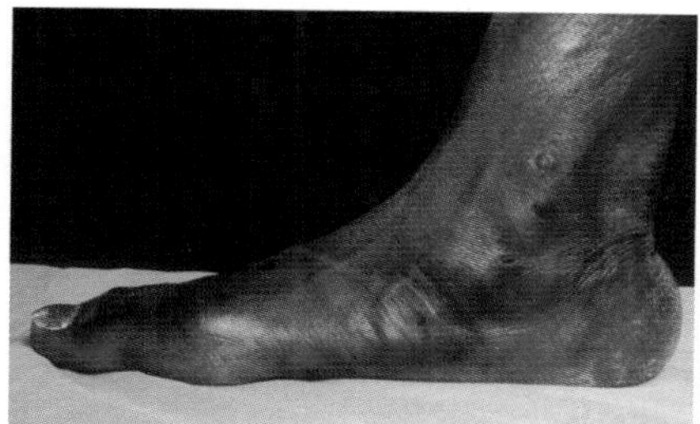

Fallen arches

Gout

This is a metabolic disease caused by a build up of uric acid crystals in the joints. Uric acid is the waste product formed from protein breakdown and is normally excreted via the kidneys. Problems may arise if there is too much protein in the diet or excretion is impaired causing a build up in the system. There is sometimes a genetic predisposition to this condition but diet and diuretic drugs may also have an effect. Its characteristics are pain, inflammation and swelling, and it mostly affects males.

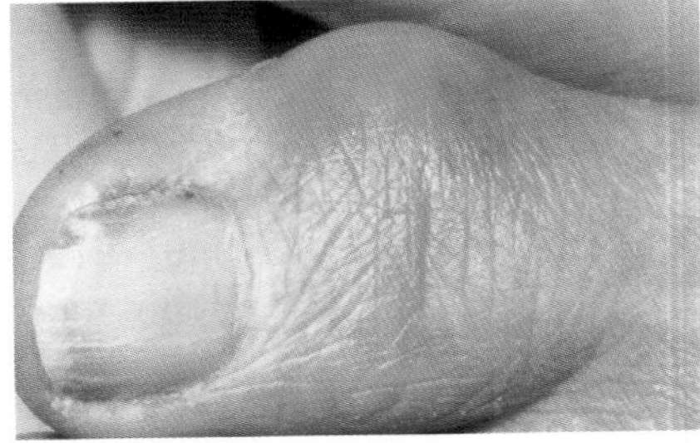

Gout

Hammer toes

This is a deformity of the middle three toes, which may lead to other problems such as painful corns, bursitis or arthritis. The condition may be hereditary, caused by ill-fitting shoes or a bunion. They become more rigid with age.

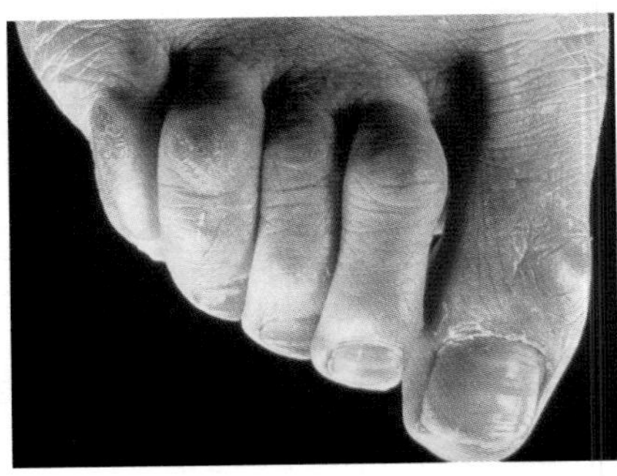

Hammer toes

Heel spurs

This is an overgrowth of bone on the heel of the foot, which builds up over a period of time. Being overweight may contribute to this condition.

High arches (pes cavus)

A high arch causes the foot to be more rigid, limiting movement, and it can pull the toes backwards in a condition known as 'clawfoot', making it more susceptible to corns and calluses. The natural shock absorption provided by the arch is reduced. Metatarsal arch supports will help to alleviate problems.

Hyperhidrosis

It is quite normal for the feet to sweat and occasionally for there to be a slight odour. For some the problem can be more persistent – there is a greater density of sweat glands in the skin of the soles of the feet than anywhere else on the body and overactivity of the sweat glands causes an abnormal amount of sweat to be produced. The feet, being enclosed for long periods of time in socks, stockings or tights and shoes, are often affected by this condition.

Ingrowing toenail (onychocryptosis)

This is a common condition of the big toe penetrating the nail wall at the side of the nail itself. It may look red and sometimes swollen and in some cases it may be extremely painful. There are several causes, such as pressure from shoes or trainers, cutting the nails too low, and imbalance when walking causing pressure on the nail and forcing it into the tissue at the side of it.

Onychomycosis

This is the name given to ringworm of the nail. The fungus enters the nail at the free edge and spreads down towards the matrix (the root of the nail). The first sign of the disease is a small patch at the side or free edge of the nail, which is white or yellowish in colour. It causes the nail to become thickened and discoloured and eventually it may become cracked and lift away from the nail bed completely. This is a progressive disease and if left untreated will spread from one nail to the next.

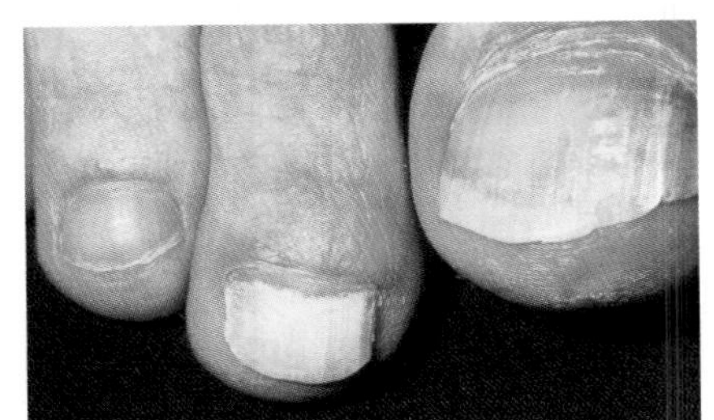

Onchomycosis

Verruca plantaris

This is a viral infection causing warts on the soles of the feet, which then become flattened with pressure. As the warts often occur on the weight-bearing part of the foot, it forces the lesion into the dermis and this puts pressure on the nerve endings thus causing pain. Verrucae appear in different forms, the most common being a single isolated lesion with defined margins and a small black dot in the central core. On non-weight-bearing surfaces they appear more like a common wart raised with a craggy appearance.

You will in the course of your work as a reflexologist see many different conditions of the feet and it is always a good idea to write notes about them as you treat them. Include the characteristics of the condition, the causes, how it affected the client and if you had to adapt treatment. Then you can use this information for future reference.

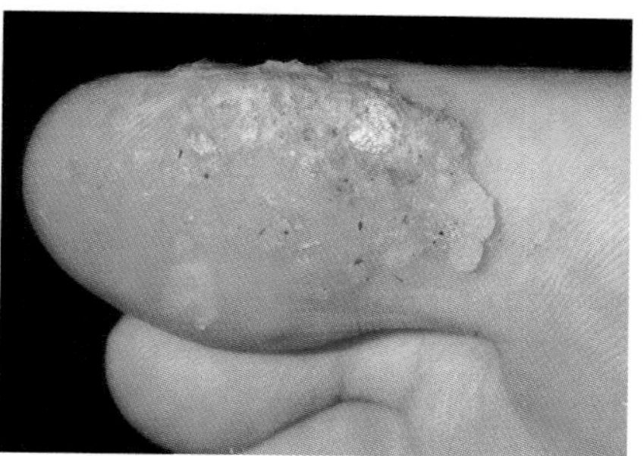

Verrucca

PRACTICE IN CONTEXT

Compile a table of different conditions which affect the feet and classify them under the following headings: permanent, temporary, muscular, skeletal, skin, nail and infectious.

ASSESSMENT OF KNOWLEDGE

1. Why is it important for the reflexologist to recognise different foot conditions?
2. What are the characteristics of athlete's foot?
3. Which part of the foot does a bunion affect?
4. What adverse effects will fallen arches have on the foot?
5. Name one viral infection of the foot.

6 Anatomy and physiology of the foot

Working on the feet requires you to be familiar with the anatomy and physiology of the foot. A thorough knowledge of the foot and how it works will allow you to offer advice with confidence when required. Knowing the positions of certain bones and tendons will help you to learn where specific reflex points are positioned, as your tutor may refer to points on the foot when providing instruction in reflexology techniques.

The following definitions will help in understanding the anatomy of the foot

Definition of terms

Anterior	At the front
Distal	Further from the point of origin or further from the point of attachment to the body
Dorsal	On the back (top of the foot is called the dorsal surface)
Dorsiflexion	Bend the foot upwards
Inferior	Below
Lateral	Away from the midline of the body
Ligaments	They hold bones together at joints
Medial	Near to the midline of the body
Plantar	On the front (the sole of the foot is called the plantar surface)
Plantarflexion	Straightens the ankle bends the foot downwards
Posterior	At the back
Proximal	Nearer to the point of origin or nearer to the point of attachment to the body
Superior	Above
Tendon	A cord of connective tissue which attaches a muscle to the periosteum of a bone

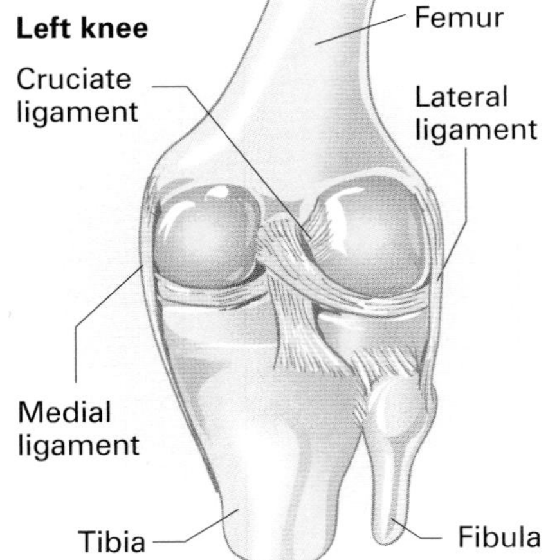

Figure 6.1 A ligament

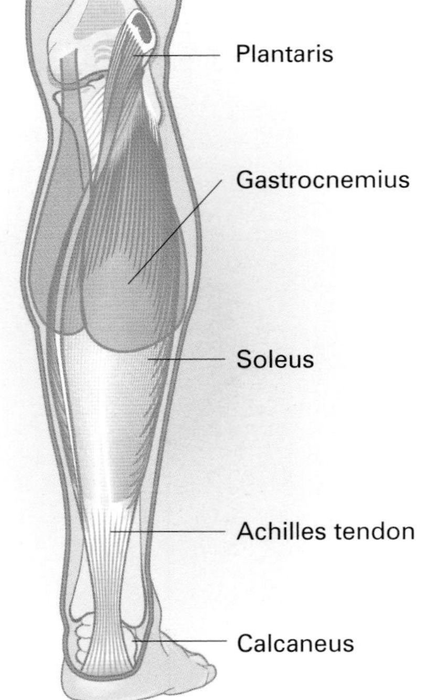

Figure 6.2 A tendon

The structure of the foot

The foot is an arched, flexible platform that supports and moves the body. It is made up of a complicated arrangement of bones, which allow us to stand firmly with ease and to walk and run while keeping our balance. To enable the foot to bear the weight of the body the bones of the toes are broader and flatter than those of the hands. The foot is extremely flexible because of the intricate anatomy, which consists of bones, ligaments, tendons and muscles.

The bones of the feet

The bones of the foot consist of the tarsals, metatarsals and phalanges.

There are seven **tarsal** or ankle bones and these are:

- **1 calcaneus** The largest and strongest of the tarsals, it is situated at the lower back part of the foot. It transmits the weight of the body to the ground and provides a strong lever for the calf muscles.

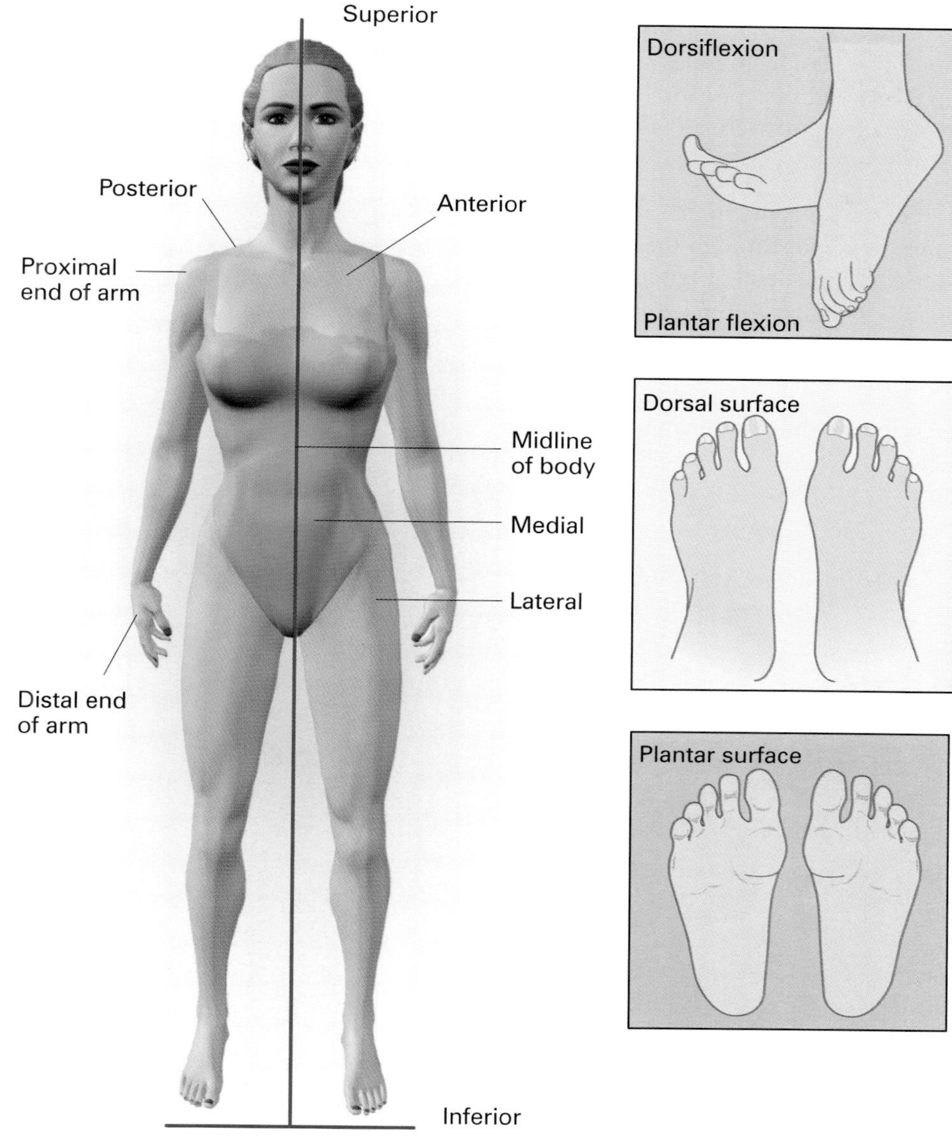

Figure 6.3 Anatomical positions

- **1 talus** This is situated above calcaneus in the posterior part of the foot, helping to support the tibia above and initially bearing the entire weight of the body during walking before transmitting half the weight to calcaneus.
- **1 cuboid** This is situated on the outer side of the foot in front of the calcaneus and behind the fourth and fifth metatarsals.
- **1 navicular** This is situated in front of talus and behind the first, second and third cuneiform bones.
- **3 cuneiform** These are bones wedge shaped and situated in front of navicular, and together with the cuboid they form the anterior row of tarsals.

There are five **metatarsals.** They are long bones that articulate with the tarsal bones at their proximal end and with the phalanges at their distal end.

There are fourteen **phalanges** altogether, two in the big toe and three in the other four toes. Each one consists of a proximal base, a shaft and a distal head.

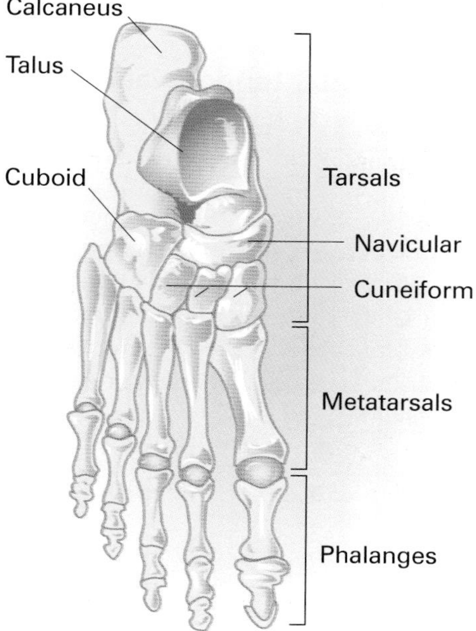

Figure 6.4 The bones of the foot

The arches of the feet

The bones are arranged in two flexible arches, supported by muscles and ligaments. These allow the weight of the body to be supported and they provide leverage when walking. They are the longitudinal arch and the transverse arch.

The **longitudinal arch** has two parts: the medial longitudinal arch and the lateral longitudinal arch. The medial longitudinal arch, which is the higher of the two, originates at the calcaneus, ascends to the talus, descends through the navicular, the three cuneiform and the three medial metatarsals. The lateral longitudinal arch also begins at the calcaneus; it rises at the cuboid and descends to the two lateral metatarsals. The talus is the key part of the medial arch and the cuboid is the key part of the lateral arch.

The **transverse arch** runs across the foot and is formed by the calcaneus, navicular, cuboid and the posterior part of the five metatarsals.

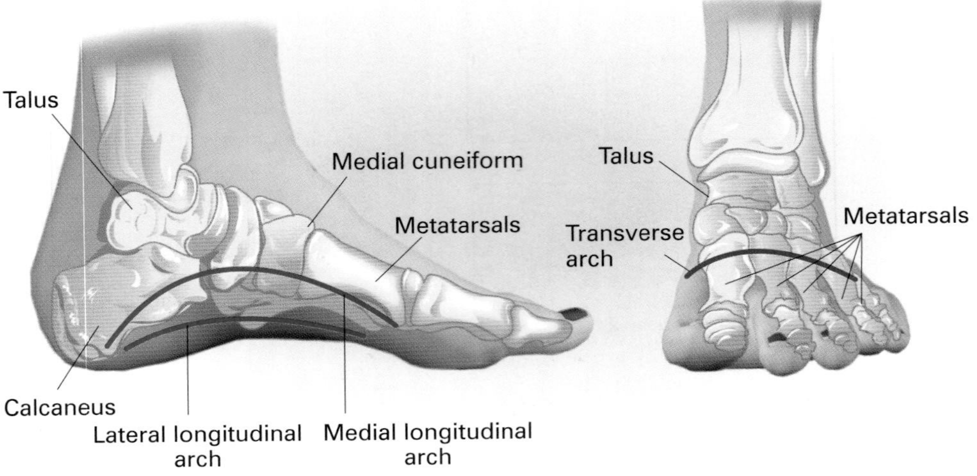

Figure 6.5 The arches of the foot

Ligaments, tendons and muscles

The foot has many movable joints between all the bones, therefore strong ligaments and muscles are necessary to maintain the power, flexibility, suppleness and stability of the foot while moving, walking, running and jumping.

Muscles are made up of a large number of muscle fibres to form contractile tissue that allows a muscle to function by alternate phases of contraction and relaxation. To work efficiently muscles require an adequate blood supply to provide oxygen and nutrients and an efficient removal of waste products via the lymphatic system. These nutrients provide the energy required by the muscles and it comes from the breakdown of carbohydrates and fat in the diet.

The muscles which plantarflex the foot are:

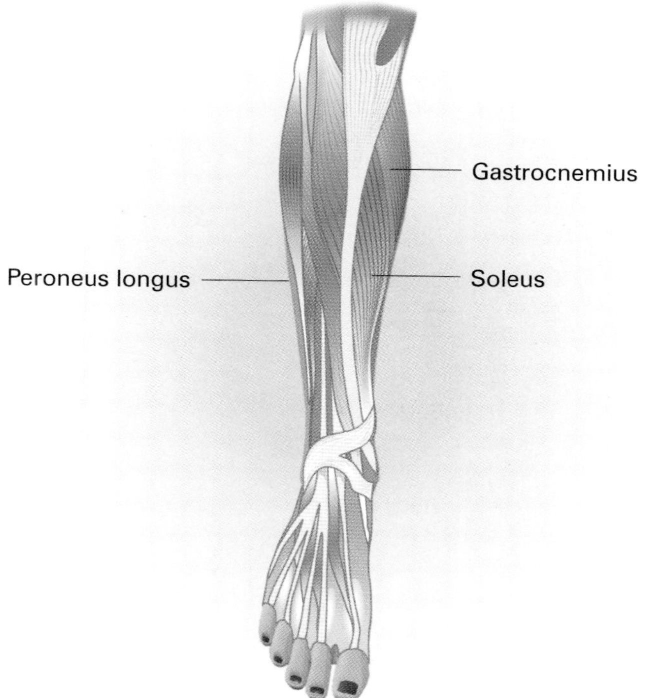

Figure 6.6 *Muscles that plantarflex the foot*

The muscles that dorsiflex the foot are :

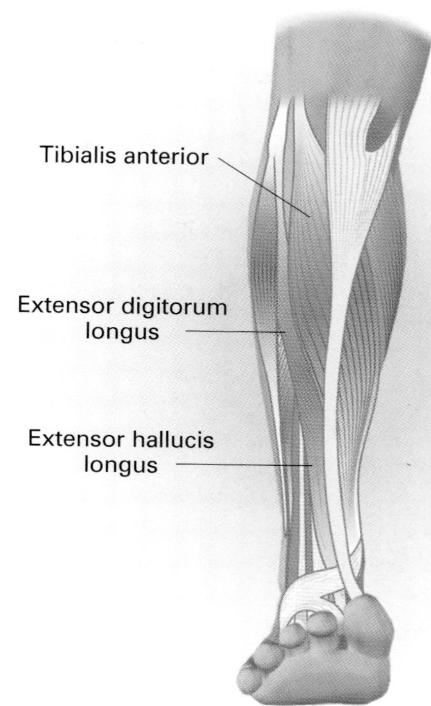

Figure 6.7 *Muscles that dorsiflex the foot*

The **Achilles tendon** raises the foot and it is attached to the soleus and gastrocnemius muscles in the back of the lower leg where it inserts into the calcaneus on the heel.

There are four ligaments in the foot which strengthen the ankle joint and these are the anterior, posterior, lateral and deltoid ligaments.

The blood supply

The **popliteal artery** begins behind the knee joint and is a continuation of the **femoral artery**. The arteries of the leg, which carry blood to the foot, are shown in the following flow chart.

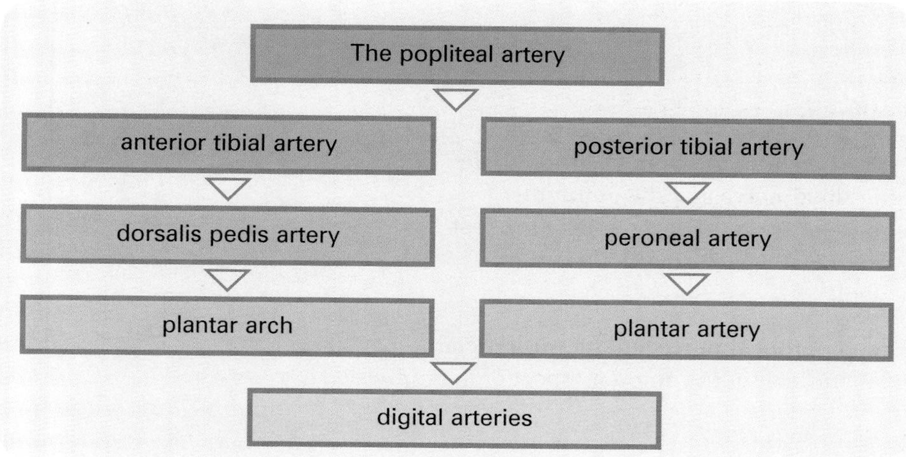

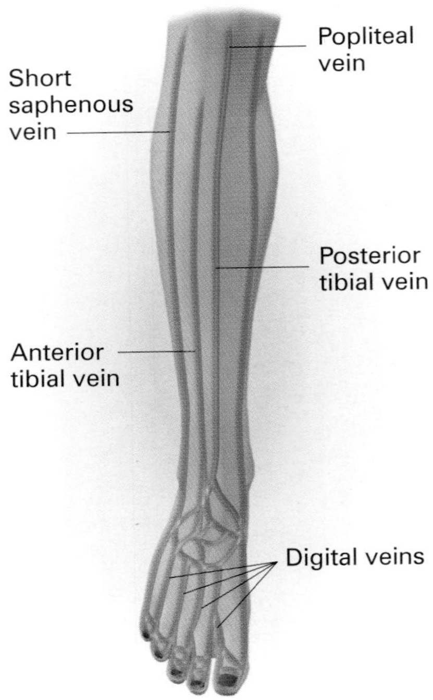

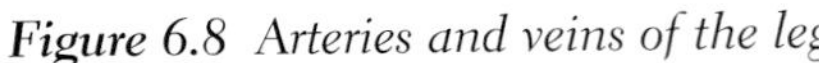
Figure 6.8 Arteries and veins of the leg

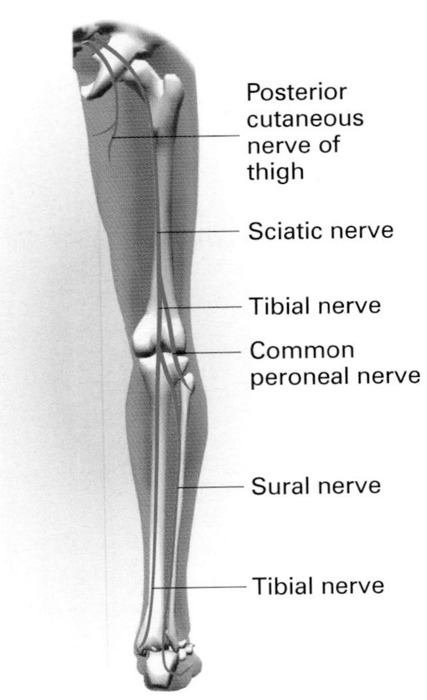

Figure 6.9 Nerve supply to the leg and foot

The veins which take blood away from the foot and back towards the heart are:

Superficial veins

- The short saphenous vein from behind the ankle joint ascends the leg to join the deep popliteal vein.
- The long saphenous vein, the longest in the body, ascends the leg past the knee to the thigh to join the femoral vein.

Deep veins

These veins accompany the arteries and their branches and they have the same names.

- Digital veins
- Plantar venous arch
- Posterior tibial vein
- Anterior tibial vein
- Popliteal vein

The nerve supply

The **sciatic nerve** is the largest in the body. It descends from the buttock, through the thigh to the hamstrings, and then divides into the **tibial nerve** and the **common peroneal nerves**. The tibial nerve supplies the muscles and skin of the sole of the foot and the toes. One of its main branches is the **sural nerve** which supplies the heel, lateral aspect of the foot and the dorsum of the foot.

The common peroneal nerve divides into the **deep peroneal nerve** and the **superficial peroneal nerve**. These nerves supply the muscles and skin of the anterior aspect of the lower leg and the dorsum of the foot and toes.

PRACTICE IN CONTEXT

Using a blank diagram of the foot, label the dorsal surface, plantar surface, the lateral aspect and the medial aspect of the foot.

Working with a partner, inspect their feet and locate the position of the phalanges, metatarsals and tarsals, then examine the arch of the foot and make a note of any irregularities overall.

ASSESSMENT OF KNOWLEDGE

1 Name the tarsal bones.
2 What is the main function of the arches of the feet?
3 Name the muscles which plantarflex the foot.
4 Name four ligaments that strengthen the ankle joint.

- Reflexology procedure
- Locating the reflex points
- Stress
- Contra-actions
- Aftercare advice

Providing **Reflexology**

7 Reflexology procedure

Now that you have completed a detailed consultation with your client and noted your findings from your visual observations, you may provide the reflexology treatment.

There are several schools of thought regarding procedure and it is up to you to decide the best method for you personally or for your client. This will often depend upon the method you have been taught. It is important however for professional development to continue, and you should endeavour to increase your knowledge, learn new techniques and keep abreast of progress made within this field. The procedure you follow may therefore change or be adapted according to your new knowledge and experience. Whatever method is chosen make sure it is professional, comfortable and appropriate for the client you are treating.

Make sure your treatment area is well prepared and you have everything to hand as you must not leave your client once you have started the treatment. Reflexology should be continuous and flowing as this contributes to the relaxing effects of treatment. This may be achieved by treating the right foot first and then the left, always keeping the foot not being worked on covered and warm.

Timing of treatment

In general, a full reflexology treatment usually lasts for approximately 45 minutes; however there are occasions when this may be adapted. It is important to assess each individual client, taking into consideration their age, physical and emotional condition, medical history, their own ability to cope with treatment and their personal attitude.

The first treatment with a detailed consultation will always be longer, approximately one hour, and there are also occasions when it may be necessary to reduce the treatment time, as in these cases.

- Small babies will only require a very short and gentle treatment, preferably using the index finger rather than the thumb only on specific areas requiring treatment, and lasting for approximately five minutes.
- Children may be treated for up to fifteen minutes as the response to treatment is much quicker and there is a danger of overstimulation causing excessive elimination of toxins.
- Elderly clients may require a shorter treatment time but this will also depend on their state of health.
- A client with a terminal illness may often benefit from a gentle short treatment as it is relaxing and may help alleviate pain and increase energy levels.
- Oversensitive clients who react very quickly to treatment or are emotionally overwrought may require less time.

Regularity of treatment

This will vary with each individual. Many people benefit from just one treatment but there are those clients who rely on a regular course. There can be a quite significant effect after one treatment but in general it usually requires three or four before the results are obvious.

For most people treatment is given weekly. This allows the body time to eliminate the toxins and restore energy levels before the next treatment. You may feel that in some cases the client requires treatment more often because of their condition or problem. In such cases make sure that there are at least three days in between and as the condition improves treatment may be applied less often.

For the best results it is ideal to have a course of six to eight full treatments and then follow with a maintenance programme appropriate to the individual's needs. There is no guarantee that all problems will disappear immediately but there will be a change in symptoms and the degree of suffering felt. The more acute problems often find quick relief but anyone with a chronic condition will need more treatment time to achieve results.

Preparation of the client

Once the client has been positioned comfortably with support for the head, back and legs if required, and a cover for warmth when necessary, you will begin by cleansing the feet with antiseptic wipes or another cleansing medium. Rose water or witch hazel may also be used to cleanse and refresh the feet as they both have a cooling effect, most pleasant on a warm summer day.

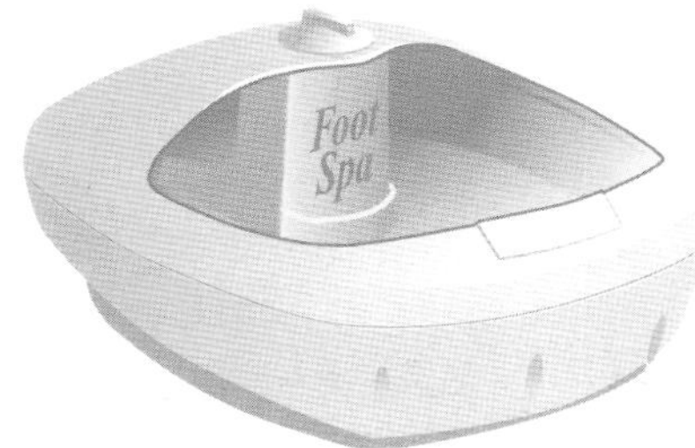

A foot spa

The use of a foot spa is also very therapeutic as it cleanses and relaxes at the same time. If a client comes to you after a hard day's work they may appreciate a relaxing soak in a foot spa before they settle onto the couch for treatment.

If you are busy, the time the client spends in the foot spa will provide you with a little extra time to organise yourself between clients. Whatever method is used always make sure that the feet are completely dry and continue with a relaxing massage of both feet. This will ensure that:

- the client begins to relax
- the feet are warmed
- circulation is increased
- muscles and ligaments are loosened
- the client becomes accustomed to your touch
- areas of hard skin are softened with the addition of a cream or oil.

The procedure

1. Ensure client is positioned comfortably.
2. Ensure you are positioned comfortably so that your own energy flow is not impeded.
3. Prepare both of the client's feet.
4. Use relaxing massage techniques on both feet.
5. Cover the client's left foot.
6. Start on the client's right foot working the reflex points of each system in the body and then continue working on the left foot.

Reflex areas on the feet

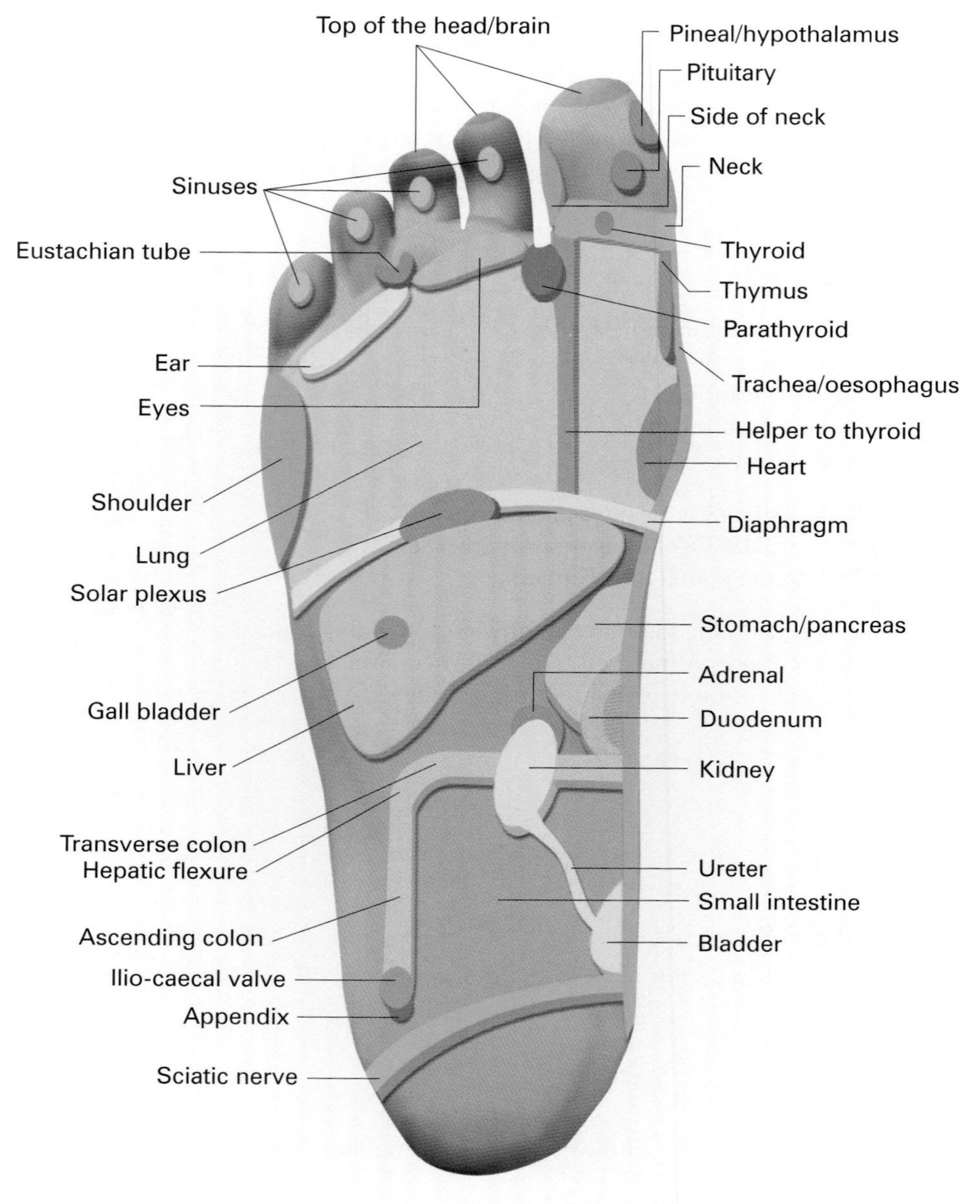

Figure 7.1 Foot map – plantar view of right foot

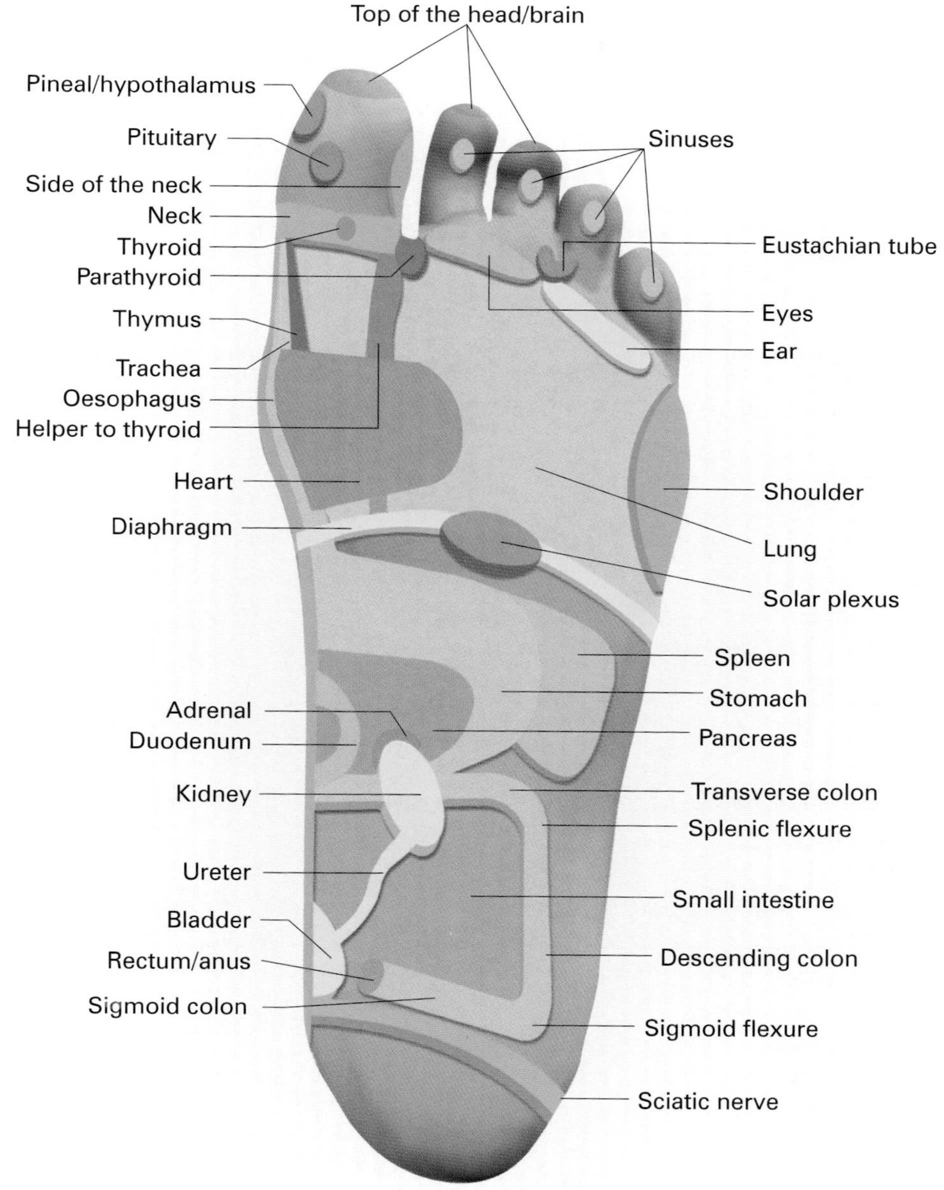
Top of the head/brain
Pineal/hypothalamus
Pituitary
Side of the neck
Neck
Thyroid
Parathyroid
Thymus
Trachea
Oesophagus
Helper to thyroid
Heart
Diaphragm
Sinuses
Eustachian tube
Eyes
Ear
Shoulder
Lung
Solar plexus
Spleen
Stomach
Pancreas
Adrenal
Duodenum
Kidney
Transverse colon
Splenic flexure
Ureter
Small intestine
Bladder
Rectum/anus
Sigmoid colon
Descending colon
Sigmoid flexure
Sciatic nerve

***Figure** 7.2 Foot map – plantar view of left foot*

This order of work is based upon treating the reflex points of each system on one foot and then the reflex points of each system on the second foot. In the practical procedure, there are certain reflex points which are not part of the body system in which they appear but they are treated because they are located in the area being worked. For example, when treating the skeletal system, the spine head and neck is treated but in addition the thyroid reflex – part of the endocrine system – is also treated, as it is just beneath the neck reflex. The adrenal gland is treated when you are working the urinary system as the adrenal reflex is located just above the kidney reflex. These reflexes are indicated in the table in ***bold italics***.

Order of work

CLIENT'S RIGHT FOOT	CLIENT'S LEFT FOOT
Skeletal system	
Spine/head and neck, ***thyroid***	Spine head and neck, ***thyroid***
Head/brain, ***pineal***, ***pituitary***, ***hypothalamus*** and ***face***	Head/brain, ***pineal***, ***pituitary***, ***hypothalamus*** and ***face***
Shoulder	Shoulder
Arm	Arm
Elbow	Elbow
Hand	Hand
Hip	Hip
Knee	Knee
Leg	Leg
Respiratory system	
Sinuses	Sinuses
Eyes, ***ear***	***Eyes***, ***ear***
Eustachian tube	***Eustachian tube***
Trachea ***thymus***	Trachea ***thymus***
Lungs/bronchioles, ***heart***, ***helper to thyroid*** and ***parathyroid***	Lungs/bronchioles, ***heart***, ***helper to thyroid*** and ***parathyroid***
Diaphragm	Diaphragm
Solar plexus	Solar plexus
Digestive system	
Oesophagus	Oesophagus
Stomach/***pancreas***	Stomach/***pancreas***
Duodenum	Duodenum
Small intestine	Small intestine
Appendix	Transverse colon
Ileo-caecal valve	Descending colon
Ascending colon	Sigmoid colon/ rectum, anus
Hepatic flexure	Spleen
Transverse colon	Liver
Liver	
Gall bladder	
Urinary system	
Bladder	Bladder
Ureter	Ureter
Kidney	Kidney
Adrenal	***Adrenal***
Sciatic nerve	***Sciatic nerve***

CLIENT'S RIGHT FOOT	CLIENT'S LEFT FOOT
Lymphatic system	
Upper and lower lymph areas of neck and groin Breast/mammary	Upper and lower lymph areas of neck and groin Breast/mammary
Reproductive system	
Ovaries/testes Uterus/prostate Fallopian tubes/vas deferens	Ovaries/testes Uterus/prostate Fallopian tubes/vas deferens

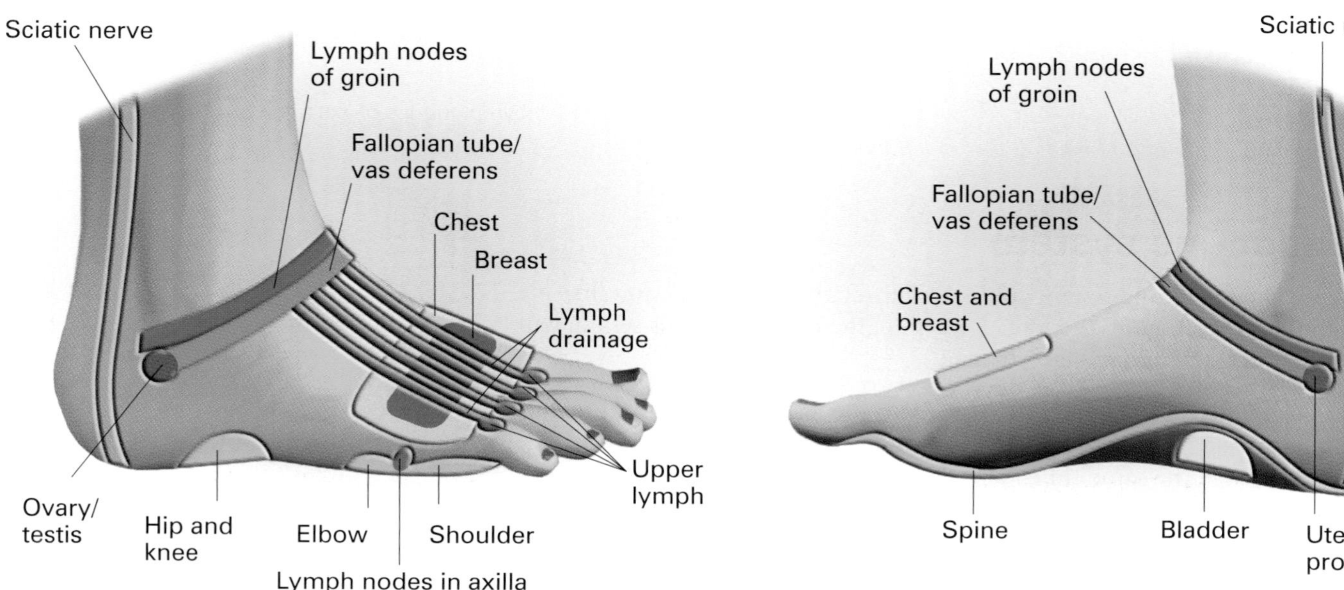

Figure 7.3 Foot map – lateral and medial view of right foot

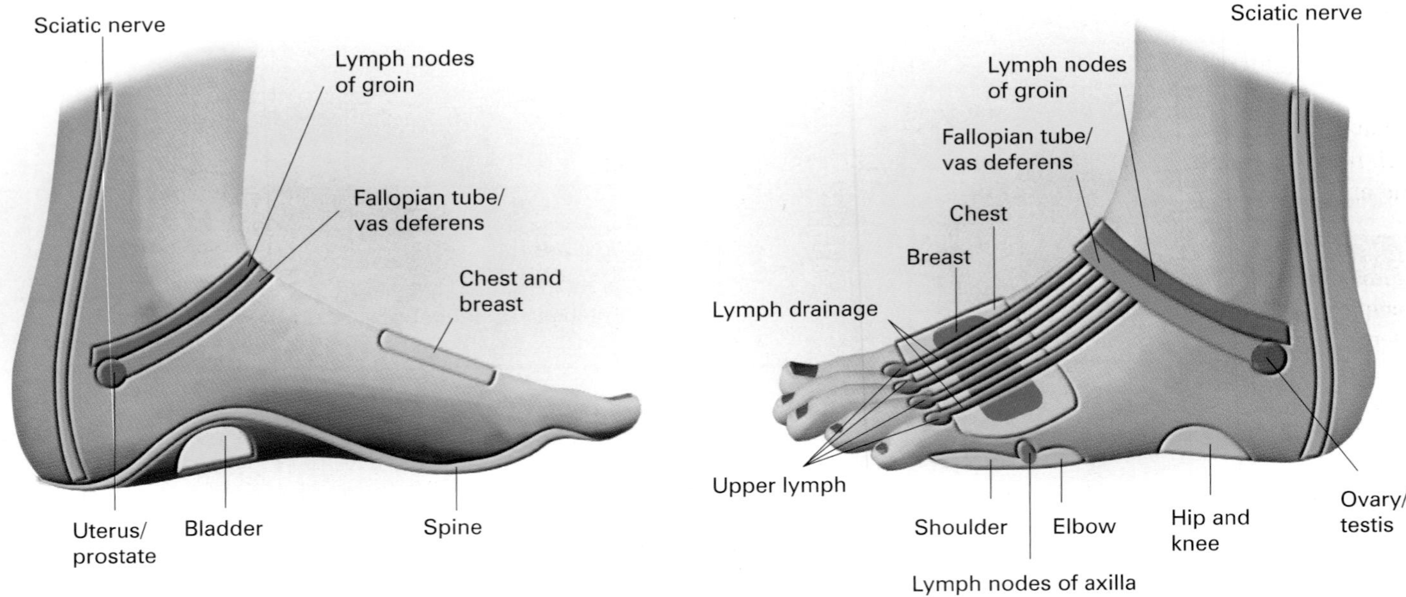

Figure 7.4 Foot map – lateral and medial view of left foot

The endocrine system

The glands of the endocrine system are located throughout the body and they are in the corresponding position on the foot. Therefore, the reflexes for this system will be treated when other systems are being treated.

Pituitary, pineal and hypothalamus are located on the back of the big toe and are treated when the head and brain reflexes are worked. The thyroid is in the neck area and may be treated at the same time. The parathyroid reflex is situated between the big toe and second toe and may be treated when working on the eye reflex. Helper to thyroid would be worked whilst treating the heart reflex. The thymus is situated on the ball of the foot beneath the big toe in the area of the trachea reflex and may be worked at the same time. The adrenals are situated just above the kidney reflex and worked at the same time. The pancreas is situated just below the stomach reflex and may be treated at the same time.

The cardiovascular system

The cardiovascular system consists of the heart, the blood and all the vessels that transport the blood around the body. There are no particular reflexes specifically for the circulation, therefore when the other systems of the body are treated during a general reflexology session, the circulatory system will also benefit.

The heart reflex is found mainly on the client's left foot between the shoulder line and the diaphragm line in the thoracic area and less so on the right foot under the shoulder reflex. The heart reflex may therefore be treated at the same time as the lung reflexes are worked.

The face

The reflex points for the face are worked on the front of the big toe and the teeth on the front of the four smaller toes. The sinuses, eyes, ears, eustachian tube and teeth may all be worked at the same time by thumb and finger walking on both sides of the toes.

Treatment reference chart

As reflexology is a holistic treatment it always includes working the reflexes of the whole body. You may then concentrate on associated reflexes or return to certain reflexes that you have recognised as requiring additional treatment. There are specific reflex points which may be most beneficial to some disorders. The following chart provides a list of some of the disorders most often seen and the systems and areas to work.

CONDITION	SYSTEMS AND AREAS TO WORK
Acne	Endocrine, liver, kidney, large intestine and adrenals
Allergies	The problem area, lymphatic, circulatory, adrenals and liver
Alzheimer's disease	Spine and brain
Amenorrhoea	Reproductive, pelvic and lumbar spine
Anaemia	Thyroid, helper to thyroid, heart, spleen and liver
Angina	Respiratory, circulatory and oesophagus
Ankylosing spondylitis	Spine, joints and adrenals
Arthritis	Area which is painful, adrenals, endocrine and digestive
Asthma	Lungs, heart, diaphragm, thoracic spine, adrenals and ilio caecal valve and digestive (excessive mucus)
Bowel disorders	Ilio caecal valve and colon
Bursitis	The inflamed joint and the area of spine supplying nerves to the joint
Candida	Intestines, spleen and reproductive
Cataract	Eyes, sinuses and cervical spine
Cerebral palsy	Spine and brain
Colitis	Digestive, adrenals and lumbar spine
Conjunctivitis	Eye, sinuses, lymphatic and cervical spine
Constipation	Intestines, liver, gall bladder, adrenals and lumbar spine
Crohn's disease	Intestines, adrenals and lymphatic
Cystitis	Urinary, adrenals, coccyx, pelvic and lumbar spine
Depression	Endocrine and solar plexus
Diabetes	Pancreas, pituitary, eyes, circulatory, respiratory, adrenals, spleen and kidney
Diarrhoea	Intestines, liver, adrenals, solar plexus
Diverticulitis	Digestive, sigmoid colon and lumbar spine
Dysmenorrhea	Reproductive, urinary, coccyx, pelvic and lumbar spine
Ear disorders	Ears, face, head, cervical spine and adrenals
Eczema	Adrenals, digestive, liver and lungs
Emphysema	Heart, lungs, thoracic spine, adrenals and digestive system (excessive mucus)
Endometriosis	Reproductive, endocrine and spine
Epilepsy	Brain and spine
Eye disorders	Eyes, neck and cervical spine
Fibroids	Reproductive
Fibromyalgia	Problem area, adrenals and spine
Gall stones	Liver, gall bladder, thyroid and parathyroid
Glandular fever	Endocrine, respiratory, lymphatic, spleen and circulatory
Glaucoma	Head, spine, eyes and solar plexus
Gout	The affected joints and the corresponding spinal area, endocrine and circulatory
Hay fever	Sinuses, ears, eyes, liver and adrenals
Haemorrhoids	Solar plexus, diaphragm, liver, gall bladder, descending colon and rectum
Headaches	Spine, brain, liver to detoxify and endocrine
Hepatitis	Liver, lymphatic, stomach, small and large intestines
Hiccups	Diaphragm, lungs, thoracic spine and solar plexus
Hypertension	Circulatory, respiratory and kidneys (avoid adrenals)
Hypotension	Circulatory, respiratory, kidneys and adrenals
Incontinence	Urinary, intestines, coccyx, pelvic and lumbar spine
Indigestion	Digestive and intestines

CONDITION	SYSTEMS AND AREAS TO WORK
Infertility	Uterus or prostate, ovaries or testes, fallopian tubes or vas deferens and pituitary
Insomnia	Head, brain, pineal and solar plexus
Kidney stones	Kidneys, ureter, bladder, lymphatic, pituitary and adrenals
Lumbago	Lumbar spine, coccyx and pelvic
Mastitis	Endocrine, breast, shoulder and lymphatic
Meniere's disease	Head, sinuses, neck and cervical spine
Menopause	Endocrine system and solar plexus
Migraine	Head, neck, spine, liver, and endocrine for pmt.
Multiple sclerosis	Spine, brain and adrenals
Nephritis	Urinary system, spleen (to help immune system) and lumbar spine
Neuralgia	Face, sinuses and cervical spine
Oedema	Circulatory and kidneys
Osteoarthritis	The joint affected, spine and urinary system
Phlebitis	Circulatory and respiratory
Premenstrual tension	Hypothalamus/pituitary, ovaries, sacral and lumbar spine and circulatory
Prostate conditions	Prostate, bladder, rectum, groin lymph, lumbar and sacral spine and adrenals
Psoriasis	The area affected, adrenals, solar plexus
Retinitis	Eyes, sinuses, neck
Sciatica	Lumbar spine, coccyx, pelvis, hip and sciatic nerve
Seasonal affective disorder	Brain, pineal
Sinusitis	Sinuses, eyes, ears, face, lymphatic and cervical spine
Sports injuries	Area of injury, circulatory, spinal area relating to injury, adrenals
Stroke	Spine, brain, circulatory, respiratory and kidneys
Tennis elbow	Shoulder, elbow, cervical spine
Thyroid imbalance	Thyroid, parathyroid, neck and pituitary
Tinnitus	Head, neck, ears, eustachian tube, sinuses and cervical spine
Tonsilitis	Throat, neck, head, sinuses, lymphatic and cervical spine
Vertigo	Ear, sinuses and cervical spine
Whiplash	Neck, cervical spine and solar plexus

PRACTICE IN CONTEXT

It is important to be focused on your client during treatment and create an atmosphere conducive to their own self-healing. No matter how busy or stressful your own life is, it is essential that you put this to one side and approach your client free from personal thoughts and problems. To prepare yourself practise some deep breathing exercises as conscious breathing deepens your awareness and keeps your mind free of distraction.

Sit comfortably with your back straight and your hands resting in your lap, and breathe slowly in through the nose allowing the breath to completely fill your lungs. This will make you feel relaxed and energised. Then exhale slowly, out through the mouth, releasing any tension in the body. Repeat this several times. This exercise can be repeated before treating each client.

ASSESSMENT OF KNOWLEDGE

1. How can the reflexologist make the treatment relaxing for the client?
2. How long is a reflexology treatment with a detailed consultation?
3. Which clients may require a shorter treatment time?
4. How many treatments would you recommend to obtain noticeable results?
5. How would you prepare the client's feet for treatment?

8 Locating the reflex points

Relaxing the foot

Massage is always used prior to treatment to prepare the feet and relax the client. It also helps to improve the mobility of the foot and stimulate the energy flow.

There are several massage techniques that may be used prior to treatment to relax the foot, improve flexibility, and allow the client to become accustomed to your touch.

The general effects on the body of massage are:

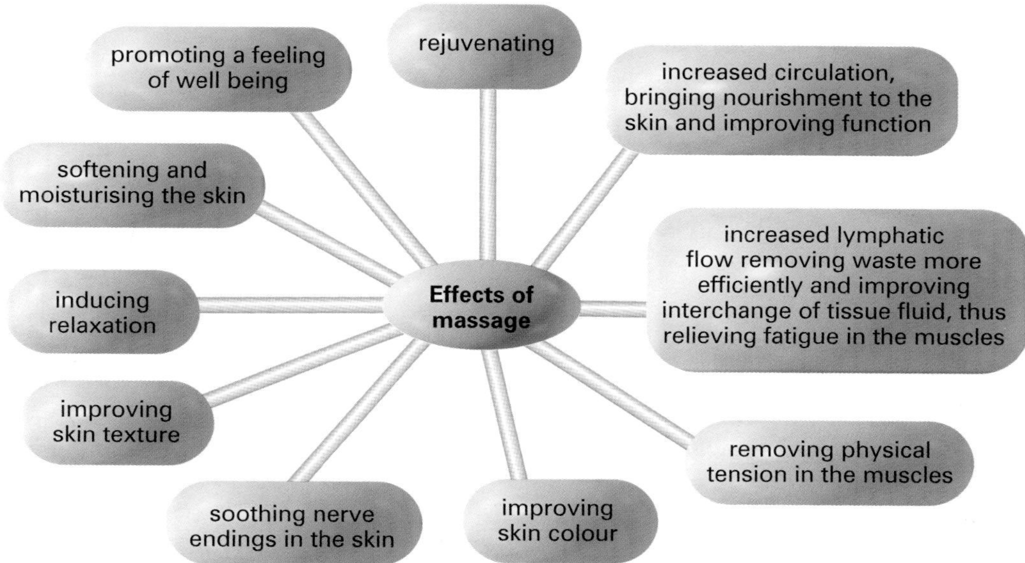
Effects of massage
rejuvenating
increased circulation, bringing nourishment to the skin and improving function
increased lymphatic flow removing waste more efficiently and improving interchange of tissue fluid, thus relieving fatigue in the muscles
removing physical tension in the muscles
improving skin colour
soothing nerve endings in the skin
improving skin texture
inducing relaxation
softening and moisturising the skin
promoting a feeling of well being

Massage techniques

Effleurage

This is a soothing stroking movement performed with both hands. Using a comfortable pressure, slide the hands from the tips of the toes down to the ankle, around the joint and then glide back up without exerting much pressure. This movement is always used to begin and end any massage.

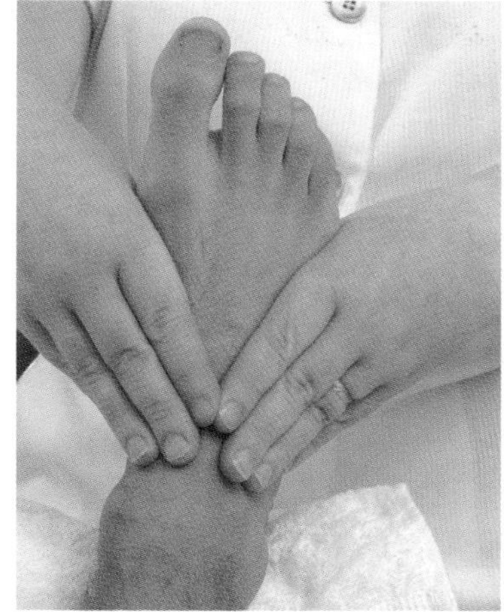

Effleurage

Thumb kneading

This is applied to the sole of the foot from the heel using small circular movements. With the fingers supporting the dorsal surface of the foot, place the thumbs together on the heel, move upwards and outwards in small circular movements, moving slowly up the foot to the toes, making the circulations bigger as you proceed. This movement helps to open the foot and release tension.

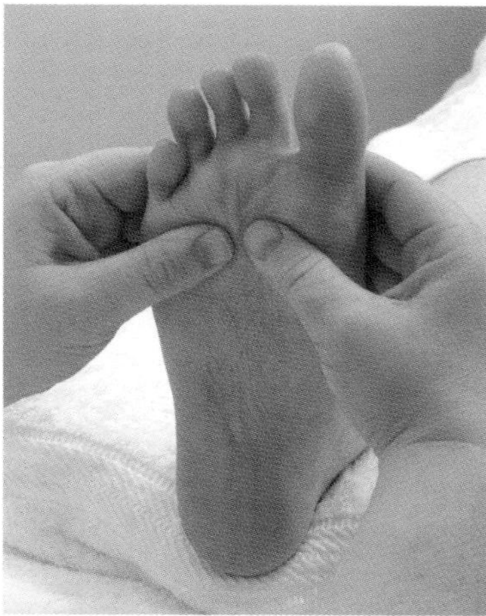

Thumb kneading

Palmar kneading

This is performed by using the padded palmar surface of your hand on the sole of the foot whilst supporting the dorsal surface with your other hand. Apply pressure in circular movements to cover the whole of the foot.

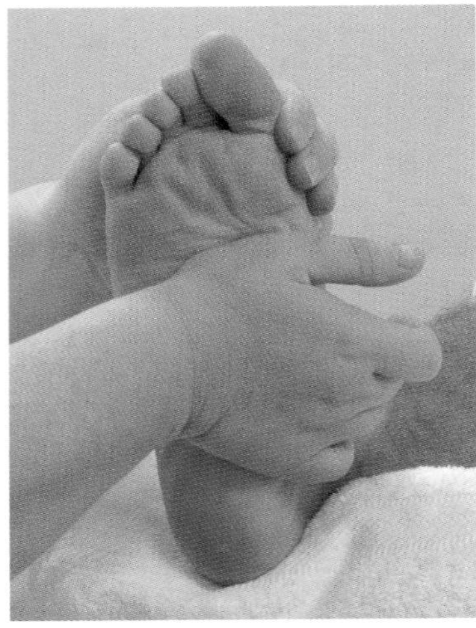

Palmar kneading

Finger kneading

Using the padded surface of the tips of the fingers, massage in small circular movements applying comfortable pressure.

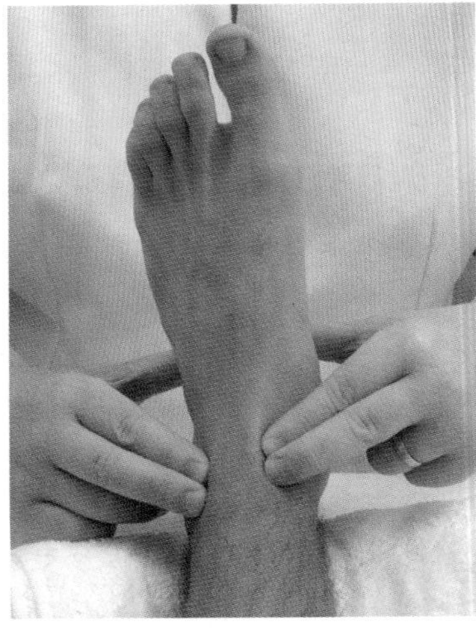

Finger kneading

Wringing

This is performed by wrapping the hands around the foot and then gently twisting the hands away from each other and back again. This stretches the foot and increases flexibility.

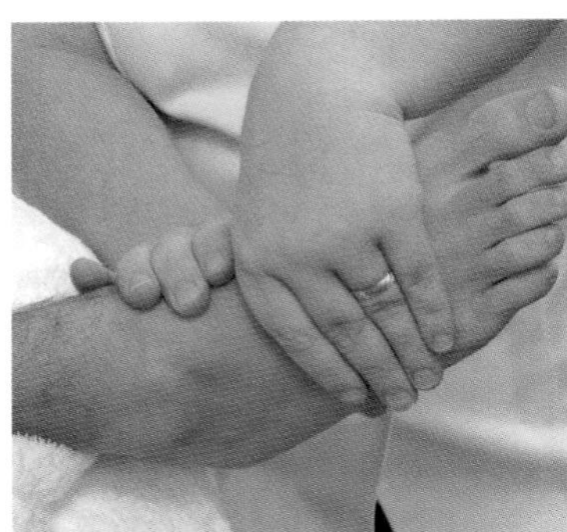

Wringing

Foot rocking

Placing both hands palmar surface up at either side of the foot, move them alternately and quickly from side to side up and down the foot.

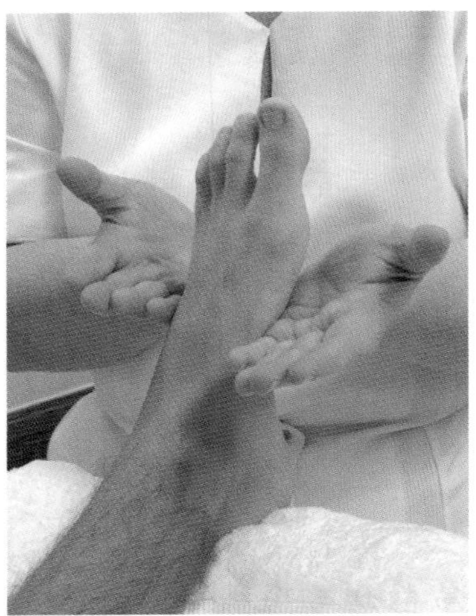

Foot rocking

Extension and flexion

Supporting the foot under the heel with one hand, gently extend and flex the foot, within the range that is comfortable for the client, with the other hand.

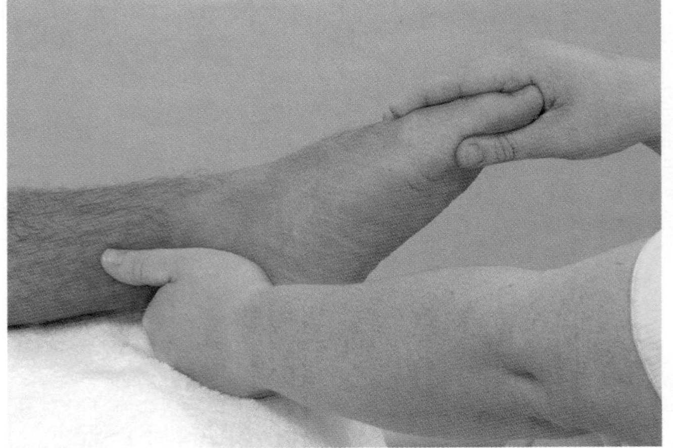

Extending the foot

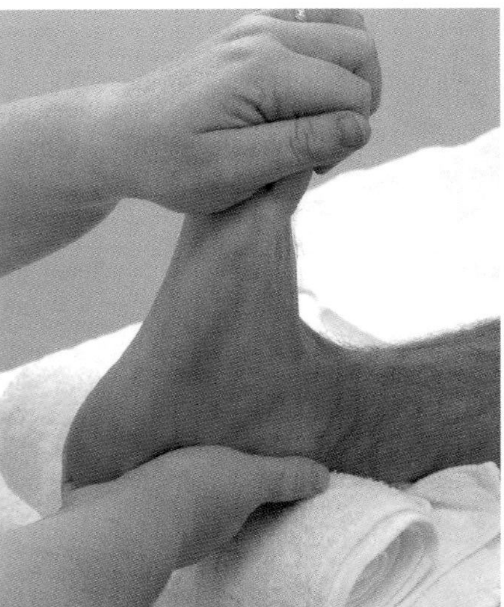

Flexing the foot

Toe rotation

Support the foot with one hand and gently rotate the toe in one direction and then in the opposite direction.

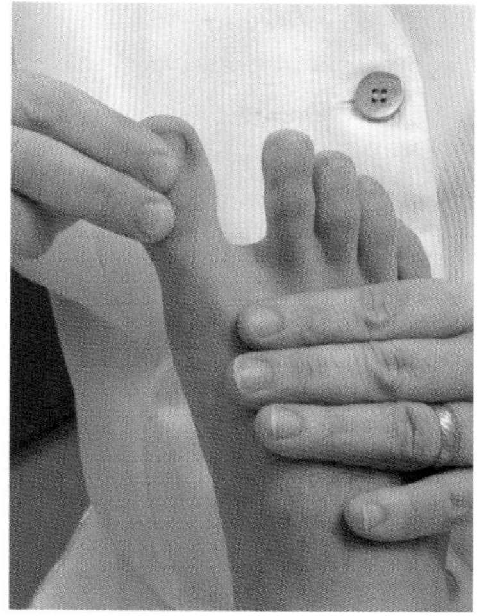

Toe rotation

Ankle rotation

Support the foot under the heel and hold the toes firmly with the other hand gently rotating the ankle first in one direction and then in the other.

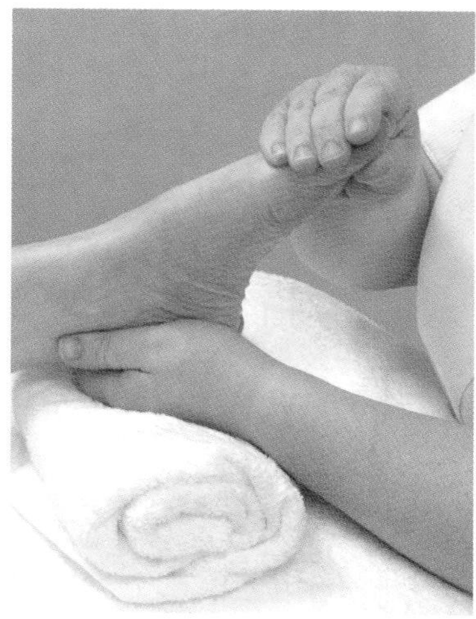

Ankle rotation

Locating reflex points

Client comfort

The final stage in the reflexology procedure is locating and working each of the reflex points. Reflexology is performed using specific massage techniques over the reflex areas, and for client comfort it is essential that the foot is treated in a gentle manner. Hold firmly and apply a pressure that is comfortable for the client. It is important to explain what you are doing at each step in the procedure, particularly with a new client. When providing treatment one hand is always used to support the foot whilst the other hand works the reflex points. Different techniques are used and they may include:

- **Thumb walking** – the thumb walks lightly over the skin in tiny steps with the thumb bent at the first joint. Used when working larger areas.

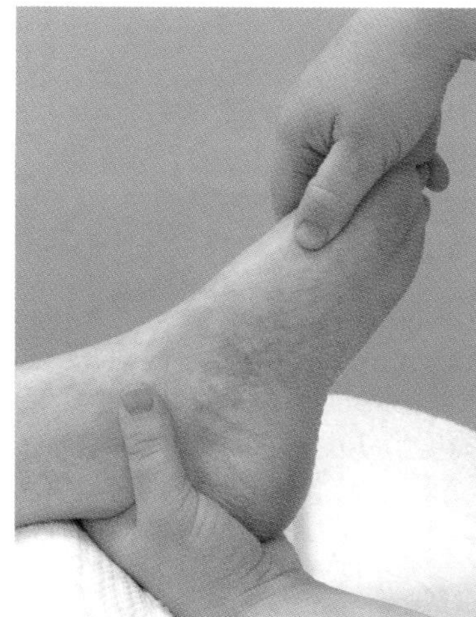

Thumb walking

- **Finger walking** – one or more fingers walk lightly over the skin. It is useful when working over bony or sensitive areas. It is applied mainly on the dorsal surface of the foot, the sides of the toes and around the ankle. Depending on the size of the reflex area being treated, one, two or more fingers may be used.

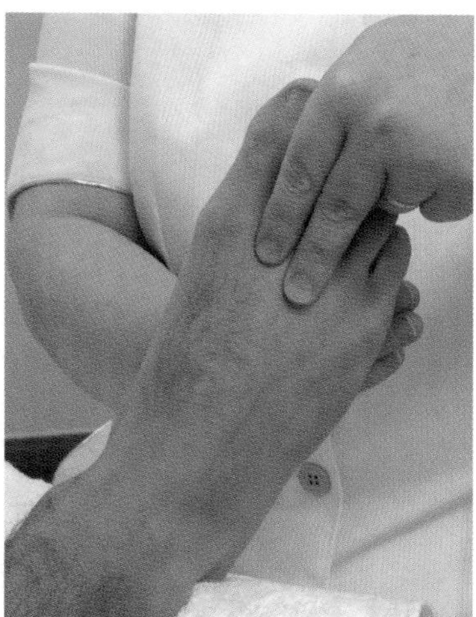

Finger walking

- **Thumb pressure** may be used statically using the padded part of the thumb to exert pressure over the reflex point. This technique is recommended for working tender or sensitive reflexes. It may also be applied, with small circular movements, over the reflex point.

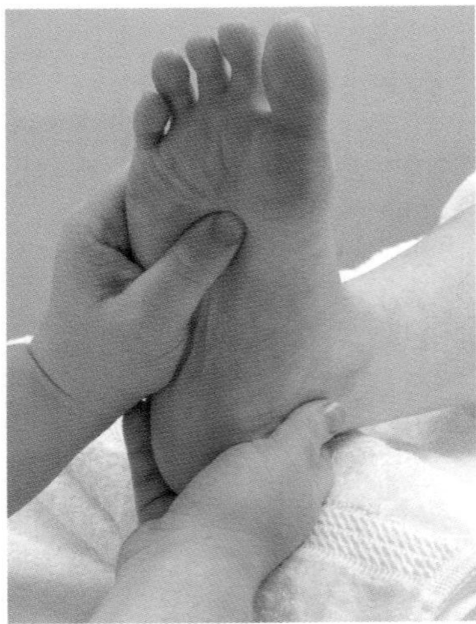

Thumb pressure

- **Finger pressure** is used in the same manner but when it is more comfortable than using the thumb, possibly on the joints.

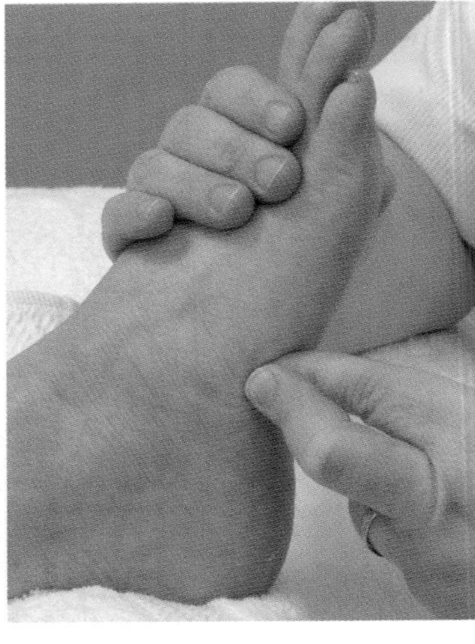

Finger pressure

- **Sliding** is performed using the thumb to slide over the surface of the skin whilst exerting a gentle pressure. This helps to break down crystal deposits and is used mainly on the soles of the feet. Both thumbs may be used alternately over the reflex area.

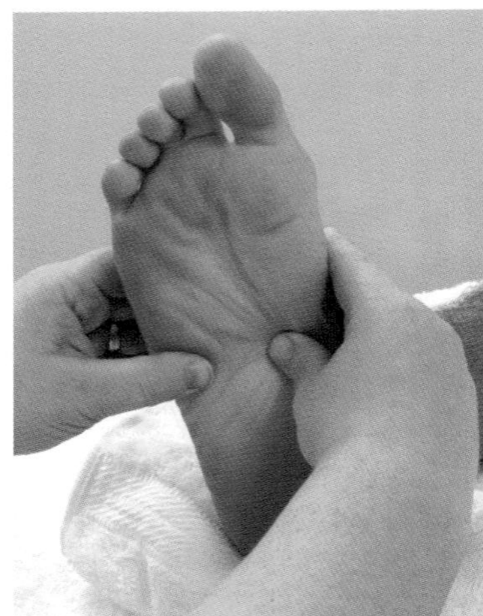

Sliding

- **Hooking** is used when locating reflex points more accurately, when they are too deep or very small. Place the thumb over the reflex point, apply pressure, then pull the thumb back across the point, push in and back up.

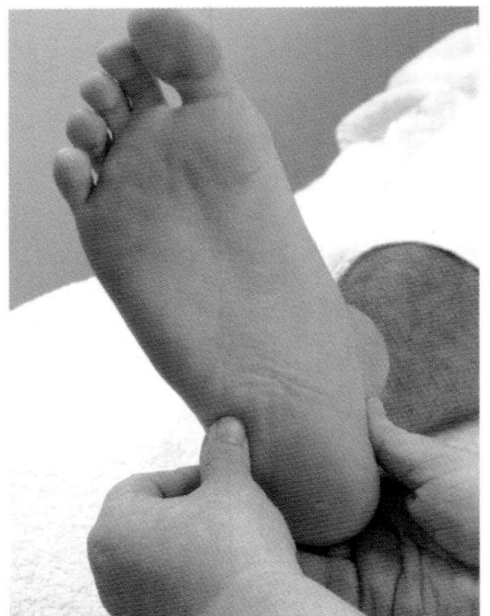

Hooking

The position of the working thumb or fingers should always be pointing in the direction in which you are moving. The movement should be in tiny steps to ensure that full contact is made with each reflex point. Practise using both hands as this will provide a more efficient treatment and allow you to work comfortably on either foot.

The reflex points and working them

Spine

Located on the medial aspect. Support the foot and thumb-walk up the spine from the lumbar area on the calcaneus to the cervical area at the base of the big toe nail.

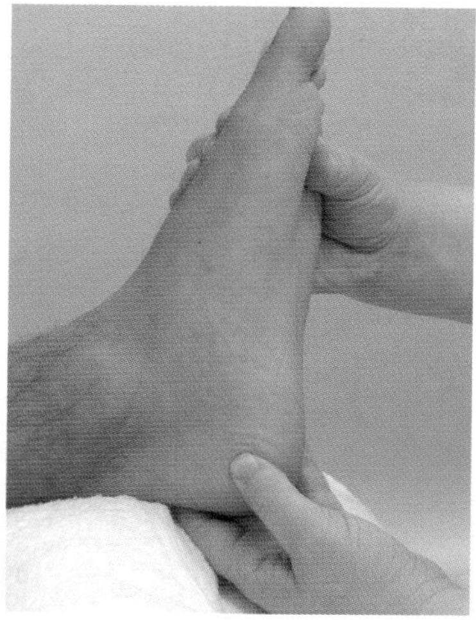

Spinal reflex – up

This move may be repeated in reverse from the big toe to heel.

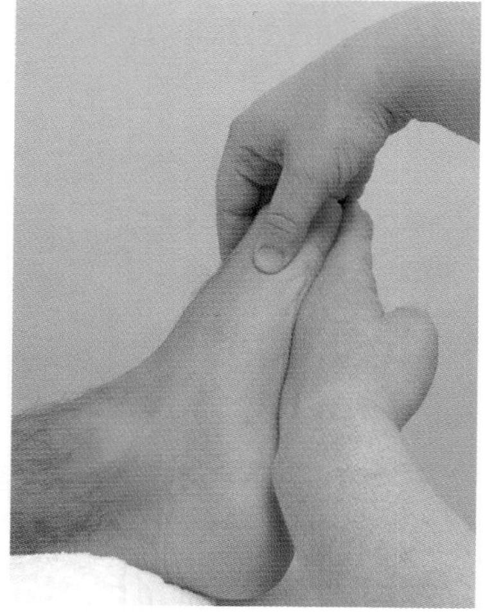

The spinal reflex – down

Back of the head

Located on the back of the big toe. Support the toes from behind, thumb-walk from the base to the top of the big toe in parallel lines to cover the whole area.

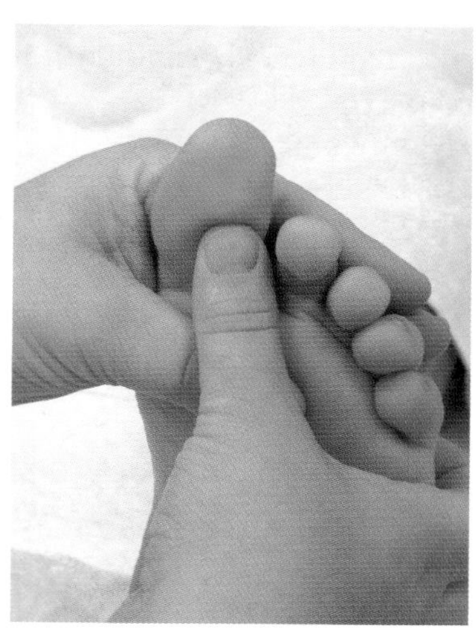

The back of the head

Side of the neck and top of the head

Located on the medial and lateral aspect and top of the big toe. Finger-walk or thumb-walk up the side of the big toe, across the top and down the other side of the toe.

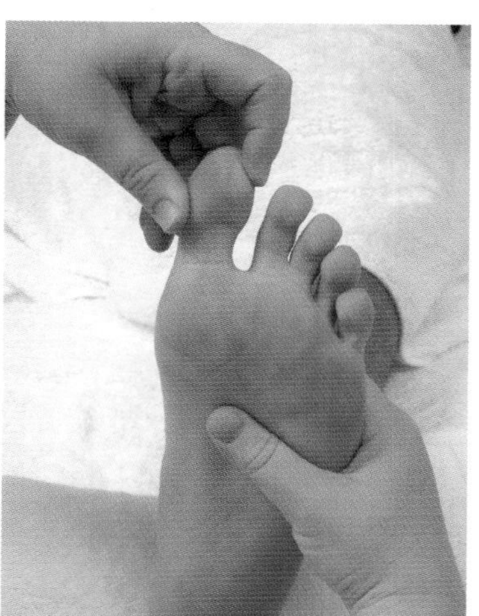

The side of neck

Pineal/hypothalamus

Located near the top, towards the medial aspect of the big toe. Gently rotate the thumb over the reflex and support the toe joint with your fingers.

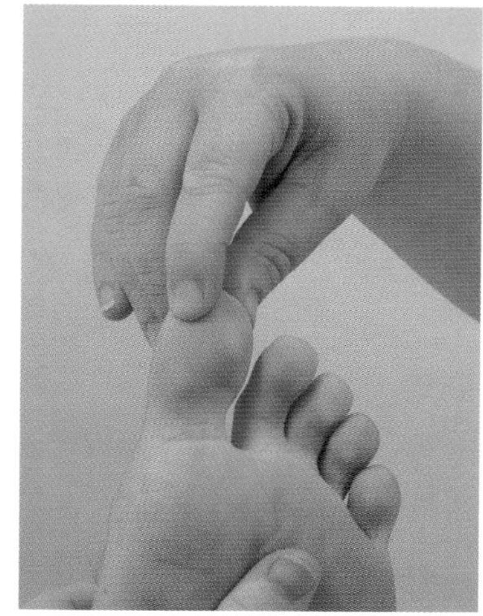

The pineal

Pituitary

Located in the centre of the fleshy pad of the big toe. Support the foot with one hand and the front of the toe with the fingers of your working hand and gently apply a rotating pressure.

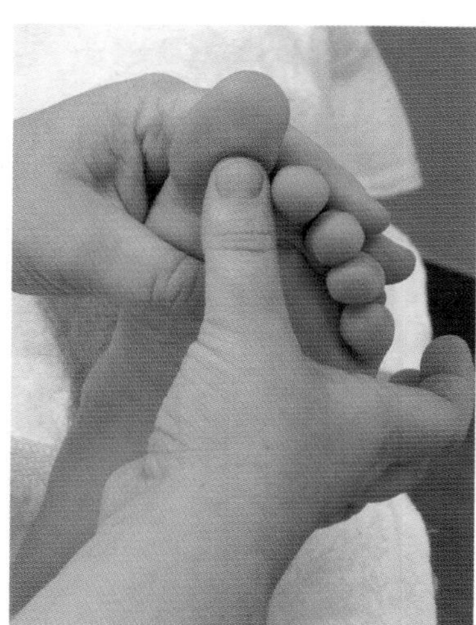

The pituitary

Neck

Located at the base of the big toe. Thumb-walk across from the medial to the lateral aspect.

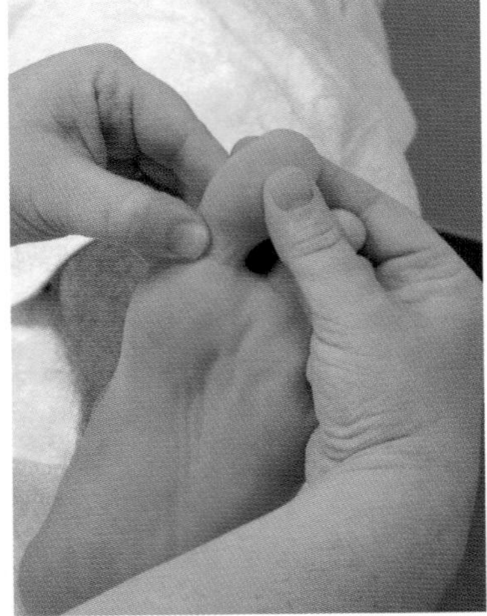

The neck

Thyroid

Located on the top half of the ball of the foot under the big toe. Thumb-walk over the whole area in semi-circular movements whilst supporting the top of the foot.

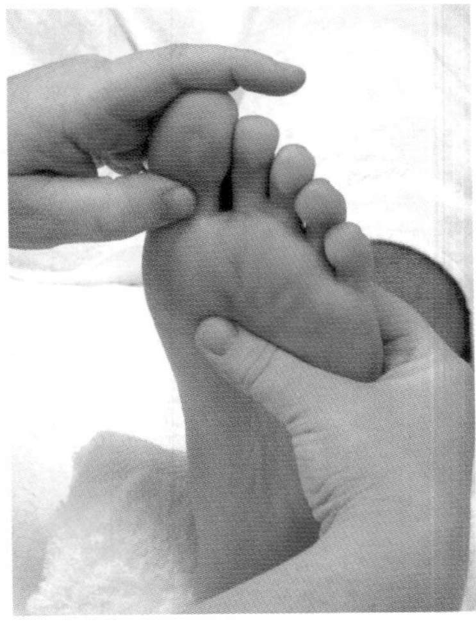

The thyroid

Parathyroid

Located on the lateral aspect of the base of the big toe.

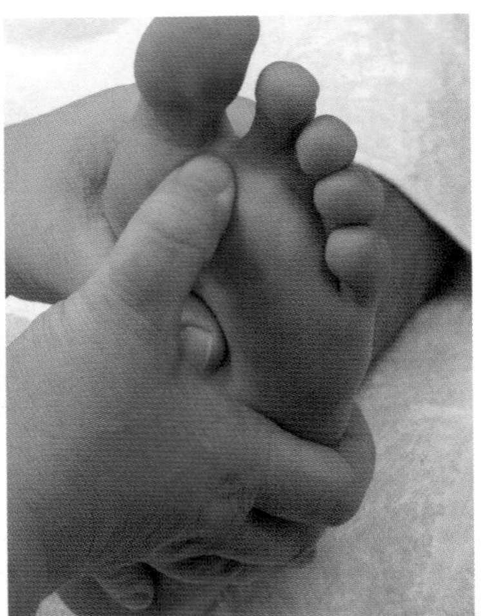

The parathyroid

Helper to thyroid/parathyroid

Located on the lateral side of the thyroid reflex. Thumb-walk up towards the parathyroid reflex.

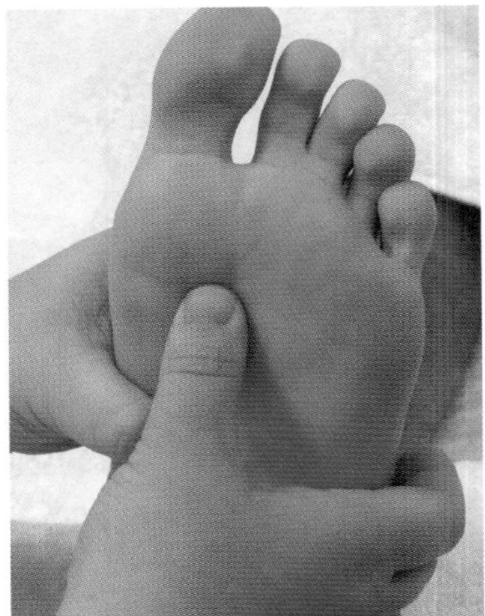

Helper to thyroid/parathyroid

Thymus

Located on the medial side of the thyroid reflex, slightly lower and close to the spinal reflex. Thumb-walk or circle over the area.

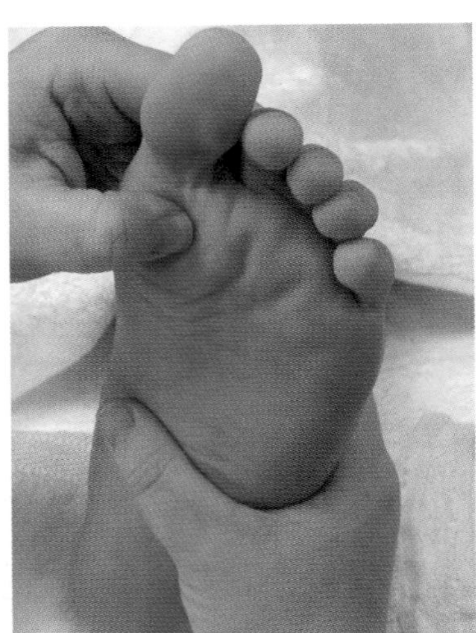

The thymus

Face

Located on the front of the big toe. Use two or three fingers of your working hand to walk across, the working thumb or other hand supporting the back of the big toe.

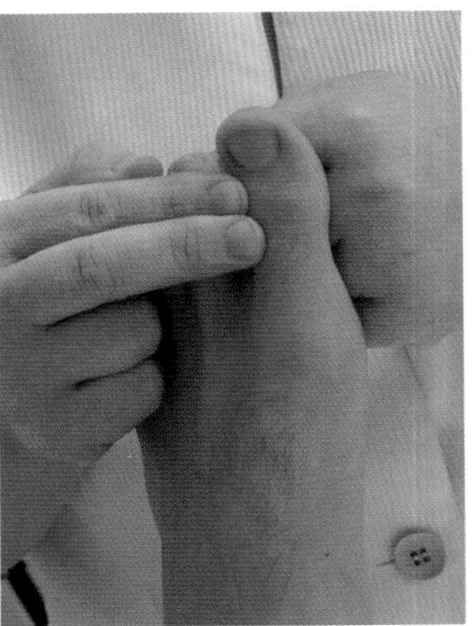

The face

Teeth

Located on the front of all four toes. Finger-walk to the base of each toe.

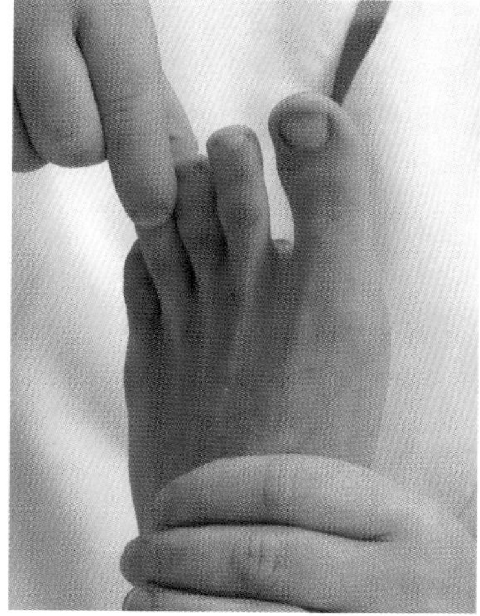

The teeth

Shoulder

Located on the lateral aspect of the base of the little toe. Support the foot, thumb-walk and finger-walk in semicircles, covering the plantar and dorsal surfaces.

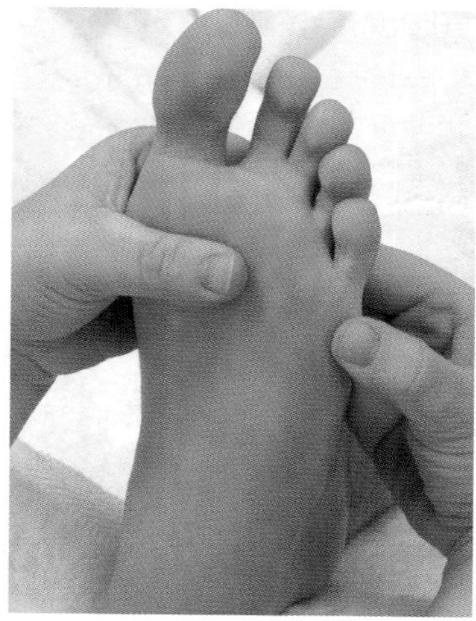

The shoulder

Arm and elbow

Located just below the shoulder reflex. Thumb-walk down and back up, or apply pressure in small circular movements.

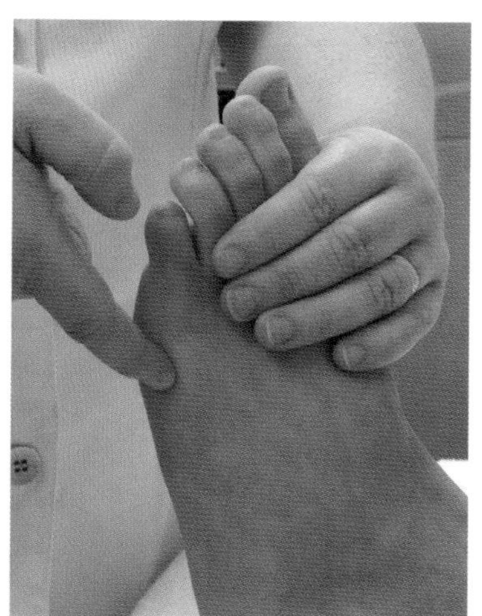

The arm/elbow

Hip and knee

Located on the lateral side of the foot, the knee is just below the elbow reflex at the end of the metatarsal and the hip is just below that to a third of the way along the calcaneus. These reflexes may be worked together.

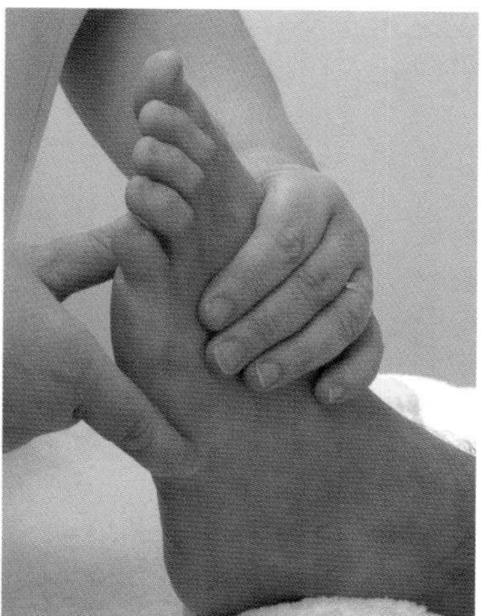

The hip and knee

Sinus

Located on the back of the toes. Support the foot and thumb-walk up or down the back of each toe in turn.

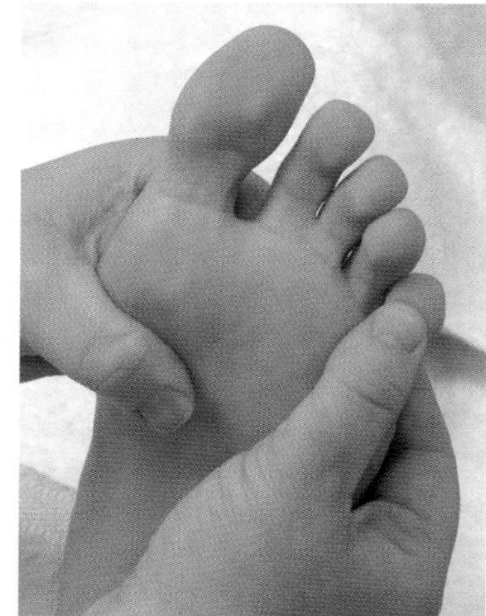

The sinuses

Eye

Located at the base of the second and third toes.

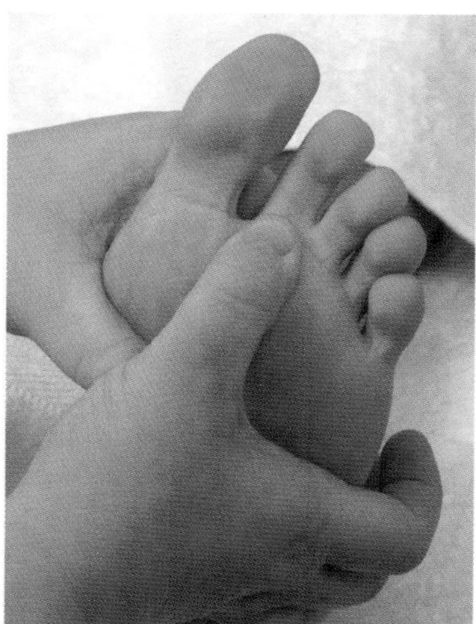

The eyes

Eustachian tube

Situated between the third and fourth toes. Gently rotate your working thumb.

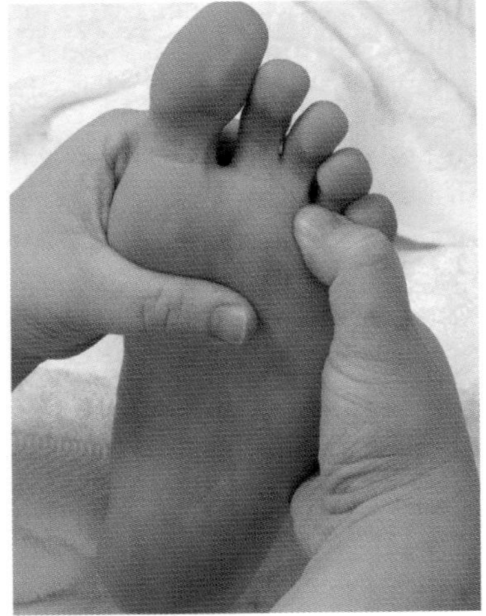

The eustachian tube

Ear

Located across the base of the fourth and fifth toes.

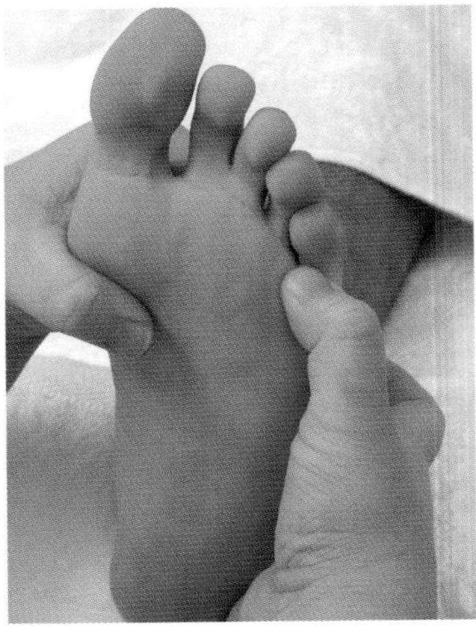

The ear

Trachea

Located at the base of the medial side of the big toe. Thumb-walk down and slightly inwards.

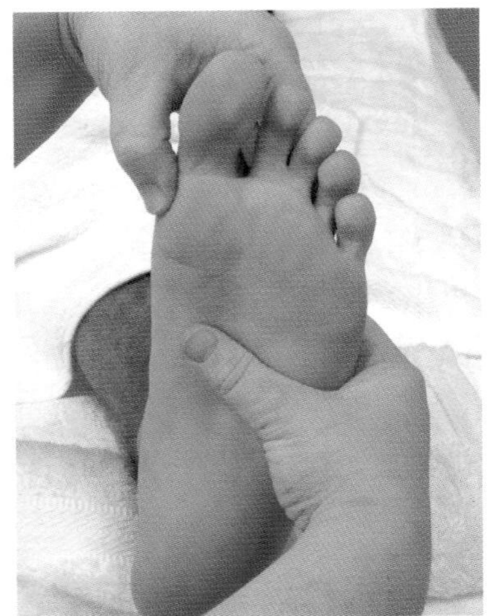

The trachea

Lung

Support the foot and with the working hand, thumb walk in horizontal and vertical lines across the ball of the foot.

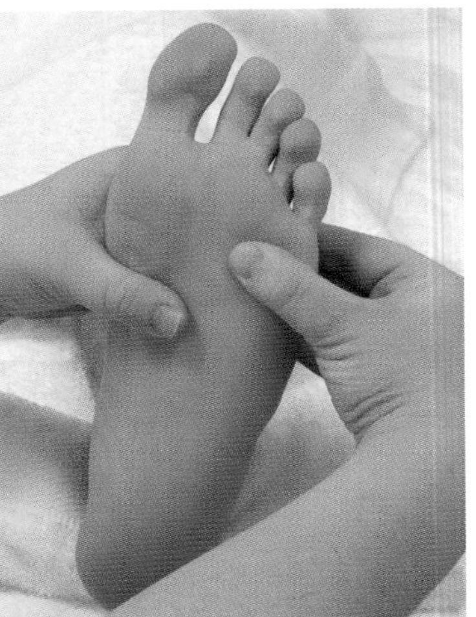

The lung

Heart

Located on the left foot in zones 1 and 2, above the diaphragm line. On the right foot there is a small reflex area in zone 1.

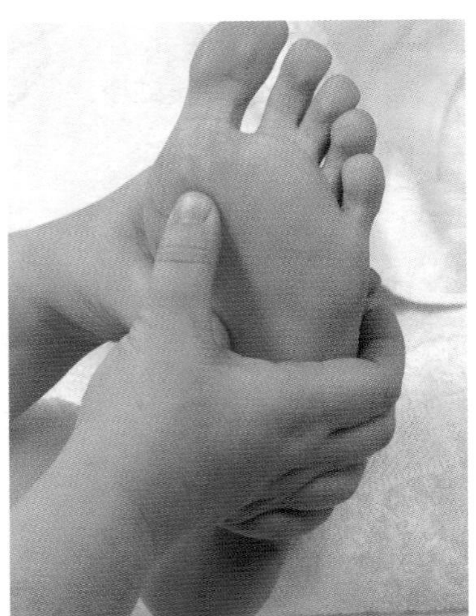

The heart

Diaphragm

Located just below the ball of the foot. Thumb-walk across the diaphragm line, supporting with your other hand.

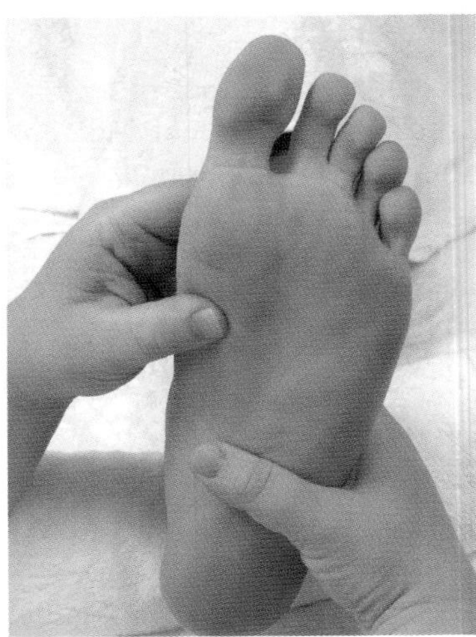

The diaphragm

Solar plexus

Located just on the diaphragm line between the zones 2 and 3. Work gently over this area in small circular movements.

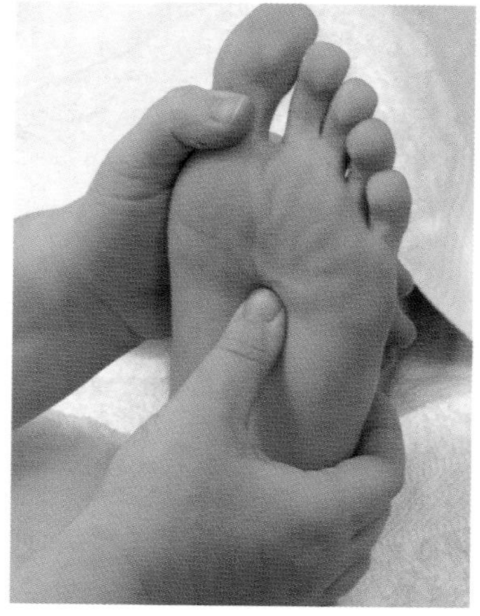

The solar plexus

Liver

Located on the right foot, it's longest side is just below the diaphragm and it's shortest side on the lateral aspect is between the waist and diaphragm line. A small area of the liver reflex is found in zones 1 and 2 on the left foot. The gall bladder reflex is situated between zones 4 and 5 in the middle of the liver.

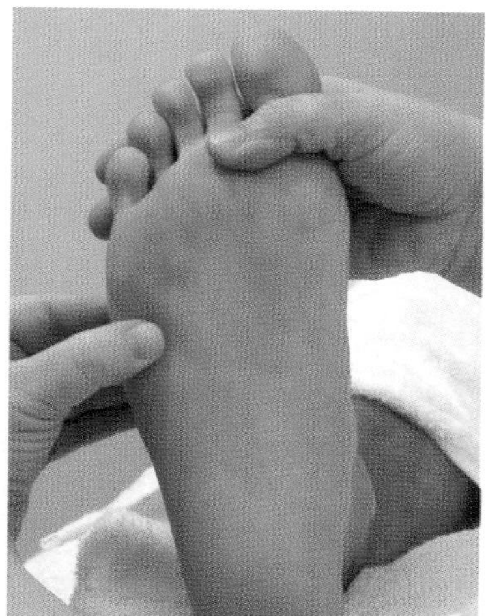

The liver

Oesophagus

Located on the medial side of the foot in zone 1, from the base of the big toe to just below the diaphragm line.

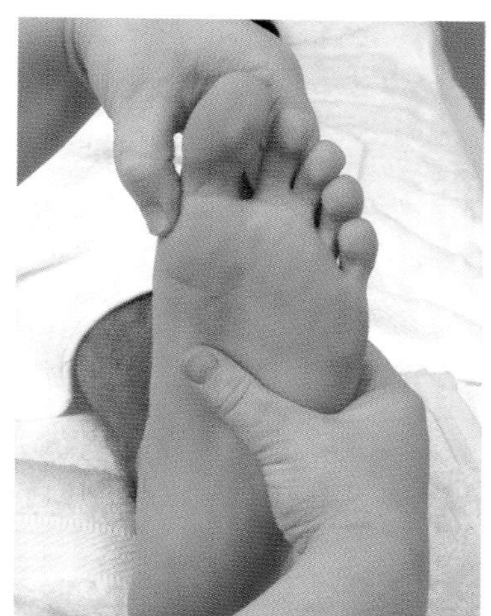

The oesophagus

Stomach

Located between the diaphragm and waistline it is larger on the left foot, covering zones 1, 2 and 3. There is a small reflex area in zone 1 on the right foot.

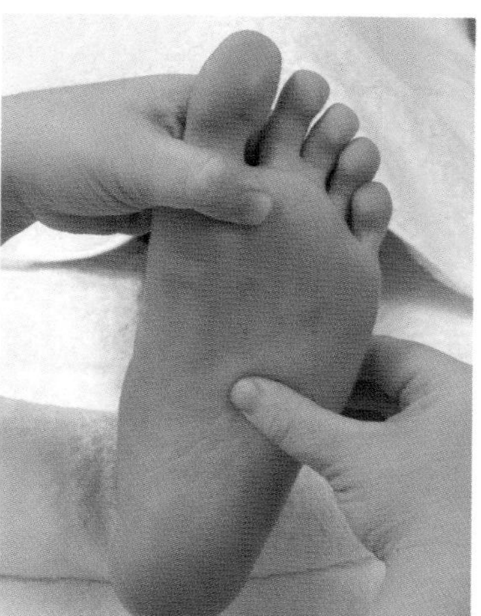

The stomach

Spleen

Located on the lateral aspect of the left foot, above the waistline in zones 4 and 5.

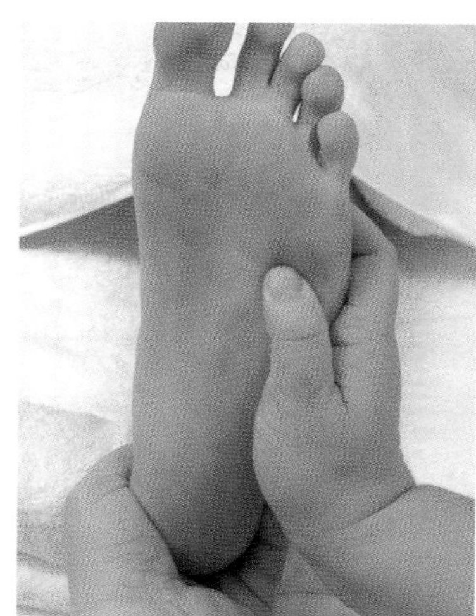

The spleen

Pancreas

Located in zones 1–3 on the left foot, 1–2 on the right, a thumb width below the ball of the foot.

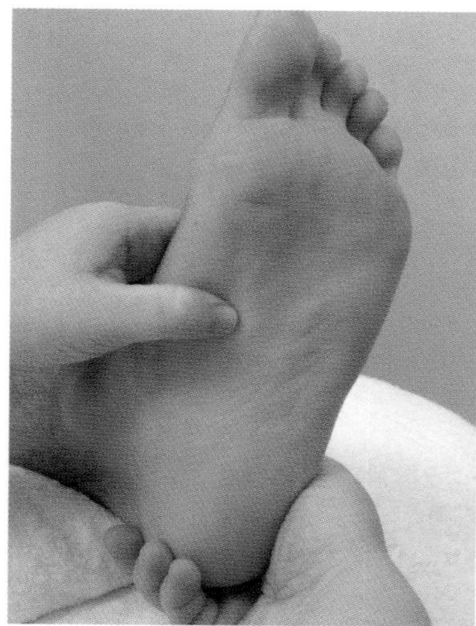

The pancreas

Duodenum

Located on the medial aspect of the foot slightly above the waistline in zone 1.

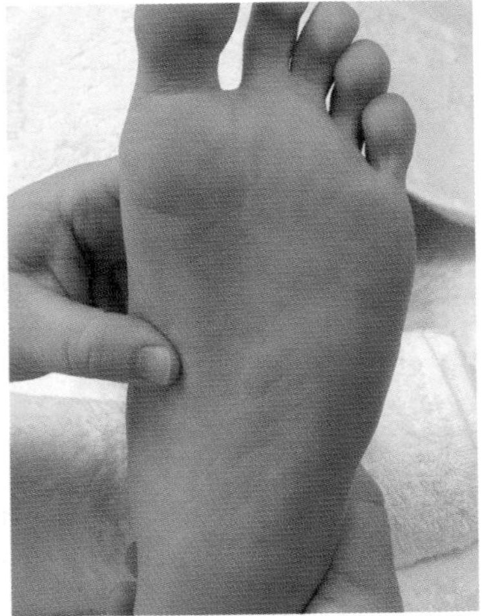

The duodenum

Small intestine

Located on the medial side of the foot, below the waistline, covering zones 1–4. Thumb-walk in both directions to cover this reflex.

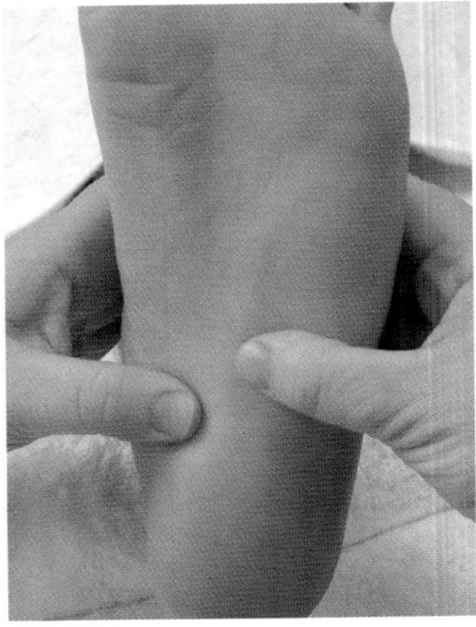

The small intestine

Appendix

Located in zones 4 and 5 only on the right foot just above the pelvic area. Use small circular kneading over this point.

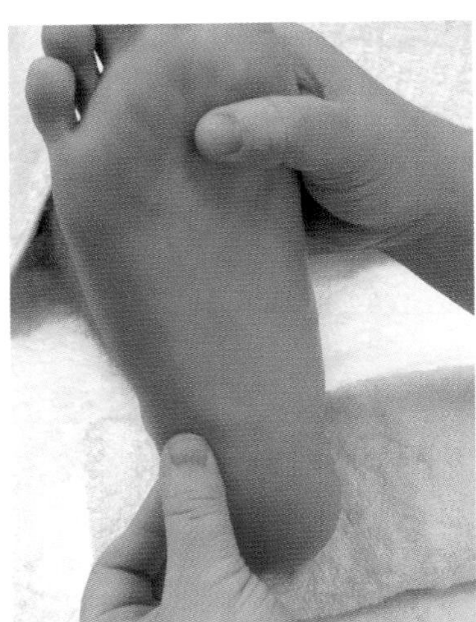

The appendix

Ilio-caecal valve

Located slightly above the appendix only on the right foot, in zones 4 and 5, at the base of the ascending colon.

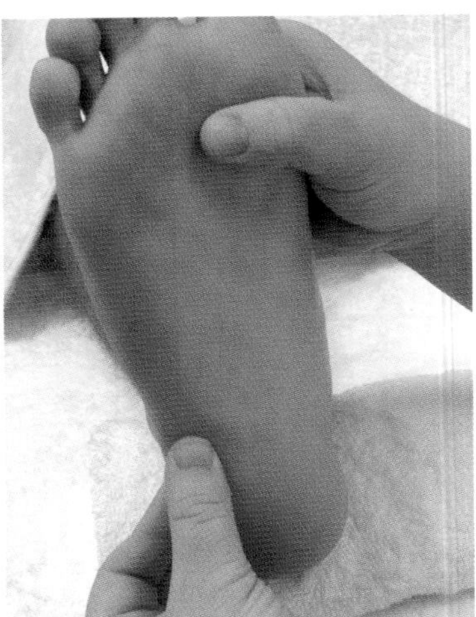

The ilio-caecal valve

Ascending colon

Located from the appendix up to the waist line only on the right foot.

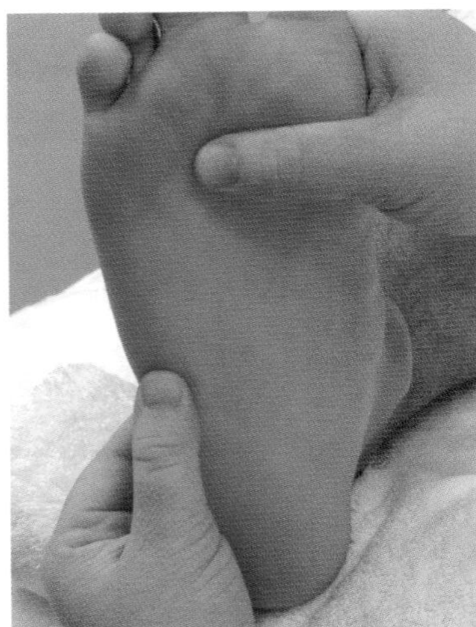

The ascending colon

Transverse colon

Located on both feet, at waist level in zones 1–4.

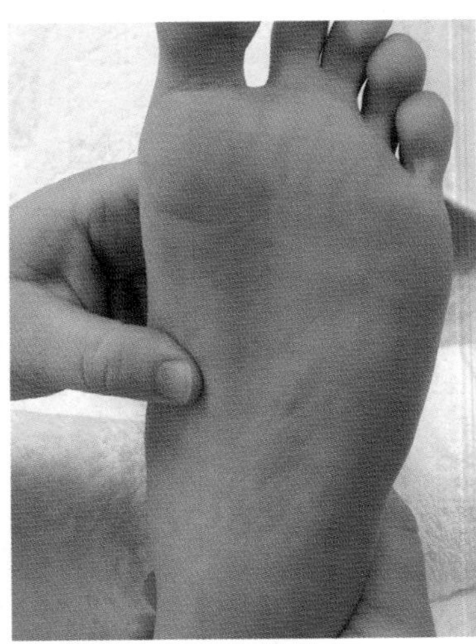

The transverse colon

Descending colon

Located in zones 4 and 5 from the waist line down to the base of the calcaneus, only on the left foot.

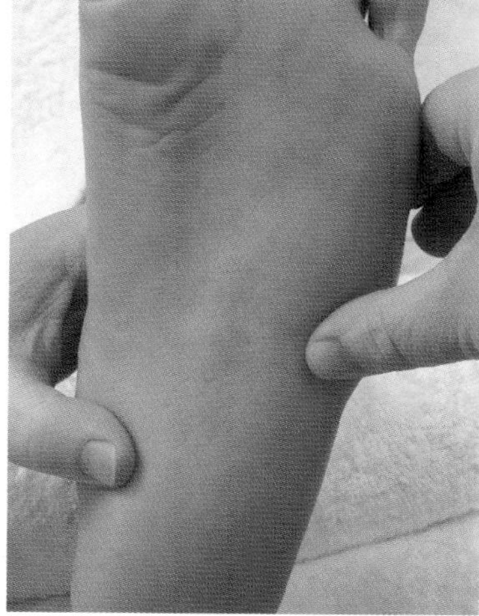

The descending colon

Sigmoid colon

Situated at the base of the descending colon. Thumb-walk and slight pressure may be applied on this reflex point before continuing to rectum/anus.

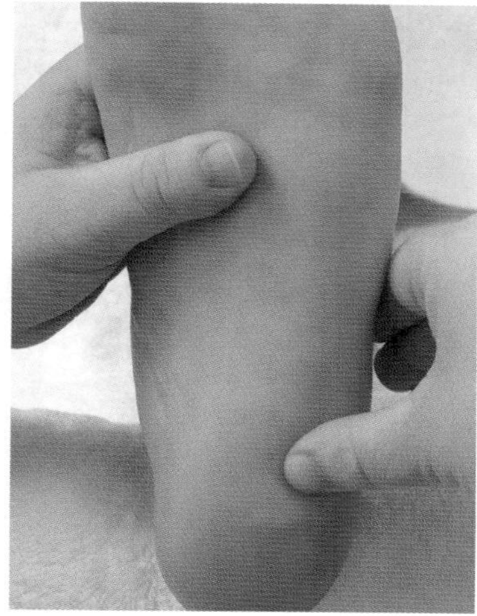

The sigmoid colon

Bladder

Located on the medial aspect of the foot, a slightly puffy area just above the pelvic line.

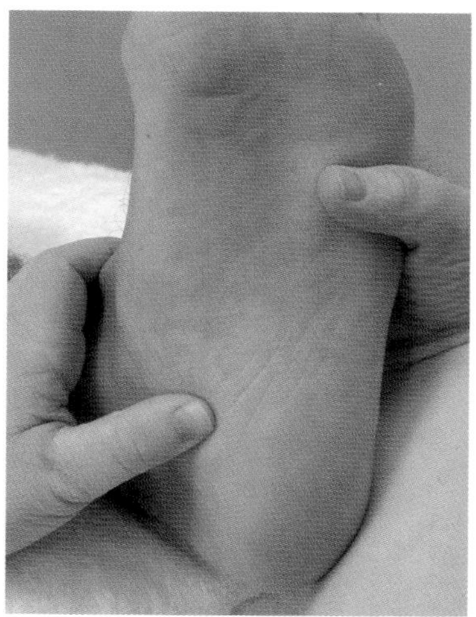

The bladder

Ureter

Located from the bladder reflex diagonally up across zones 3 and 3 to the waist line.

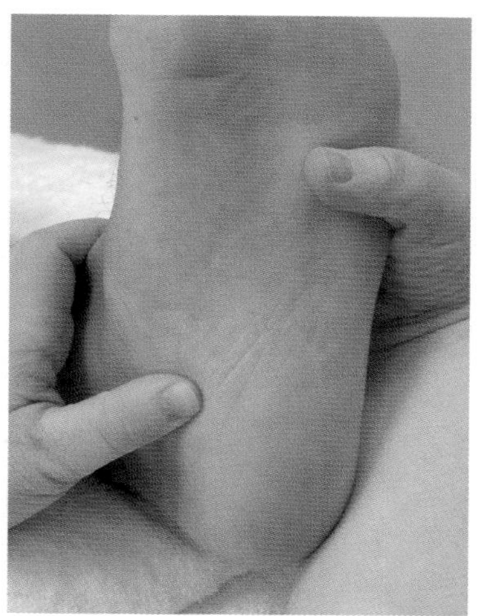

The ureter

Kidney

Located at the end of the ureter reflex at the waist line in zones 1 and 2. Gently use circular pressure movements over this reflex.

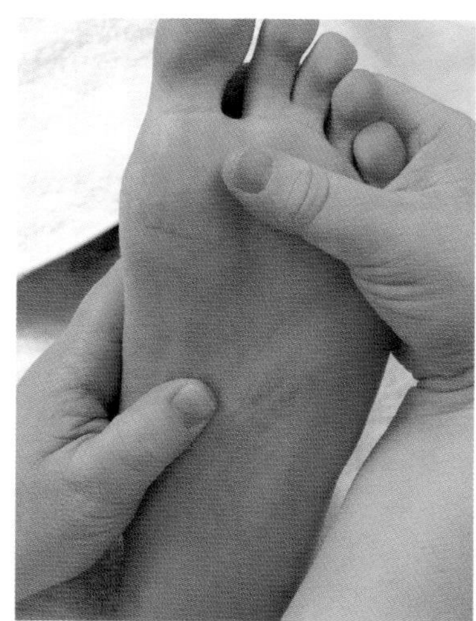

The kidney

Adrenal

Located slightly above and behind the kidney reflex in zone 2 just above the waistline.

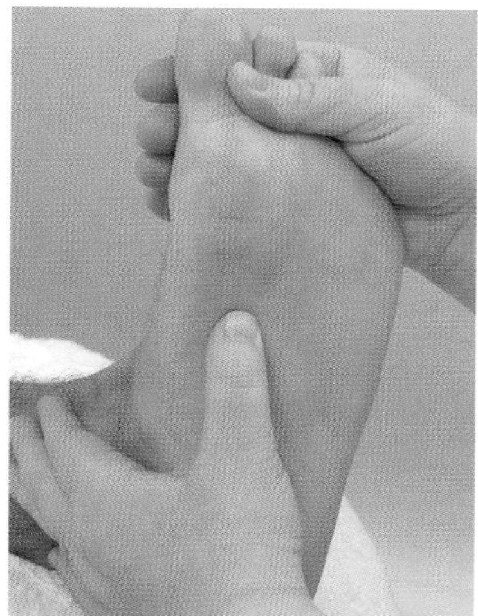

The adrenal

Sciatic

Located one-third of the way down the pad of the heel. Supporting with one hand and the fingers of the working hand and thumb-walk across the heel.

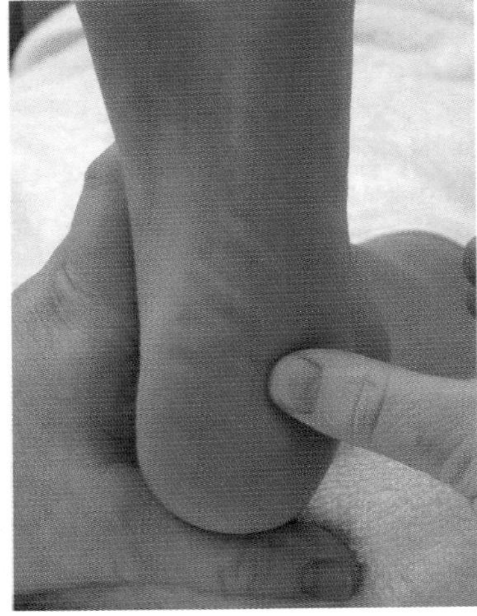

The sciatic

Medial sciatic

Support the foot and with the working hand, thumb-walk up or down the medial side of the achilles tendon.

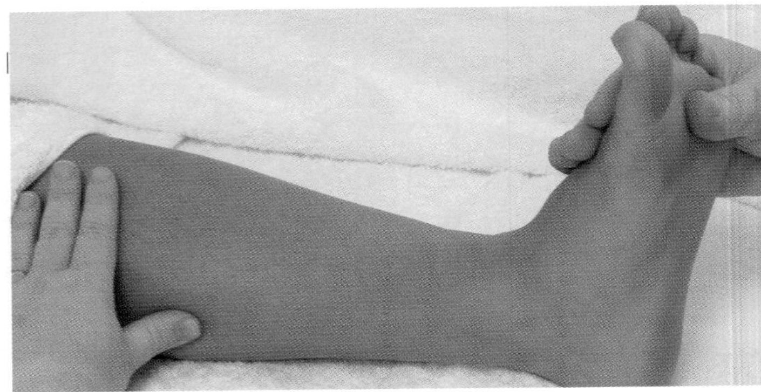

The medial sciatic

Repeat the previous movement up or down the lateral side of the achilles tendon.

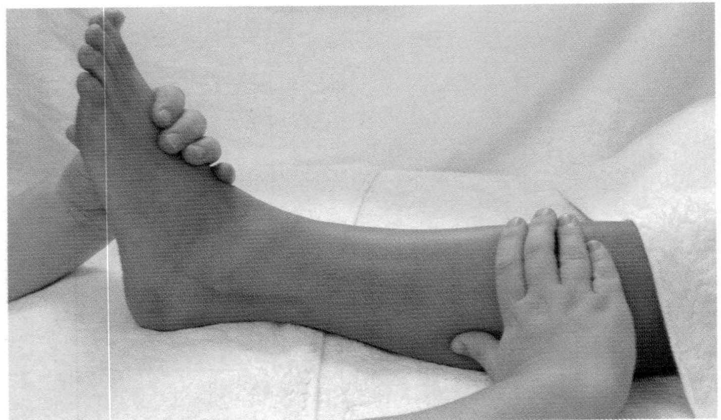

The lateral sciatic

Lateral and medial

To finish work back down to the heel squeezing gently with fingers and thumbs both lateral and medial aspects.

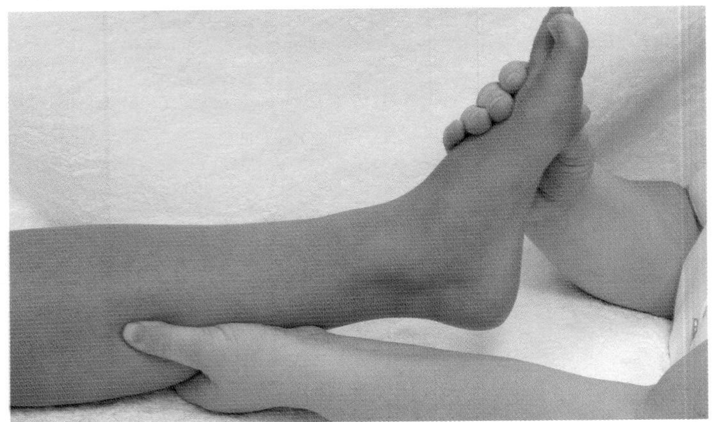

The lateral and medial aspects

Ovary/teste

Located on the lateral aspect of the foot midway between the ankle bone and the back of the heel.

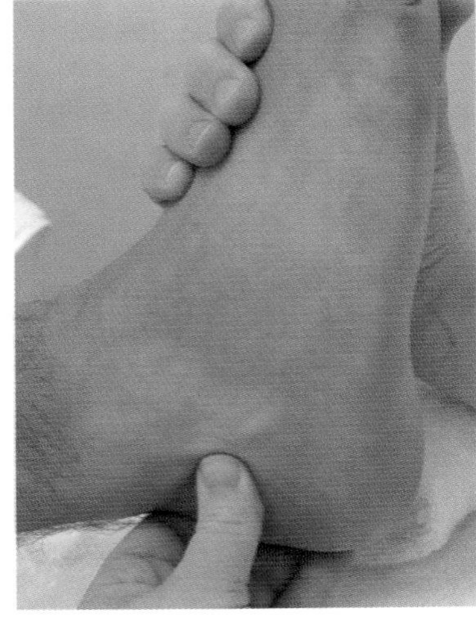

Ovary/teste

Fallopian tube/vas deferens

Located across the dorsal surface of the foot, from the ovary/teste on the lateral aspect to the uterus and prostate reflex on the medial aspect of the foot.

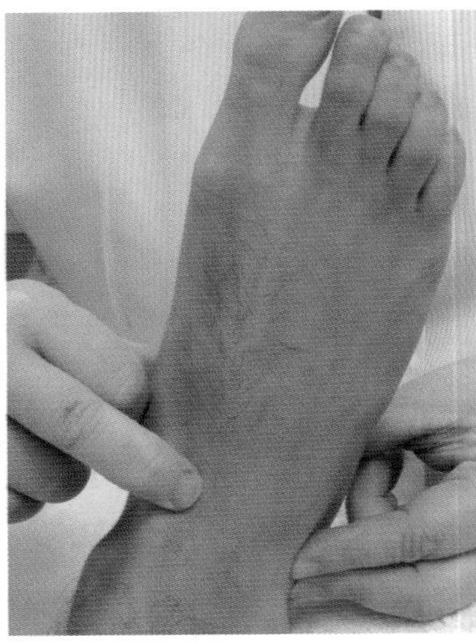

The fallopian tube

Uterus/prostate

Located on the medial aspect of the foot midway between the ankle bone and the back of the heel.

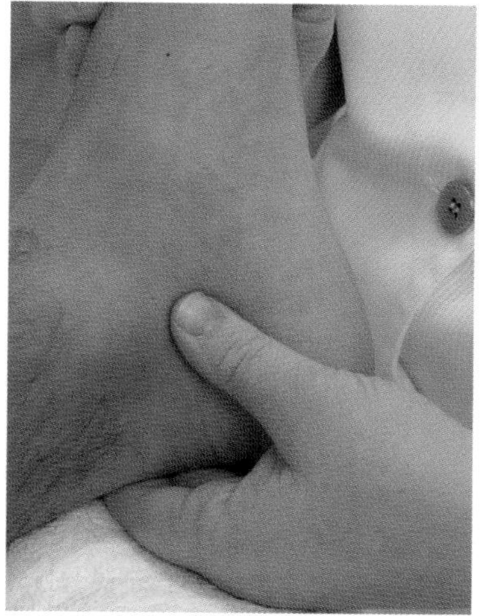

The uterus/prostate

Breast/mammary

Located in all five zones on the dorsal aspect of the foot, covering the area between the base of the toes and the diaphragm line.

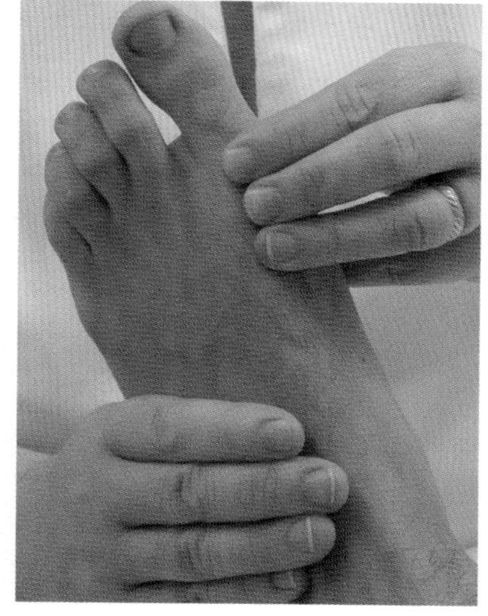

The breast

Groin lymph

Located across the dorsal surface of the foot from beneath the ankle bone on the medial aspect to the same point on the lateral aspect.

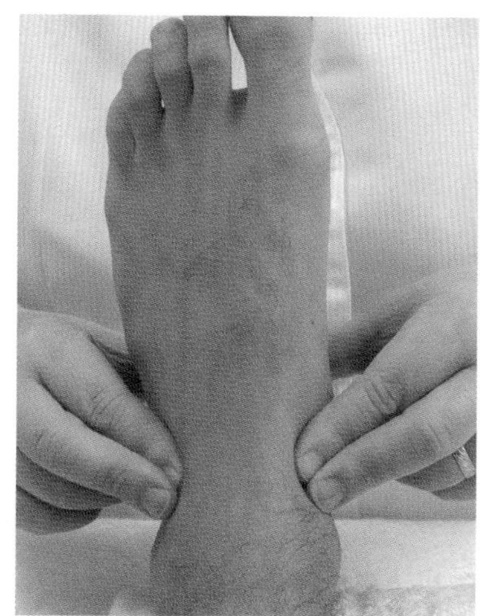

The groin lymph

Lymphatic system

Located on the dorsal surface of the foot, from between the webs of the toes to the ankle. Thumb-walk or finger-walk down these reflexes.

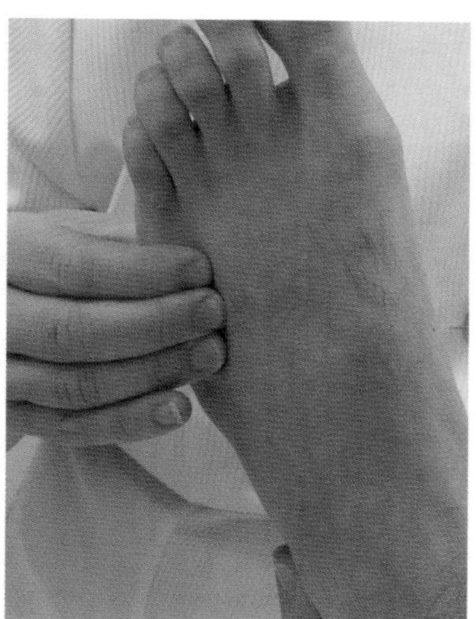

The lymphatic system

Finishing movement

Using the whole palmar surface of the hands apply slight pressure against the soles of the feet.

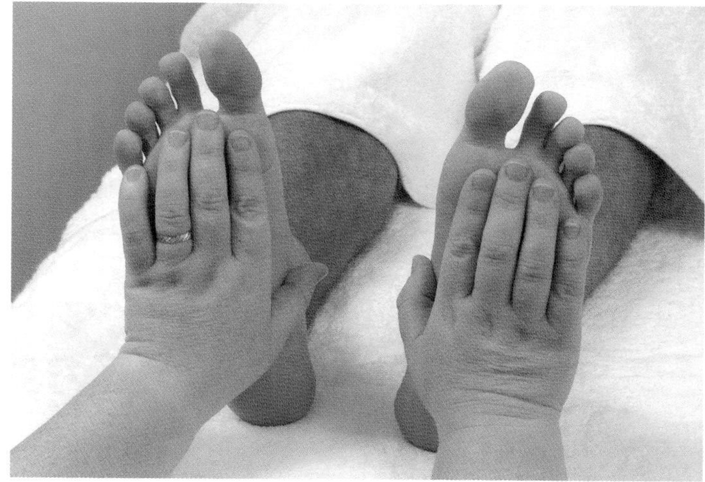

Finishing movement

PRACTICE IN CONTEXT

1 Practise the different reflexology techniques of thumb and finger walking firstly on your own hand and arm. When you feel comfortable and relaxed and the movement is flowing, practise on a partner's foot varying the pressure and working with and without a massage medium. Obtain feedback from your partner about the pressure, the sensations she is feeling and the benefit of treatment with or without a massage medium.

2 Using your foot maps of the systems and organs of the body and photographs of reflex points, practise locating specific reflex areas on the feet. Use as many different size feet as possible until you become proficient at locating individual reflex points.

Using a water soluble marker pen practise drawing the systems and organs on the feet.

3 Practise the routine you have been taught by your tutor until you can treat the whole foot confidently.

ASSESSMENT OF KNOWLEDGE

1 When is the massage technique of effleurage used?

2 How is the massage technique of wringing performed?

3 Between which transverse lines on the sole of the foot are the reflex points of the liver, the bladder, the lung, the transverse colon, the spleen and the pituitary gland?

4 When would the 'hooking' technique be used?

5 Where is the location for the following reflex points: the shoulder, the sinuses, the solar plexus and the ilio-caecal valve?

6 When treating a client who has constipation and recurring headaches, which reflex points would you work?

7 When treating a client who has cystitis and is asthmatic, which reflex points would you work?

9 Stress

It is believed that stress is a trigger to many diseases and disorders, insomnia, high blood pressure, asthma, gastric ulcers, irritable bowel syndrome and migraine to name but a few. Each individual has the ability to train themselves to release excessive nervous tension and reduce the effects of stress. They can do this in many ways but a simple solution is relaxation. Learning to relax for some people is quite difficult and that is where the reflexologist can help by providing a therapy which can deal with both the physical and emotional aspects of stress.

The problems of stress

During the consultation it is important to be aware of some of the physical or physiological problems which may be linked to, or aggravated by, stress. Examples are digestive disorders such as ulcers, indigestion, irritable bowel syndrome, diarrhoea or constipation; and emotional problems such as low self-esteem, depression or anxiety. The lungs may be affected by stress and conditions such as asthma may worsen. Severe, recurring headaches or migraine and even hair loss may be a result of stress.

Stress may be defined as 'a response by the body to a situation, which is perceived as threatening' and this may then have an adverse effect on any of the systems of the body. **Homeostasis** is when the internal environment of the body is maintained in a relative state of balance. *Homeo* means 'the same' and *stasis* means 'standing still'.

The systems of the body are working constantly to achieve this state of balance; however, stress is constantly challenging and altering this balanced state, though the body is able to fight back by utilising homeostatic mechanisms to redress the balance. Homeostasis is controlled mainly by the nervous and endocrine systems.

We all experience stress to some degree and a healthy amount of stress can be a powerful motivating force on which some people positively thrive. However, having more stress than we can handle is one of the greatest threats to our health, as the positive effects are replaced by exhaustion and we may find it difficult to cope. A great deal of stress over a long period can lead to illness, burn out or eventual breakdown.

Causes of stress

The causes of stress are many and varied. Some of the more common stressors are:

- The increasing pace at which we live
- The complexity of the work we do or the profession we are in
- Being a working mum or single parent
- Marriage, divorce or separation
- Loss of a parent or child
- Relationship problems
- Arguments
- Financial worries/debt
- Death in the family
- Moving house
- Taking on too much responsibility
- Caring for the elderly
- Job insecurity
- Long term unemployment
- Retirement
- Lack of stimulation
- Lack of success
- Illness
- Giving up an addiction
- Emotional trauma
- Unpleasant physical environment
- Bullying

Negative effects of stress

The negative effects of stress can be mental, physical, emotional, or behavioural.

The following table shows the effects of stress on the body.

Mental	Physical	Emotional	Behaviour
Poor memory	Headaches	Crying easily	Aggressive
Lack of sensitivity	Backache	Low self esteem	Obsessive
Poor concentration	Muscular tension	Poor self image	Compulsive
Indecision	Heart palpitations	No enthusiasm	Hyperactive
Inability to complete tasks	High blood pressure	Loss of confidence	Loss of appetite or comfort eating
Negativity	Stomach upsets	Depression	Smoking to excess
Putting tasks off	Constipation	Mood swings	Drinking to excess
Feeling inadequate	Passing urine often	Cynicism	Neglectful
	Indigestion	Irritability	Working too hard
	Irritable bowel	Nervousness	Not relaxing
	Diarrhoea	Anxiousness	Loss of libido
	Skin conditions	Vulnerability	Lethargy
	Low fertility	Feeling rejected	Clumsiness
	Severe PMS	Insecurity	Panic attacks
	Thyroid dysfunction		Becoming withdrawn
	Muscular cramps		Impatience
	Difficulty sleeping		Frustration
	Waking early		Hostility
	Inability to relax		Hypercritical
	Exhaustion		Inflexibility
	Weakening of the immune system		Unreasonable

Stress is an individual response internally to external factors that threaten our security. It is not always caused by traumatic events, as even good experiences such as planning a holiday, party or wedding can prove stressful. In small amounts stress is a normal part of life but when stress builds up to such a degree that it changes to distress, it becomes a negative and destructive force. Every person is different however, and a source of stress to one person could be a motivating factor for another. Some people need to create a small amount of stress in their lives to help them achieve a goal or rise to a challenge. Each individual will react differently to a given situation or experience so the stress level and the reaction to it will vary in every case.

Dealing with stress

The fight or flight response/alarm reaction response

The body has an in-built alarm system to prepare for action if it perceives a situation to be threatening. The response by the body will be to deal with the threat or run away from it. This is commonly referred to as the 'fight or flight' response or 'alarm reaction'.

Whichever response is chosen the body will provide the necessary conditions to effectively deal with the threat or run away from it. The body responds by secreting the hormone adrenalin from the adrenal medulla. It is sometimes referred to as the fight or flight hormone, as once released its effect on the body is instantaneous. Adrenalin is carried via the bloodstream to all the vital organs and systems of the body. The physical and physiological effects that occur in response are:

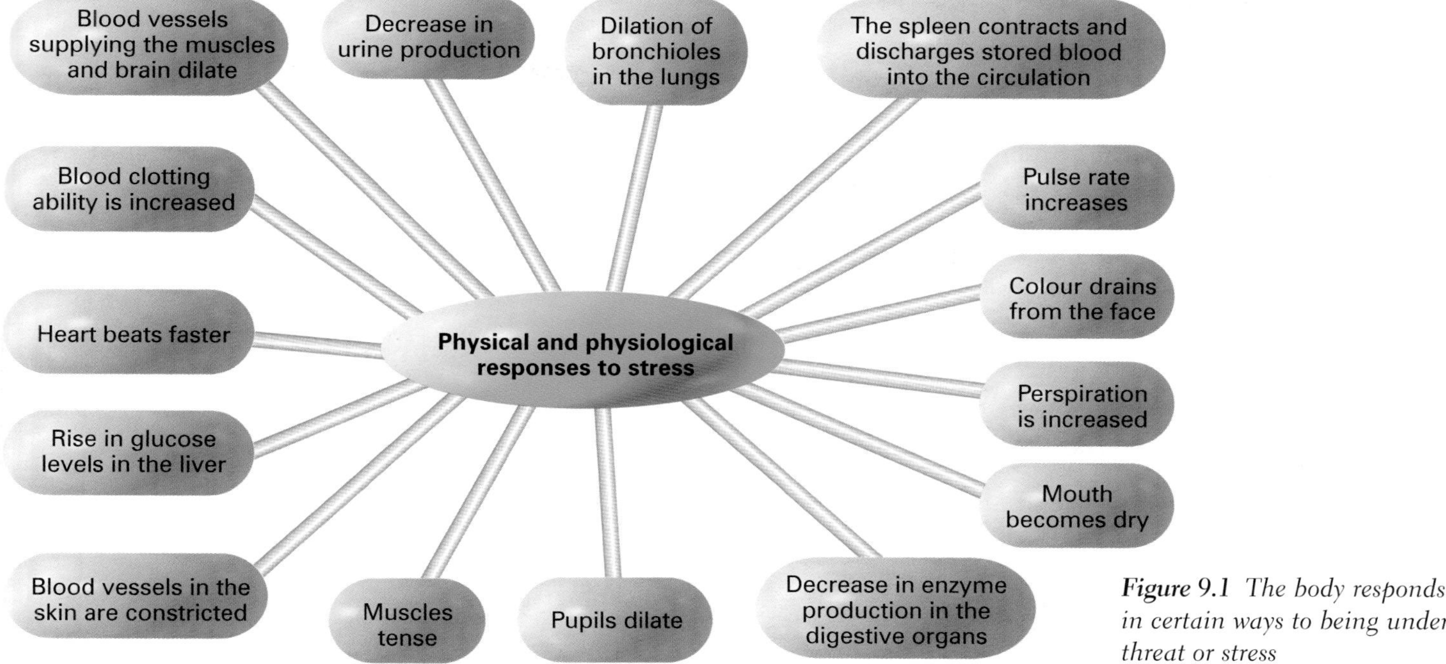

Figure 9.1 *The body responds in certain ways to being under threat or stress*

All these responses to stress are part of the 'alarm reaction' which allows the body to deal immediately with a threatening or stressful situation. The following is an outline of what happens in the alarm reaction.

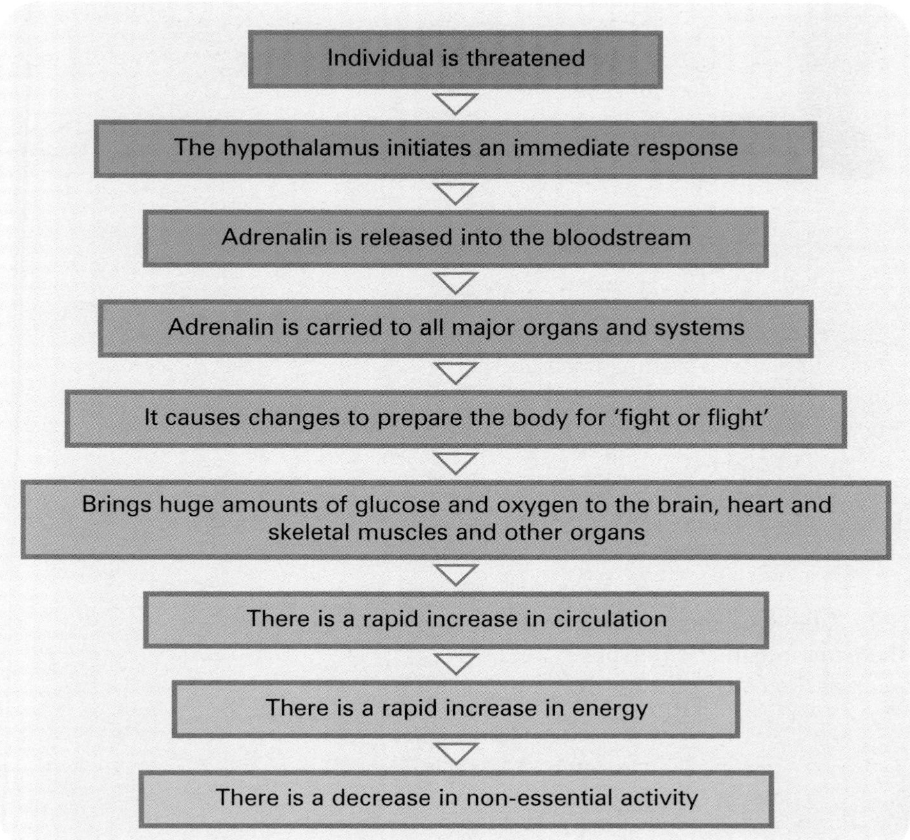

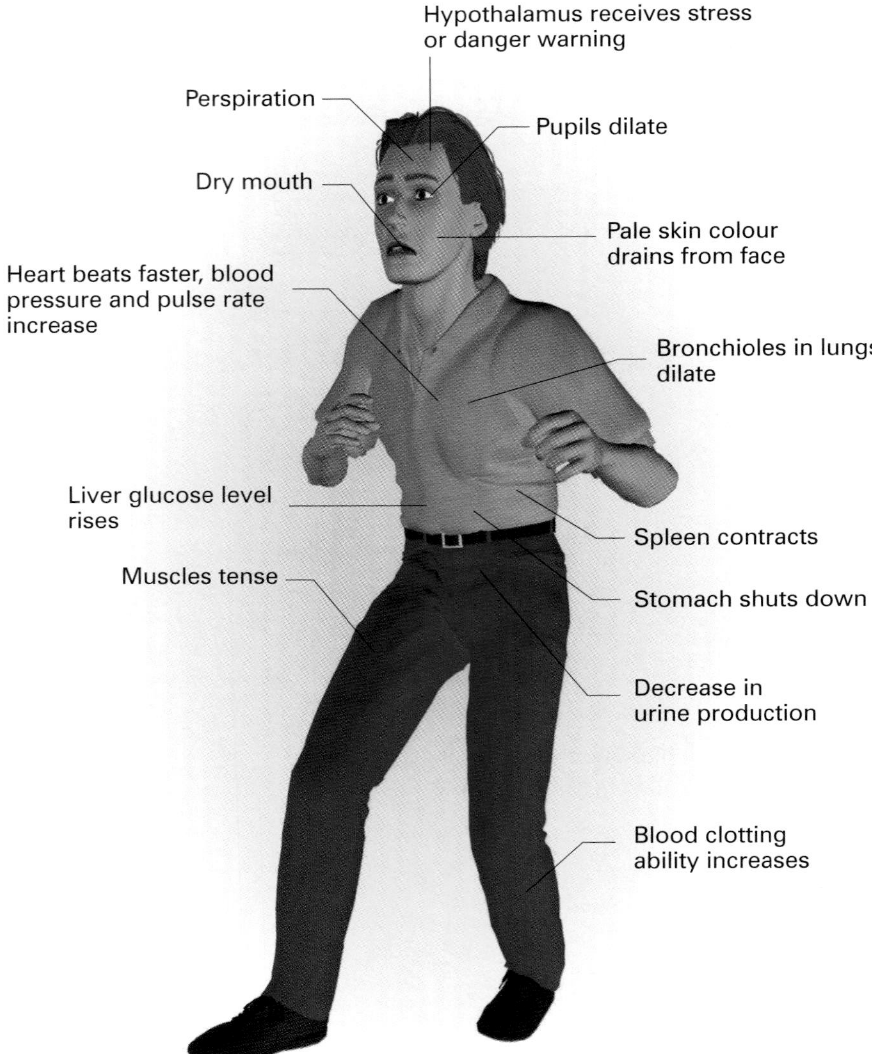

Figure 9.2 The 'alarm reaction' to stress

> **Reflection**
>
> We have all experienced stress to some degree even if we weren't aware of it. Competing in a sporting event, the mouth is dry, the heart is beating faster and our muscles tense. As soon as we start playing the adrenalin takes over and we are superhuman, nothing can stop us and our energy is boundless! There are many occasions that can be stressful; for example, when our children are ill or late coming home and we can't contact them, or when we have to meet deadlines or are just about to give a speech for the first time in front of fifty people.

The effects of the alarm reaction are short-lived to allow the individual to deal immediately with danger or stress, and then the parasympathetic nervous system comes into play and relaxes the body. In some cases the cause of stress may remain so the body does not experience this relaxation stage.

Resistance reaction

The continuous exposure to the stressor leads to the next stage in dealing with stress – this is called the 'resistance reaction'.

This response is also activated by the hypothalamus and is longer lasting, allowing the body to continue fighting the stressors. This stage will help most people continue to deal with the stress; however, it does lower the energy levels and the immunity, causing illness to occur or last longer. Clients may complain of one or several of the symptoms listed in the negative effects of stress table on page 80. In most cases these problems will be overcome and the body will then return to a more balanced state.

Prolonged adrenal stimulation will begin to deplete the body's systems and the organs will not function as efficiently as normal, if stress is not dissipated by physical activity. Blood pressure may also be affected. In some circumstances, the body is not able to overcome the stressors and it 'gives up', reaching the stage of exhaustion. This final stage has a detrimental effect on vital organs if it persists for a long period of time.

The ability of the body to handle stressors is largely determined by the individual's general state of health and well-being. Each individual also has the ability to minimise the effects of stress by their own positive attitude, their response to any challenges, adapting their lifestyle and investigating other means of combating stress.

Ways of dealing with stress

There are different methods of coping with stress. You should assess your current lifestyle and identify the causes of stress in your life. Make a detailed list and decide which of them you can control and make a note of how you can overcome the problem. Then identify the causes of stress which are out of your control. Try to think of how you can tackle these problems to reduce your level of stress. The following are some of the ways of coping with stress.

Relaxation

Taking time to relax is easier said than done if you have a career, look after a large family or care for sick relatives or are in full-time education. Relaxation can take the form of sleeping, resting, meditating, taking up a hobby or sport, or simply sitting and reading a book. It is all about making time for yourself to do as you please and put your needs first.

Exercise

Exercise is wonderful for eliminating pent-up energy. It also oxygenates the blood and burns up excess adrenaline in the body. It does not have to be rigorous; a brisk walk or a gentle exercise session a couple of times a week will help. It is important to consider your level of fitness before taking any strenuous exercise. If you are not used to taking exercise, start slowly and build up the time and effort you spend gradually, and always warm up the muscles first to prevent injury.

Alternative therapy

Finally, investigate the different forms of alternative therapy which may help to reduce stress. Here are some that may help.

Body massage

This is the manual manipulation of the muscles that provides relaxation and helps to remove tension in the muscles, as well as easing aches and pains often caused by stress. Aromatherapy is another form of massage, which also includes the use of essential oils blended together to achieve different effects.

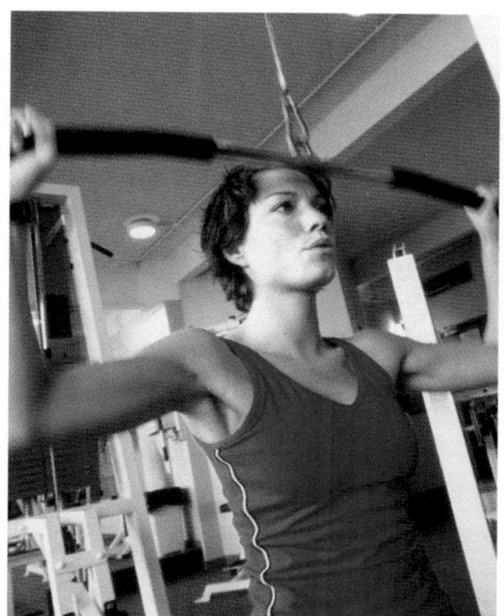

Exercise can help reduce stress levels

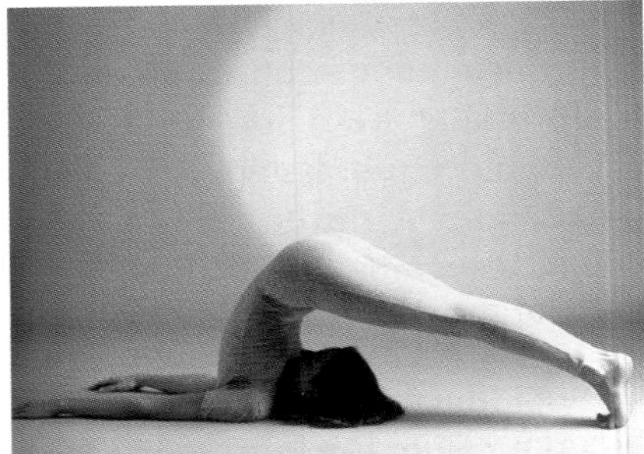

A yoga position

Tai chi and yoga

Tai chi and yoga are gentle forms of exercise which relax the body physically and have a calming effect on the mind, as does meditation. Shiatsu, from the Japanese word, may help to release tension in the body. It is derived from acupuncture and pressure is applied to points throughout the body by the finger, thumb or palm of the hand.

Bach flower remedies

Bach flower remedies can be taken to try to counteract stress and other problems. They are freely available in many chemists and health stores, and are derived from natural ingredients and have different effects.

Oils/herbs for stress-related ailments

There are many books available that discuss the beneficial effects of the use of essential oils. In addition to having a professional aromatherapy massage, these oils can be used at home to help relieve the symptoms of stress. They can be used in an aromatherapy burner, in the bath, added to a bowl of pot pourri or sprinkled onto your pillow at night. Manufacturers are aware of the potential benefits of essential oils and are now incorporating many of these oils in candles, bath, hair and skin care products. The following are some of these oils and the effects they have.

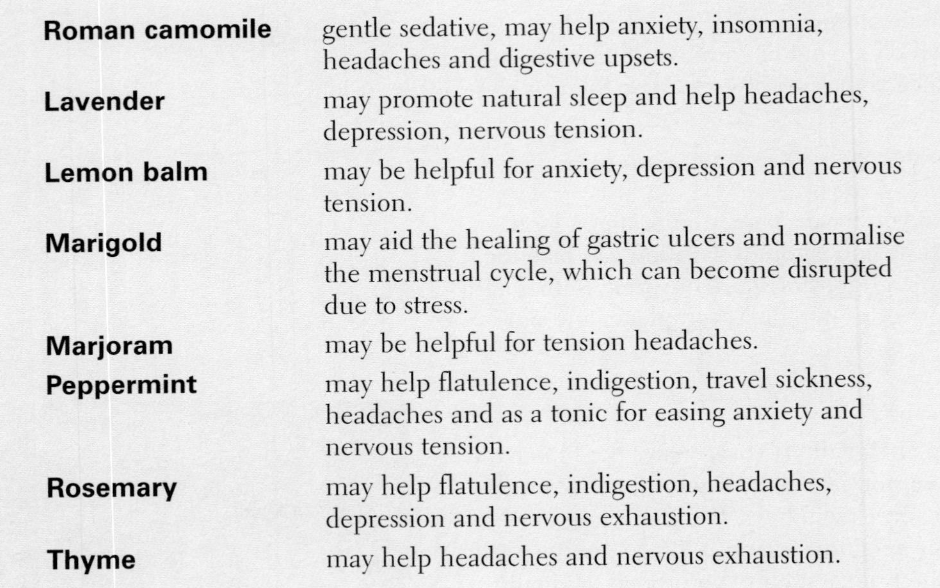

Roman camomile	gentle sedative, may help anxiety, insomnia, headaches and digestive upsets.
Lavender	may promote natural sleep and help headaches, depression, nervous tension.
Lemon balm	may be helpful for anxiety, depression and nervous tension.
Marigold	may aid the healing of gastric ulcers and normalise the menstrual cycle, which can become disrupted due to stress.
Marjoram	may be helpful for tension headaches.
Peppermint	may help flatulence, indigestion, travel sickness, headaches and as a tonic for easing anxiety and nervous tension.
Rosemary	may help flatulence, indigestion, headaches, depression and nervous exhaustion.
Thyme	may help headaches and nervous exhaustion.

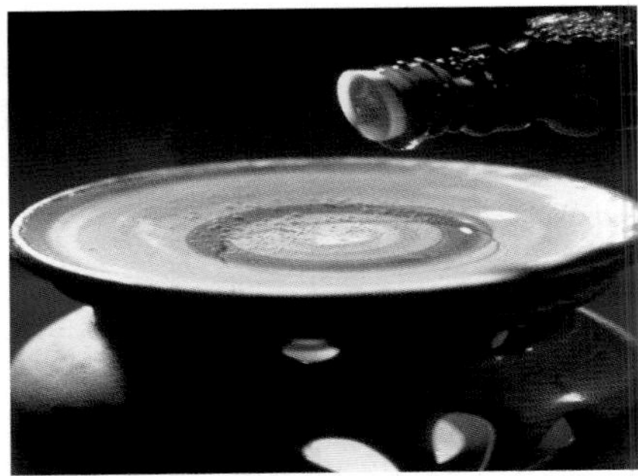

Essential oil burner/oils

Before recommending or using essential oils it is advisable to seek professional advice. Avoid using any oils during the first four-and-a-half months of pregnancy.

Herbal and fruit teas, tisanes or infusions are refreshing, caffeine-free drinks which may also provide the healing benefits of many different plants. Taken as an alternative to tea, coffee and carbonated drinks they may help in counteracting stress in producing a calming and soothing effect as well as being refreshing and invigorating.

Teas that may reduce stress by calming and soothing are camomile, peppermint, ginger, orange and honey. Teas that can refresh and revive, picking you up when you are suffering from stress, are citrus fruits, raspberry, loganberry and elderflower. These teas are all readily available in specialist shops, health food stores and most major supermarkets.

How reflexology helps in coping with stress

Many disorders are stress-related and increasing numbers of people are suffering from such disorders. Depending on the individual, stress-related illnesses may present in different forms. Some of the more common are hypertension, high blood pressure, coronary thrombosis, heart attack, allergies, anorexia, ulcers, indigestion, constipation, palpitations, migraine and depression.

Continuous stress may cause an energy blockage within the body and reflexology can be used to relax a client, release the energy blockage and improve the client's own energy levels. It may also induce a sense of well-being and help the body to heal itself, as well as balancing hormone levels and stabilising metabolism.

Stress causes tension, which causes the muscles to become tight, in particular those of the spine and back, and this will in turn have an effect on the nervous system of the body, so creating pain. The blood vessels constrict and reduce the amount of oxygen and nutrients reaching vital organs and systems.

The changes that occur to the body during a reflexology treatment that help to combat stress are both physical and mental:

- The eyes close and the head relaxes.
- The shoulders are lowered as muscular tension is released.
- Breathing becomes even.
- Mood becomes lighter as serotonin, a transmitter substance released by the brain and thought to be involved in inducing sleep, is released into the body.
- A feeling of deep relaxation is experienced.
- A feeling of revitalisation develops.

Effects of treatment

Reflexology causes the muscles to relax, physical tension to be released and the nervous system to function normally. This may have a beneficial effect on all the other systems of the body and the way in which they function.

- The blood vessels relax and this allows the blood carrying the required oxygen and nourishment to the vital organs and tissues of the body to flow more freely.
- The lymphatic system is also working more effectively and this will help in the elimination process by ridding the body of more toxins and waste products.
- The respiratory system relaxes and breathing becomes deeper and more even. This contributes greatly to relaxation but it also increases the amount of oxygen reaching the tissues.
- There is a balancing effect on the hormones and this will have an effect on all the systems in the body, as they are responsible for maintaining homeostasis, by changing the chemical activities of cells.
- Most importantly, reflexology may re-energise someone suffering from stress, as it helps to remove blockages in the energy flowing around the body, thus improving the client's own energy levels. The client may feel uplifted and calmer, symptoms of stress may be alleviated and this provides ideal conditions to allow the body to heal itself and achieve a state of homeostasis.

PRACTICE IN CONTEXT

Make a list of current stressors in your life and divide them into groups under the headings: 'positive stressors', 'stressors that may be eliminated' and 'stressors you need to take action to reduce'.

ASSESSMENT OF KNOWLEDGE

1 What is homeostasis?
2 Give examples of ten common stressors.
3 How do the negative effects of stress affect the body?
4 What is meant by the term 'fight or flight'?
5 What is the name of the hormone secreted from the adrenal glands as a response to stress?
6 Give six examples of the physical and physiological responses of the body to stress.
7 How will exercise reduce stress?
8 How does reflexology reduce stress?

10 Contra-actions

Each individual will respond to reflexology treatment in a way that is unique to them and their response to each treatment may also vary. The contra-actions to reflexology are the physical and emotional responses that occur during treatment, immediately after treatment or the time in between treatments. These reactions are a natural outcome of reflexology and form part of the 'healing process'.

During the consultation, it is advisable to discuss with your client the possible reactions or responses that she may experience from the treatment. These may vary depending on age, fitness level, physical and emotional problems and the personality of the client. Many clients may actually be unaware of the physical responses occurring, as they can be very subtle.

The reactions to treatment

Most of the reactions to reflexology are pleasant, others not so pleasant. However even the unpleasant ones can be just as beneficial, as they form a necessary part of the healing process. Because this treatment is activating the body's own healing powers, there may be occasions when a more intense reaction to treatment occurs. This is known as '**the healing crisis**', which occurs when the body is cleansing itself both physically and emotionally. Some clients may find that they feel worse before they get better. The client's reaction to treatment will vary depending on the imbalance within the body.

Some immediate responses to treatment are:

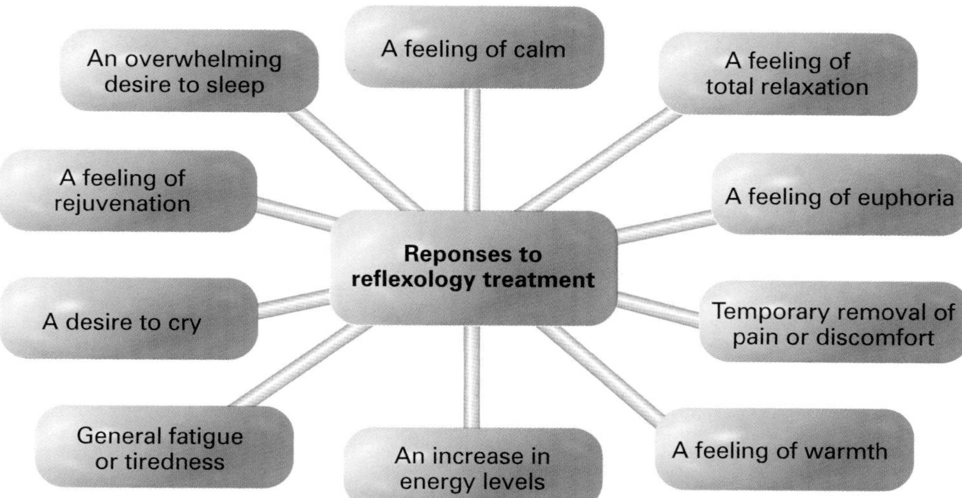

Figure 10.1 Clients may respond in various ways when they are treated by reflexology

As a response to treatment the body will start to eliminate toxins through the kidneys, bowels, lungs and skin, therefore some of the following physical reactions may be experienced by most clients to some degree.

- The natural elimination processes are stimulated therefore the client may experience an increase in urination, increased flatulence and more frequent bowel movement.
- There may be an increase in sweat production.

- These may be an increase in the secretions from the mucous membrane – in the nose, mouth and respiratory tract.
- These may be a worsening of a skin condition, spots or pimples.

The client should be advised to drink more water to assist the removal of toxins from the body and this advice can be provided immediately after treatment.

During the treatment when nerve stimulation occurs there may be a response in the part of the body corresponding to the area being worked. These responses may be feelings such as twitching or visible contracting of the muscles. A tingling sensation may occur in the limbs, often a result of the releasing of blocked up energy, or there may be an initial feeling of warmth. On some occasions there may be a feeling of pain. A sharp pain will usually indicate an acute condition and a dull pain indicates a chronic condition. Occasionally the client may experience more unpleasant side-effects such as dizziness, headaches, nausea or fever; these, however, are quite rare.

Some clients may experience an extreme emotional response to treatment – they may break down and cry, sometimes sobbing uncontrollably. This is often referred to as a 'healing crisis'. In this case you should not break contact with the client as this provides reassurance. Adopt a sympathetic approach, listen to the client if they wish to talk about their reaction and slowly draw the treatment to an end using relaxing massage techniques.

This is a difficult situation to deal with if you have another client waiting or soon to arrive. You don't want to rush the client out but you may have to leave her to attend to your other client. You could ask her to sit in the rest area with a cup of herbal tea and to relax until you are able to return. You could ask a colleague to sit with the client until she was feeling better or tell her you will contact her later to see how she is. Make another appointment to suit the client and be as sympathetic and comforting as you can.

PRACTICE IN CONTEXT

You will have the opportunity to provide reflexology for many different clients, and you will be required to explain the different reactions they may experience after treatment. Discuss with your colleagues and tutor the different approach you would adopt with (a) a young teenager (b) a nursing sister and (c) an elderly client in a nursing home.

ASSESSMENT OF KNOWLEDGE

1. Define the term contra-action.
2. Give five examples of the immediate response of a client to treatment.
3. Why should you advise a client to drink more water after treatment?
4. What physical sensations may be felt by the client when nerve stimulation occurs?
5. What is the term used to describe an intense reaction to reflexology treatment?

11 Aftercare advice

At the conclusion of treatment you should assist the client into a comfortable position. If she is on a reclining couch adjust the back, lifting it into a sitting position. Alternatively, provide a comfortable chair where the client may sit while you discuss the treatment and interpret the results. You may also answer any questions the client may have.

Steps to follow

1. Explain to your client that results are not always achieved immediately, ensure that their expectations are realistic and that they understand that some conditions require more time to achieve results. Response to treatment also depends on how receptive the client is; sometimes it requires several treatments to build a relationship with some clients.
2. At this time you may also offer advice about further treatment and possible changes to lifestyle which may reinforce the effects of treatment.

   You may discuss the changes your client should make to her diet for example, replacing coffee and tea with fruit juice and herbal teas. Reducing the amount of processed food she eats and increasing the amount of fresh fruit and vegetables will provide her with essential minerals and vitamins and reduce the fat content of her diet. It is also believed that the antioxidant vitamins, A C and E help to slow the ageing process by reducing free radical damage.

   Advise your client to drink plenty of water to help flush toxins out of the system, rest as much as possible and abstain from alcohol.
3. Discuss with your client the sensations felt during treatment and how they feel now, after treatment. You must then discuss the findings you noted during treatment, the significance of these findings and the possible responses the client may still experience within the next twenty-four hours. It is important to be reassuring and explain the benefits of these responses in aiding the healing process.
4. The next step is to make recommendations that you feel will benefit your client personally. There may be simple lifestyle changes she needs to make that will reinforce the treatment she is having and you could suggest complementary treatment. Practical advice should only be given if it is needed. You may need to refer her to a GP or other practitioner, recommend other therapies or provide information about support groups in the area, if requested.
5. Take this opportunity to discuss with your client any revisions you need to make to your original treatment plan. This will be based on the result of treatment and the client's wishes. You may need to alter the number of treatments she will need or the regularity of treatment.
6. Finally, answer any questions the client may have, to provide reassurance, motivation or practical help and advice. At this time you can arrange further reflexology appointments to suit the client.

Homecare advice

Many problems with feet have probably been caused by abuse over many years. The ever-changing world of fashion has led most adults to squeeze their feet into different shaped and ill-fitting shoes, the worst culprit being the stiletto-heeled shoe which throws the body out of line, affecting the balance and eventually the spine.

Some people, as they rapidly grew in size, failed to change their shoe size and continued to squeeze their feet into shoes which were too small for their feet. In cases where a person has one foot slightly larger than the other, problems of the feet can arise in trying to keep on a shoe which is too large or squeezing into a shoe which is too small.

Another common cause of foot abuse is a person working in an occupation which requires long periods of standing or working in an unnatural position with their weight unevenly distributed.

Most people have, at some time in their lives, worn synthetic shoes which provide no ventilation, thus increasing the risk of fungal infection. The same applies to nylon socks and stockings, which will increase the amount of sweat produced by the feet.

Advice on caring for feet

The advice to your client should be:

- Wear the correct size and width of shoe.
- Select lower heels which will maintain the natural balance.
- Wear leather or shoes made from natural fibres, if possible sandals or open shoes to allow the skin to breathe.
- Wear 100% cotton or wool socks rather than nylon or mixed fibres.
- Have regular foot baths using additives of aromatherapy oils or herbs sealed in a muslin bag. Before using essential oils it is advisable to seek the advice of an aromatherapist or other expert and ensure that there are no contraindications to oils used. The following are oils or herbs for use with certain conditions.

  Athlete's foot – tea tree is antiseptic, peppermint is refreshing.

  Cuts or wounds – tea tree if infected, lavender, geranium, camomile.

  Fluid retention – geranium, cedarwood, juniper.

  Gout – basil, juniper, camomile, lemon, rosemary.

  Muscular pain – black pepper for its analgesic effect, juniper, rosemary, thyme.

  Perspiration – basil, cypress, lavender, neroli.

  Rheumatism – basil, eucalyptus, ginger, lavender, rosemary.

  Sprains – lavender, hyssop, nutmeg, rose otto.

  Sweaty smells – ginger, nutmeg.

  Verrucae – lemon, sweet thyme.
- Use a hard skin remover regularly to prevent an accumulation on the foot.
- Massage the feet regularly with oils or creams (preferably without strong perfume) containing healing or moisturising ingredients. Creams which contain alpha hydroxy acids are effective in preventing a build up of hard skin.
- Visit a chiropodist to treat foot disorders.
- Have a professional pedicure to keep feet and toenails in tip top condition.

- Exercising the feet will maintain their health and help to combat any deformities.
- Walking is an excellent way to exercise the feet, and do it barefoot when possible. Walking on sand provides additional exercise and helps to refine the skin tissue as the small grains of sand have an exfoliating effect on the skin.
- Specific exercises such as picking up marbles with the toes and passing them from one foot to the other will help to tone the ligaments and tendons of the feet. To strengthen the arch, place an elastic bandage six inches long in front of the foot and then, using your toes, pull it towards you making it as small as possible. Before starting any exercise loosen and warm up the foot by rotating at the ankle and plantarflexing and dorsiflexing the foot.

Finally, you may provide the client with any of the products you have recommended to improve the condition of the feet or as an antidote to stress. Escort your client to reception or allow her to wait in a rest area until she is ready to leave and make sure that you have recorded any future appointments.

PRACTICE IN CONTEXT

1. Compile a list of useful addresses and telephone numbers of other therapists and specialist organisations in your area as well as product manufacturers and distributors. This may provide a valuable source of reference when a client asks for some specific advice or recommendation.
2. Design an aftercare leaflet detailing all the advice you would offer in the care of feet. You may then give this to each client to take home after treatment.

ASSESSMENT OF KNOWLEDGE

1. What advice can you give your client to reinforce the benefits of treatment?
2. Why would you advise the client to drink plenty of water?
3. Name the antioxidant vitamins.
4. Give two causes of foot problems.
5. State three pieces of advice you can give your client to ensure healthy feet.
6. What are the benefits of exercising the feet?

- The skeletal system
- The muscular system
- The cardiovascular system
- The lymphatic system
- The respiratory system
- The skin
- The digestive system
- The urinary system
- The endocrine system
- The nervous system
- The reproductive system
- The special senses

The Body **Systems**

12 The skeletal system

A thorough knowledge of the body systems and how they work is essential to the reflexologist, not only to recognise their position on the reflex maps of the feet but also to understand how an imbalance caused by disease or injury may affect the health of the client.

The skeletal system provides the framework for the body and it consists of bones and the cartilage, ligaments and tendons that hold them together.

Bones provide support, shape and movement to the body and they provide attachment for muscles and tendons. They protect vital organs, blood cells develop in the red bone marrow, and bone also acts as a reservoir for minerals such as calcium. This is an important function, as calcium is required by nerve cells for their activities, muscle needs calcium to achieve a contraction and blood needs calcium to help with clotting.

The skeleton

The skeleton is composed of the axial skeleton and the appendicular skeleton.

The **axial skeleton** forms the centre axis of the body and is made up of: the skull – cranium, face and lower jaw – the vertebral column, the ribs and the sternum.

The **appendicular skeleton**, or the parts which are appended (joined to) the axial skeleton, is made up of: the shoulder girdle and arms and the pelvic girdle and legs.

The skeleton has about 200 bones, which vary in shape, size and function.

The bones of the skeleton

The bones of the skeleton are classified as:

Long	These form the limbs.
Short	These are found in the wrist and ankles.
Flat	These are for protection, e.g. the skull, or for attachment of certain muscles. They are made from a sandwich of hard bone with a spongy layer in between.
Irregular	These are irregular in shape to cope with the job they do, e.g. the vertebrae.
Sesamoid	These are small bones which develop in the tendons around certain joints, e.g. the patella in the knee.

Bones are active living tissues and the process by which they are formed is called ossification. Osteoblasts are bone-forming cells which, when calcified, become osteocytes. The osteoblasts secrete substances composed of collagenous fibres, forming a framework into which calcium salts are deposited. This process is called calcification. When the osteoblasts are surrounded by this calcification they are known as trabecula.

The bone develops hollow centres that contain marrow, in which the manufacture of blood cells takes place. The periosteum is a tough fibrous sheet covering the surface

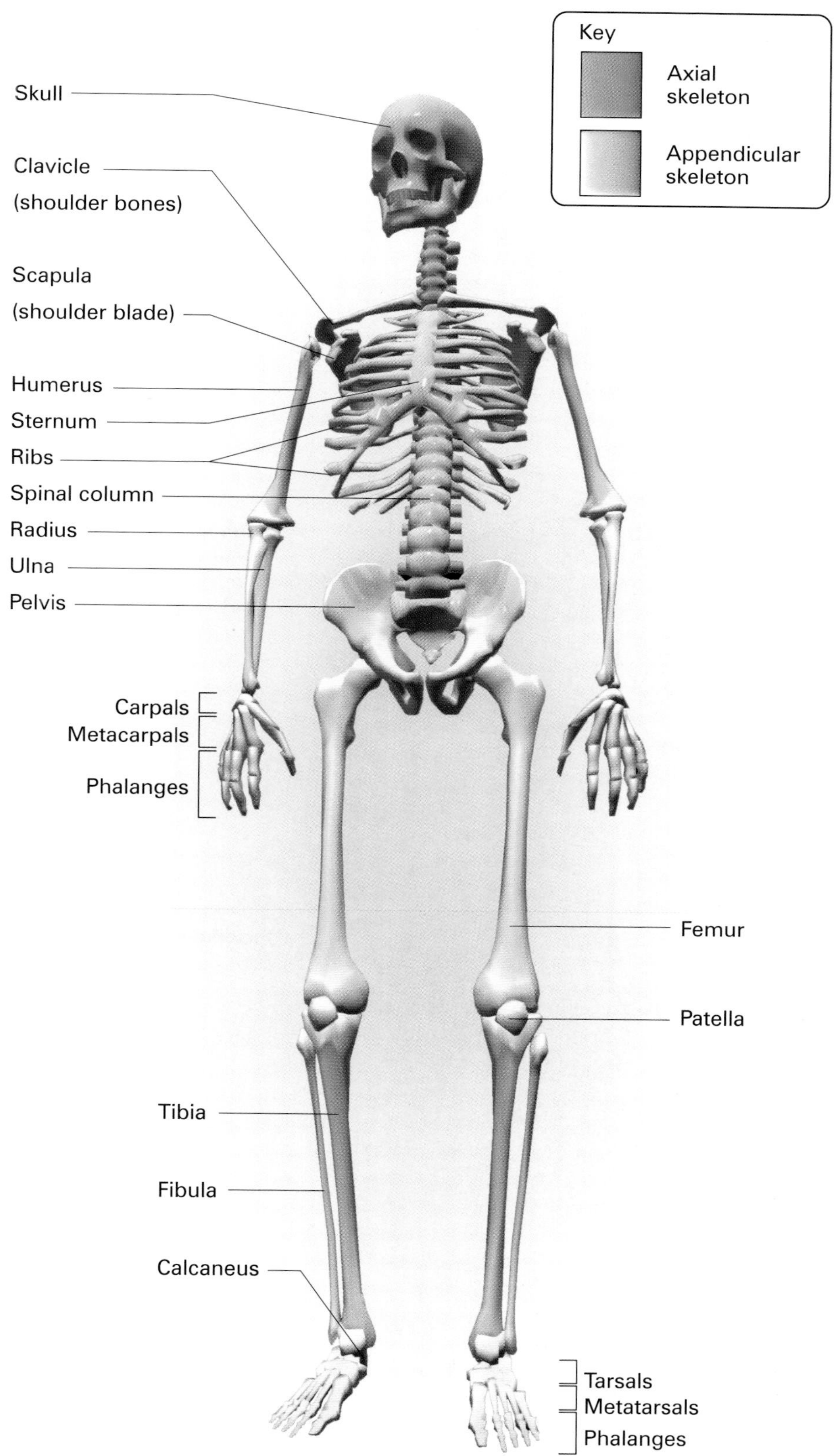
Key
Axial skeleton
Appendicular skeleton
Skull
Clavicle
(shoulder bones)
Scapula
(shoulder blade)
Humerus
Sternum
Ribs
Spinal column
Radius
Ulna
Pelvis
Carpals
Metacarpals
Phalanges
Femur
Patella
Tibia
Fibula
Calcaneus
Tarsals
Metatarsals
Phalanges

Figure 12.1 The skeleton

of bones, except where a bone forms a joint and is covered by hyaline cartilage. The blood supply to the bones is received via the periosteum on its surface and via an artery in the nutrient foramen in the shaft of the bone.

Most of the bones of the skeleton have protruberances and ridges for the attachment of muscles and tendons.

Skull

The skull is divided into the cranium and the face, and is made up of the following parts.

Cranium

The cranium is made up of:

- One frontal
- Two parietal
- Two temporal
- One ethmoid
- One sphenoid
- One occipital

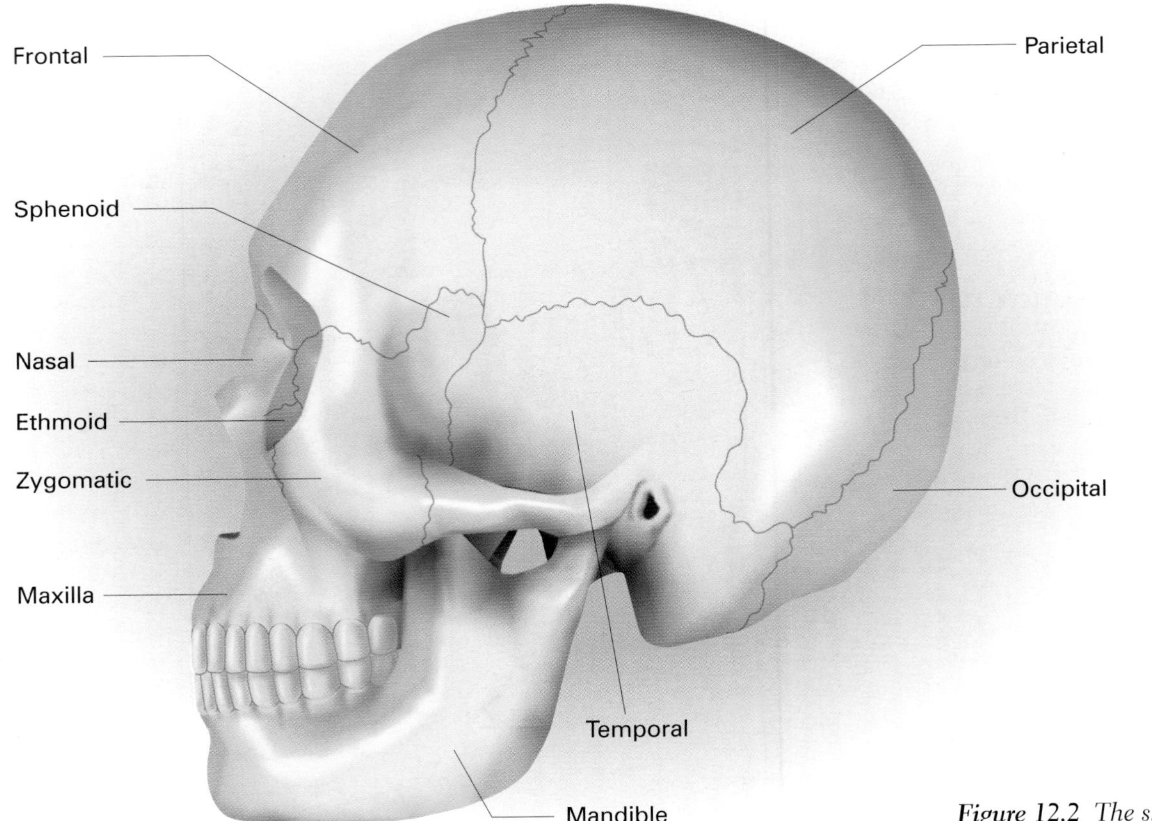

Figure 12.2 The skull

Face

The face is made up of:

- Two maxillae
- Two zygomatic
- Two nasal
- One mandible
- Two palatine
- Two inferior turbinate
- One vomer
- Two lacrimal

Trunk

The trunk comprises:

- The sternum or breast bone
- Twelve ribs
- The spinal column, which consists of:
  - Seven cervical vertebrae
  - Twelve thoracic vertebrae
  - Five lumbar vertebrae
  - Five sacral vertebrae fused together to form the sacrum
  - Four coccygeal vertebrae fused together to form the coccyx

The spinal column provides flexibility and strength to the body. The arms are joined to the spinal column by the shoulder girdle and the legs are joined by the pelvic girdle.

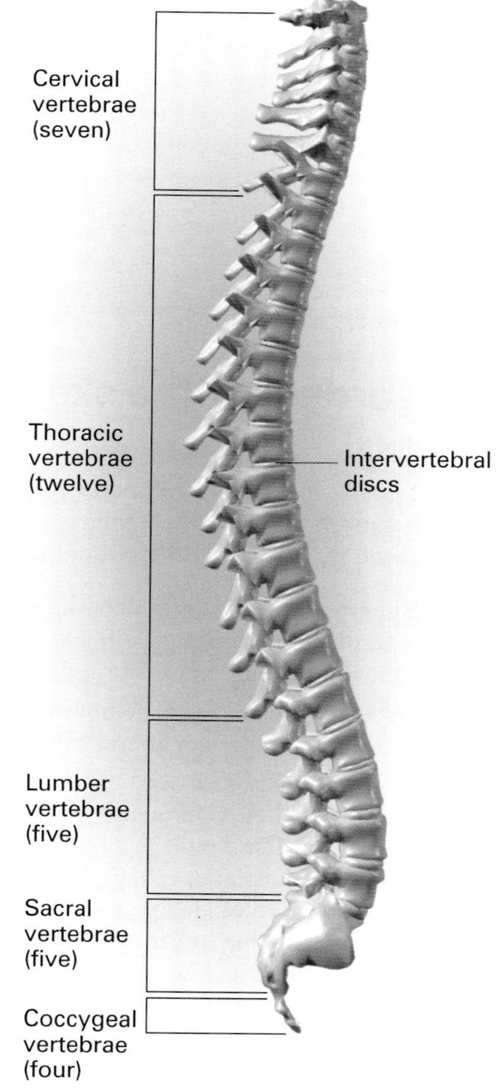

Figure 12.3 Vertebral column

Shoulder girdle and arms

The clavicles (collar bones) and scapulae (shoulder blades) form the bones of the shoulder girdle. The humerus is the long bone of the upper arm and the radius and ulna are the long bones of the forearm. The bones of the hand consist of 5 metacarpals and 14 phalanges and the bones of the wrist consist of 8 carpals.

Pelvic girdle and legs

The pelvic girdle comprises two innominate bones each consisting of three individual bones fused together. The **ilium** is the upper part, the **pubis** is the anterior part and the **ischium** is the posterior part.

The leg consists of the femur which is the thigh bone, the largest and strongest bone in the body, the patella which is a small flat bone protecting the knee joint, and the tibia and fibula which are the bones of the lower leg beneath the knee.

The foot consists of 7 tarsals, 5 metatarsals and 14 phalanges.

The joints

Bones are rigid structures and any movement that takes place occurs at the joints. A joint is the point at which two or more bones meet. There are three main types of joint in the body and these are:

1. **Fibrous** – fixed or immovable joints, which have fibrous tissue between the bones.
2. **Cartilaginous** – slightly movable with cartilage between the ends of the bones.
3. **Synovial** – freely movable joints which have particular characteristics:

- The articulating surfaces of the bones are covered with hyaline cartilage.
- A fibrous capsule supported by ligaments surrounds the joint to provide protection whilst allowing freedom of movement.
- A synovial membrane lines the capsule of the joint.
- The capsule of the joint contains synovial fluid, which is a lubricant and provides nutrients for the living cells.

Synovial joints are classified depending on their range of movement and structure.

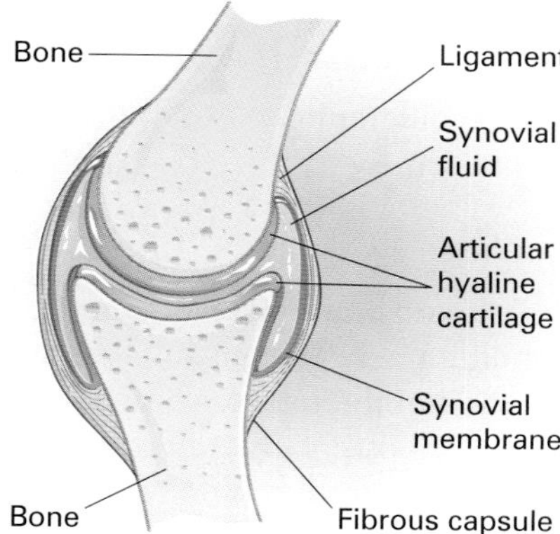

Figure 12.4 Synovial joint

Joint classification	Range of movement
Plane	Short gliding movements
Hinge	In one plane only, it will flex and extend
Ball and socket	The widest range of movement, flexion, extension, abduction, adduction, circumduction , rotation
Pivot	Rotation only
Condyloid	Movement in two planes, flexion and extension, abduction and adduction, limited circumduction
Saddle	Movement in two planes, flexion and extension, abduction and adduction and circumduction

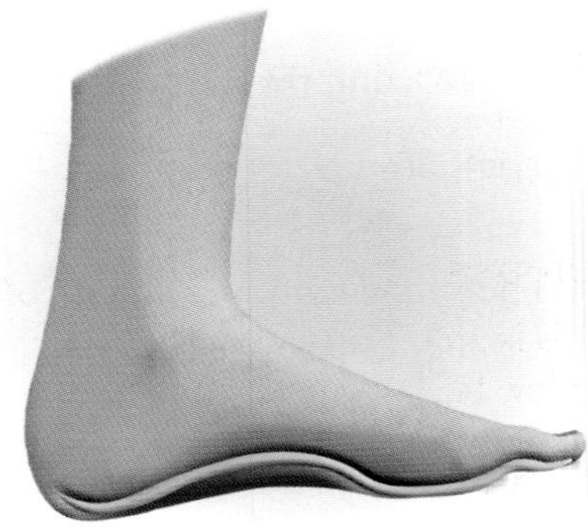

Figure 12.5 The spinal reflex

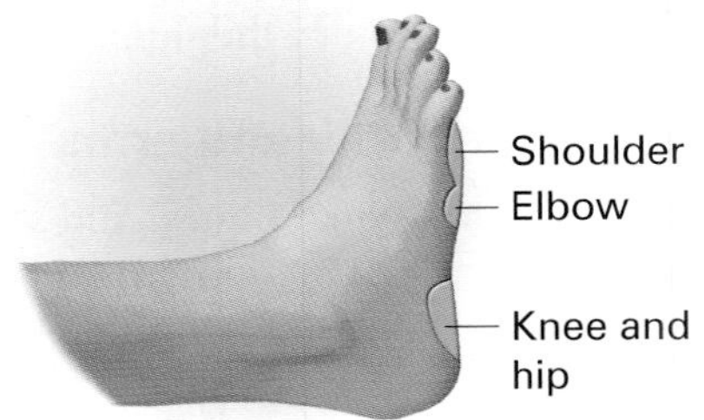

Figure 12.6 Foot map – reflex area for shoulder, elbow, knee and hip joints

Disorders of the skeletal system

Arthritis

This condition is characterised by inflammation, pain and sometimes stiffness in the joints, and it may also affect the muscles close to the affected area. The most common types of arthritis are rheumatoid arthritis, osteoarthritis and gouty arthritis.

- **Rheumatoid arthritis** is a common form of inflammatory arthritis with inflammation, swelling, pain and some loss of function in the joint. At its most extreme the joint may ossify and fuse together making it immovable.
- **Osteoarthritis** is a degenerative disease of the joint resulting from a combination of ageing, wear and tear and irritation of the joint.
- **Gouty arthritis** is caused by overproduction of uric acid (waste product produced during metabolism of nucleic acids) or an inability to excrete normal amounts from the system. This results in a build up of uric acid in the blood, which then reacts with sodium to form a salt called sodium urate, and these crystals then deposit in soft tissues which include the joints. This irritates the cartilage causing inflammation, pain and swelling. If left untreated, this results in the articulating bones of the joint fusing together and becoming immovable.

Bursitis

This is an acute chronic inflammation of a bursa (sac of synovial fluid around a joint) caused by trauma, acute chronic infection or rheumatoid arthritis. It results from prolonged excessive friction, and symptoms include, pain, swelling, tenderness and limited movement.

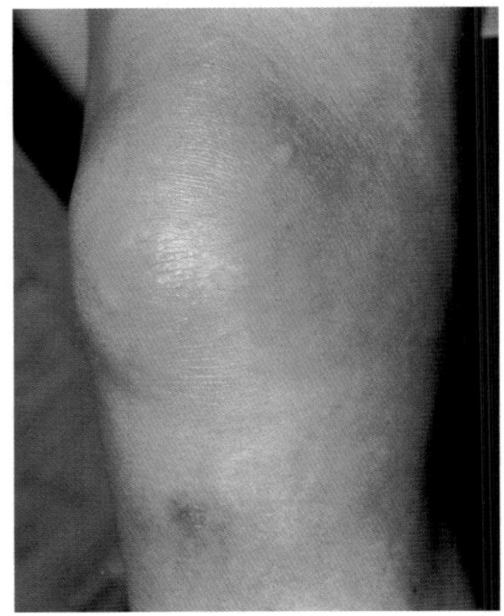

Bursitis

Curvatures of the spine

Due to different conditions the spine may become misshapen and the normal curves will become exaggerated as in the cases of scoliosis, kyphosis and lordosis.

Scoliosis

This is an abnormal lateral curvature of the spine usually in the thoracic region. This condition may be congenital or acquired from a persistent and severe sciatica. Paralysis of the muscles on one side of the body as a result of poliomyelitis may also cause scoliosis. This fault causes changes in the ligaments, bones and joints which may lead to further problems such as one leg longer than the other, uneven scapulae, pelvic tilt and one shoulder higher than the other.

Kyphosis

This causes the thoracic part of the spine to curve outwards resulting in a round shouldered or hunched back appearance. It can be caused by rickets, poor posture and in the elderly a degeneration of the intervertebral discs.

Lordosis

This is an inward curve of the spine in the lumbar region, commonly referred to as a hollow back. Causes may include, rickets, poor posture, a result of pregnancy or obesity.

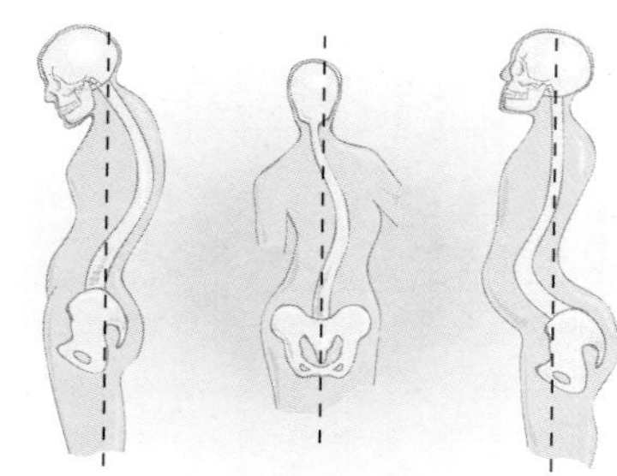

Figure 12.7 Kyphosis, scoliosis, lordosis

Herniated (slipped) disc

Intervertebral discs act as shock absorbers for the body and they are subject to wear and tear as a result of their exposure to extreme compressional force. If the disc becomes injured or weakened, the surrounding fibrocartilage may rupture and pressure may occur on the spinal nerves causing extreme pain.

Osteomalacia

In adults a deficiency in vitamin D causes the bones to give up large amounts of calcium and phosphorous. It affects the bones in the pelvis, legs and spine in particular. This condition is caused by a poor diet, devoid of milk, and little exposure to natural sunlight or repeated pregnancies that deplete the body of calcium.

Osteoporosis

This is an increased fragility of the bones which affects the middle-aged and elderly, leaving the sufferer susceptible to fractures. It is a common condition particularly among caucasian females and it affects the whole of the skeletal system, especially the spine, feet and legs. A decrease in bone mass causes the spine to collapse and curve, causing the thorax to drop and the ribs fall onto the pelvic rim. This then leads to gastrointestinal distension and an overall decrease in muscle tone.

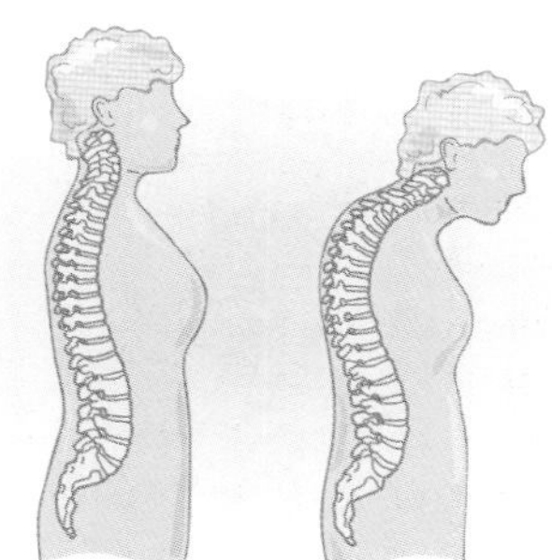

Figure 12.8 Osteoporosis of the spine

Rickets

This is a condition that affects mainly children and results from a deficiency of vitamin D. This prevents the body from transporting calcium and phosphorous from the digestive tract into the bloodstream for utilisation by the bones. The bones stay soft as the calcification process is interrupted and the weight of the body causes the bones in the leg to bow; malformation of the head, chest and pelvis may also occur.

PRACTICE IN CONTEXT

Memorise the names of the bones of the skeleton and practise working the reflexes for this system.

ASSESSMENT OF KNOWLEDGE

1. Give four functions of the skeletal system.
2. How many vertebrae are there in the spine?
3. Name five bone classifications.
4. How does the bone receive its blood supply?
5. What is the name given to the process by which bones are formed?
6. What is a joint?
7. Name the three main types of joint in the body.
8. Describe scoliosis.
9. Name three types of arthritis.
10. Which vitamin deficiency contributes to rickets?

13 The muscular system

Bones and joints form the framework of the body, but they require help to produce movement, which is an essential body function, and this is achieved by the contraction and relaxation of the muscles.

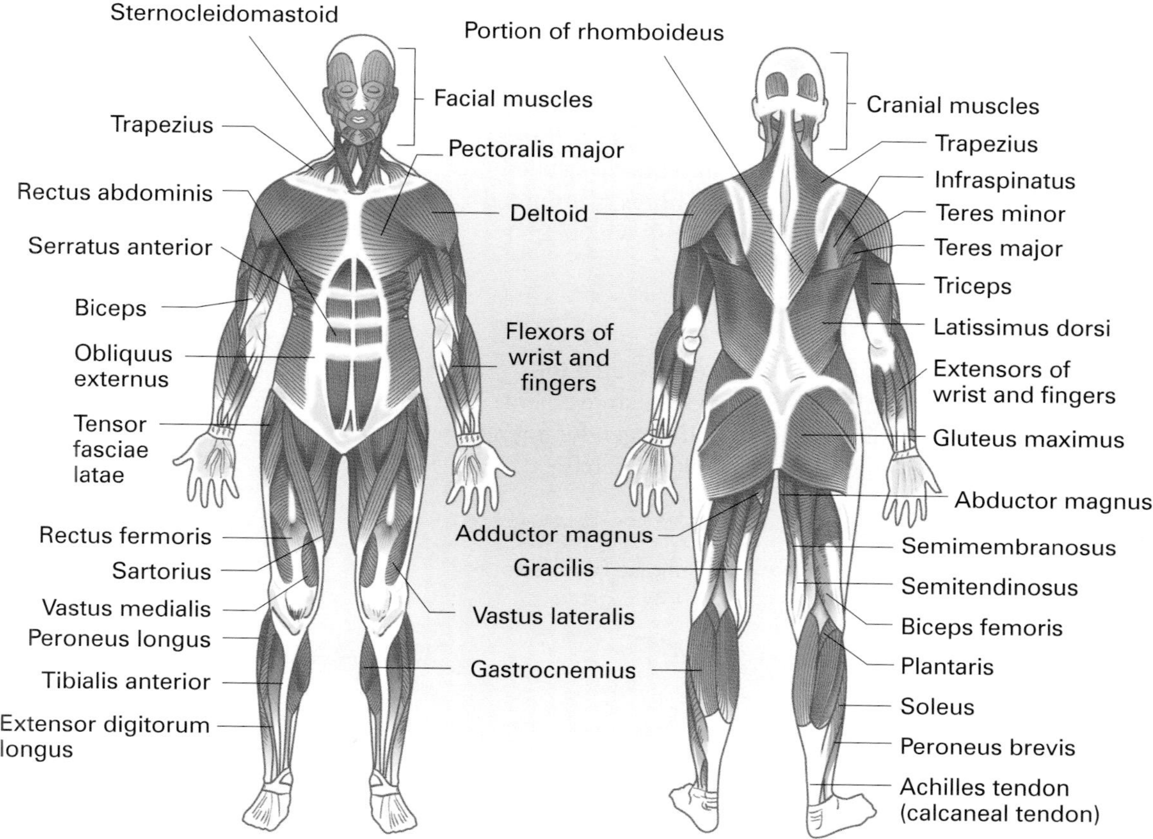

Figure 13.1 Muscles of the body – anterior view and posterior view

Muscle tissue is composed of highly specialised cells and makes up about 40% of the body's total weight. Its characteristics are important in maintaining homeostasis.

Characteristics of muscle tissue

- **Excitability** – the ability of muscle tissue to receive messages and respond to stimuli.
- **Contractability** – the ability to shorten and thicken (contract) in response to a stimulus.
- **Extensibility** – the ability of muscle tissue to stretch.
- **Elasticity** – the ability of the muscle to return to its original shape after contraction or extension.

There are three different kinds of muscle in the body:

1 **Skeletal** – voluntary, striated. These are attached to bones.

2 **Visceral** – involuntary, non-striated. These are smooth muscles located in the walls of hollow internal structures, for, eg the blood vessels, bladder and stomach.

3 **Cardiac** – involuntary, striated. These form the walls of the heart.

Skeletal muscle

Skeletal muscle is protected by **fascia**, a layer of connective tissue. Deep fascia holds muscles together, separating them into functioning groups, allowing free movement of the muscles and carrying nerves and blood vessels. The **epymisium** is an extension of deep fascia and covers the entire muscle.

This type of muscle tissue looks like a series of parallel fibre bundles, the smallest of which are called **actin** and **myosin filaments**. Made of protein, they are sometimes known as the contractile proteins. These filaments are gathered into bundles called **myofibrils**, which are gathered into further bundles called **muscle fibres** surrounded by **endomysium** and then gathered into further bundles called **fasiculi** which are surrounded by **perimysium**.

Structure of voluntary muscle

The skeletal muscles are well supplied with nerves and blood vessels essential for motion. They are stimulated by an impulse from a nerve cell to produce movement, and muscle action depends on blood supply providing nutrients and oxygen for energy and to remove the waste products in the muscle which are the result of exercise.

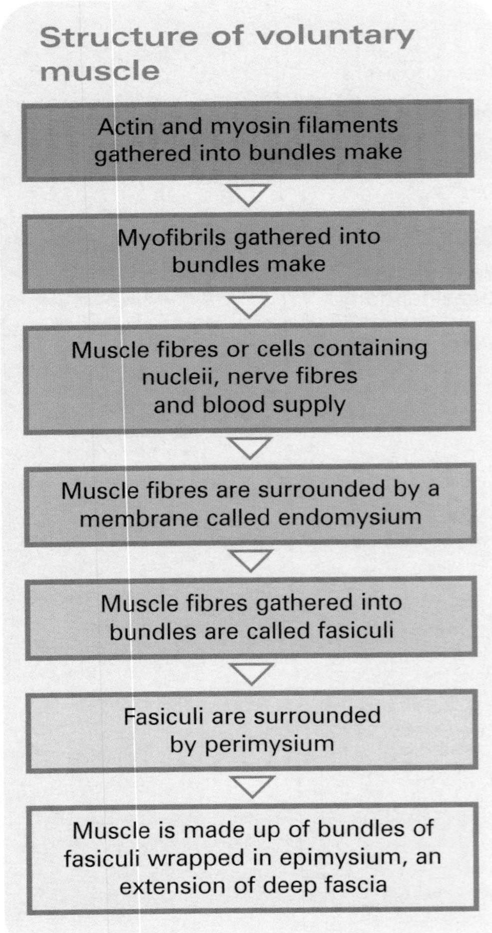

Structure of voluntary muscle
Actin and myosin filaments gathered into bundles make
Myofibrils gathered into bundles make
Muscle fibres or cells containing nucleii, nerve fibres and blood supply
Muscle fibres are surrounded by a membrane called endomysium
Muscle fibres gathered into bundles are called fasiculi
Fasiculi are surrounded by perimysium
Muscle is made up of bundles of fasiculi wrapped in epimysium, an extension of deep fascia

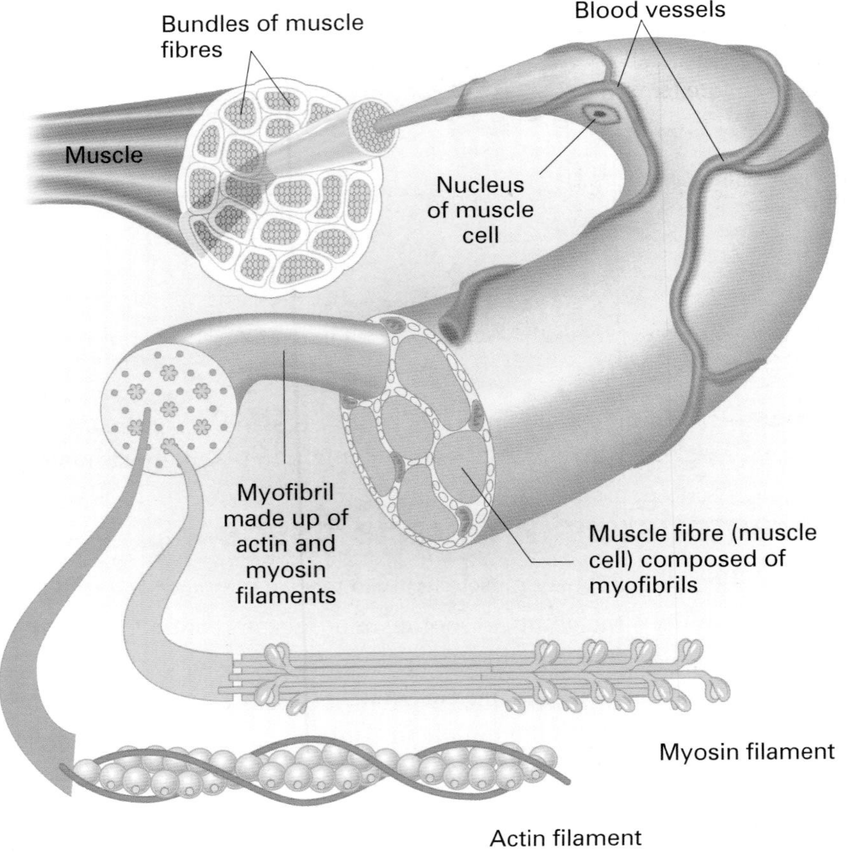

Figure 13.2 Structure of voluntary muscle

Muscle tone

This is when the muscle is in a state of partial contraction with some of the muscle fibres contracted and some relaxed. Partial contraction will tighten a muscle without actually moving it. Tone is essential in maintaining posture; if tone is lost this may cause physical problems.

Muscle fatigue

This occurs when skeletal muscle has been contracted for a long period of time. It becomes tired and weaker in response until it stops responding altogether, usually as a result of inadequate blood supply and lack of oxygen, together with a build up of lactic acid and carbon dioxide which accumulates in the muscle during exercise.

Visceral muscle

This muscle is smooth, non-striated and involuntary as its contraction is usually not under conscious control. The cells are spindle shaped with one central nucleus and are bound together in sheets by areolar connective tissue. It is not under the control of the will and is found in the walls of blood and lymph vessels, the stomach, the alimentary canal, the respiratory tract, the bladder and the uterus. These muscles do not become fatigued.

Cardiac muscle

This muscle is only found in the heart and is striated in appearance like skeletal muscle, with fibres that are short and thick, forming a dense mass. However, unlike skeletal, it is involuntary muscle tissue, not under the control of the will. The cardiac muscle cells have one nucleus and very little connective tissue. Cardiac muscle contracts rhythmically even without nervous stimulation and it does not tire easily, but could if the heartbeat was raised considerably for a long period of time without enough rest between contractions.

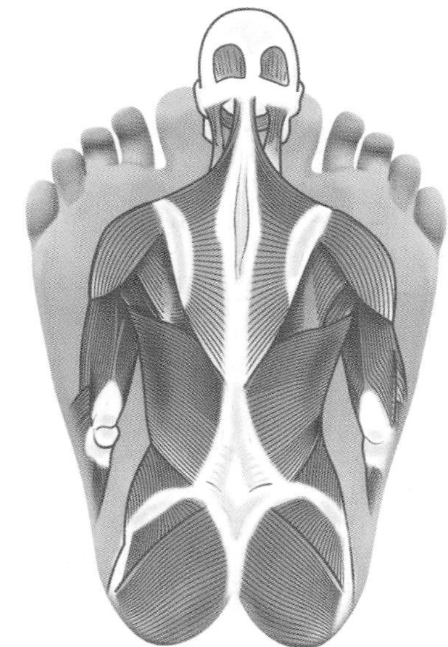

Figure 13.3 The muscles of the body will all be treated when you work each different reflex area during a reflexology treatment

Disorders of the muscular system

Fibrositis

This condition is an inflammation of fibrous tissue causing pain and stiffness, in particular the muscle covering. This may often follow an injury, repeated strain of a muscle or prolonged muscular tension.

Lumbago

Low backache caused by inflammation and pain in the muscles in the lumbar region of the spine may be a result of incorrect lifting or bending, slipped disc or strained muscle or ligament.

Muscular dystrophy

This is a muscle-destroying disease characterised by degeneration of muscle cells, which in turn results in atrophy of the muscle. The causes are genetic, faulty metabolism of potassium, protein deficiency or the inability of the body to utilise creatine.

Repetitive strain injury (RSI)

This is becoming increasingly more common, in particular among those people who use computer keyboards. It is the overuse or overstretching of muscles or ligaments which results in injury or damage to a particular muscle or group of muscles.

Sports injuries

Common areas affected are the ankle and knee joints, back and shoulder. Injury may be due to muscle fatigue, not warming up sufficiently, excessive stretching or overworking the muscles.

Tendonitis

Inflammation of a tendon often occurs after excessive overuse. Achilles tendonitis is common amongst sports men and women as a result of incorrect footwear or insufficient preparation when competing.

Tennis elbow

This is inflammation around the elbow joint caused by overworking the muscles through a particular sport or RSI.

PRACTICE IN CONTEXT

Memorise the names of the muscles of the body. Research the diseases which affect the muscular system and note the effects they will have on the body.

ASSESSMENT OF KNOWLEDGE

1. What is the main function of a muscle?
2. What is the name of the shoulder muscle?
3. What does the term excitability mean in relation to muscle tissue?
4. How many types of muscle are found in the body?
5. What is the difference between voluntary and involuntary muscle?
6. Where is cardiac muscle found?
7. What is fibrositis?
8. What are the causes of muscular dystrophy?
9. What advice would you give to a client suffering from lumbago?
10. What is a common condition amongst sportsmen, which affects the foot?

14 The cardiovascular system

The cardiovascular system consists of:

- The heart
- Blood
- Blood vessels.

The heart provides the power to pump the blood around the body through the blood vessels. The blood is the vehicle by which the circulatory system conveys oxygen, nutrients, hormones and other substances to the tissues, carbon dioxide to the lungs and other waste products to the kidneys.

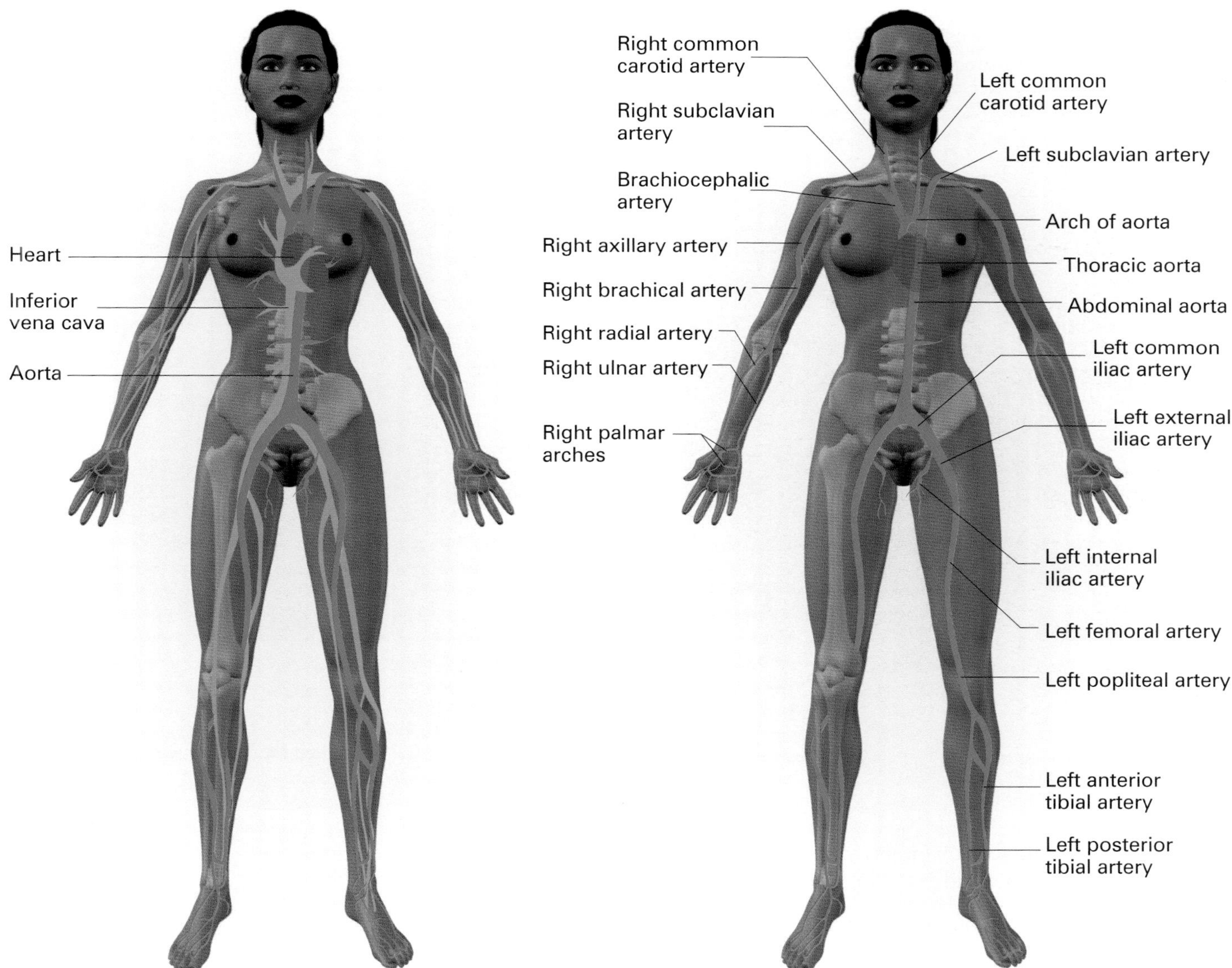

Figure 14.1 *The cardiovascular system*

The heart

The heart is the centre of the cardiovascular system. It is a large muscular organ and it beats over 100,000 times a day to pump the blood through the blood vessels. The blood vessels are a network of tubes that transport blood from the heart to the tissues and then back to the heart again.

The heart is located between the lungs in the thoracic cavity, with about two-thirds lying to the left of the body's midline. It is enclosed in a loose-fitting serous membrane called the **pericardial sac**.

The wall of the heart is divided into:

- The **epicardium**, or external layer, which is thin and transparent.
- The **myocardium**, or middle layer, composed of specialised cardiac muscle, which makes up the bulk of the heart and is responsible for the heart contraction.
- The **endocardium**, or inner layer, which lines the inside of the myocardium and covers the valves of the heart and tendons that hold them open. It is made up of a thin layer of endothelium, which lies over a thin layer of connective tissue.

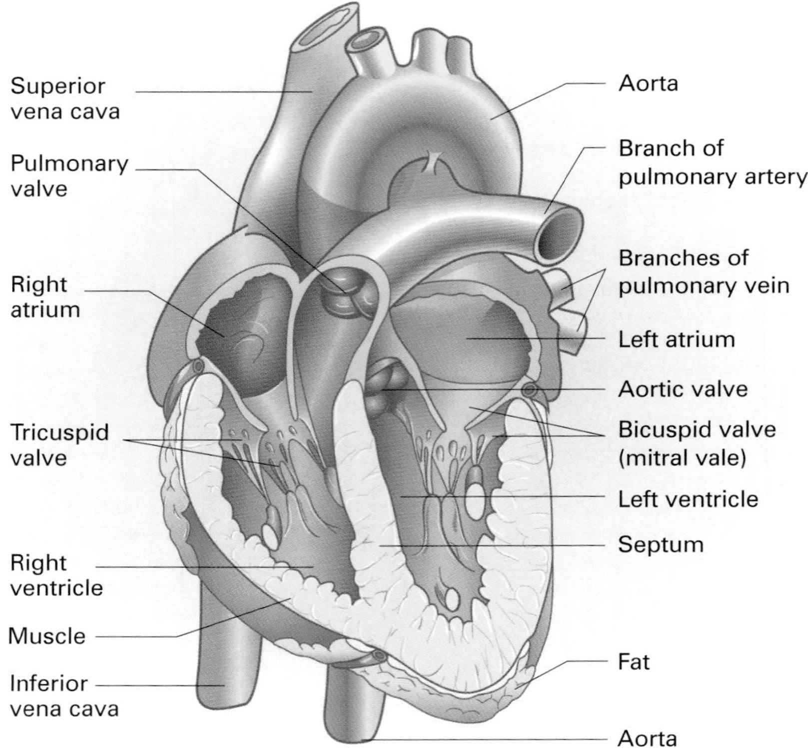

Figure 14.2 The heart

The heart is divided into four chambers, or cavities, and each chamber is a muscular bag with walls that contract and push the blood through:

- The two upper chambers are called **atria**.
- The two lower chambers are called **ventricles**.

Each atrium has an appendage called an **auricle** which increases its surface area.

The right and left sides of the heart are separated by the **septum**, a solid wall which prevents venous blood from the right side coming into contact with the arterial blood from the left side of the heart.

The passage of blood through the heart

Blood circulates from the heart through the organs and tissues, delivering nutrients and oxygen. The blood then returns to the heart in the veins, having had all the oxygen absorbed from it. The heart then pumps blood on its second circuit to the lungs to replace oxygen, returning with its oxygen supply renewed.

The heart receives blood via the right atrium from all parts of the body except the lungs, through three veins (see Figure 14.2):

1. The **superior vena cava**, which transports blood from parts of the body that are superior to the heart.
2. The **inferior vena cava**, which transports blood from parts of the body that are inferior to the heart.
3. The **coronary sinus**, which drains blood from most of the vessels which supply the walls of the heart.

The blood from the right atrium is delivered to the **right ventricle** through the **triscupid valve**.

Blood is then pumped into the **right** and **left pulmonary arteries** and transported to the lungs where it has its oxygen renewed and releases carbon dioxide.

It returns to the heart via four **pulmonary veins** which empty into the **left atrium** and then pass through to the **left ventricle**.

The blood is then pumped into the **ascending aorta** and then passed into the **coronary arteries, arch of the aorta, thoracic aorta and abdominal aorta**, which transports the blood to all parts of the body but the lungs.

Valves of the heart

The heart depends on a series of valves to function efficiently. They open and close automatically to receive and send out blood to and from the four chambers of the heart, ensuring the blood flow is in one direction only and preventing it from flowing backwards. These valves are:

- The **pulmonary** and **tricuspid** valves on the right hand side.
- The **aortic** and **mitral** valves on the left hand side.

The pulmonary semilunar valve lies where the pulmonary trunk leaves the right ventricle. It consists of three semilunar (half-moon-shaped) cusps.

The tricuspid valve is situated between the right atrium and the right ventricle and consists of three cusps or flaps.

The aortic semilunar valve lies at the opening between the left ventricle and the aorta. This is also made up of three semilunar cusps.

The mitral or bicuspid valve is situated between the left atrium and the left ventricle and it consists of two cusps or flaps.

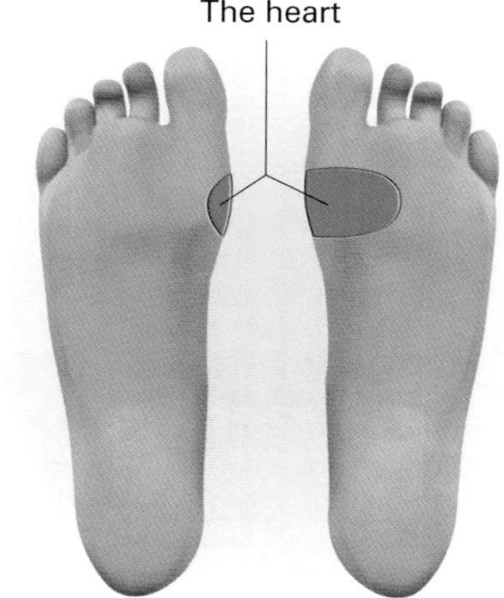

Figure 14.3 *Foot map – reflex area for heart on plantar surface of the foot*

Blood

Blood is a viscous fluid, which circulates through the heart and blood vessels and constitutes about 8% of the total body weight. It has a number of critical functions, as shown below:

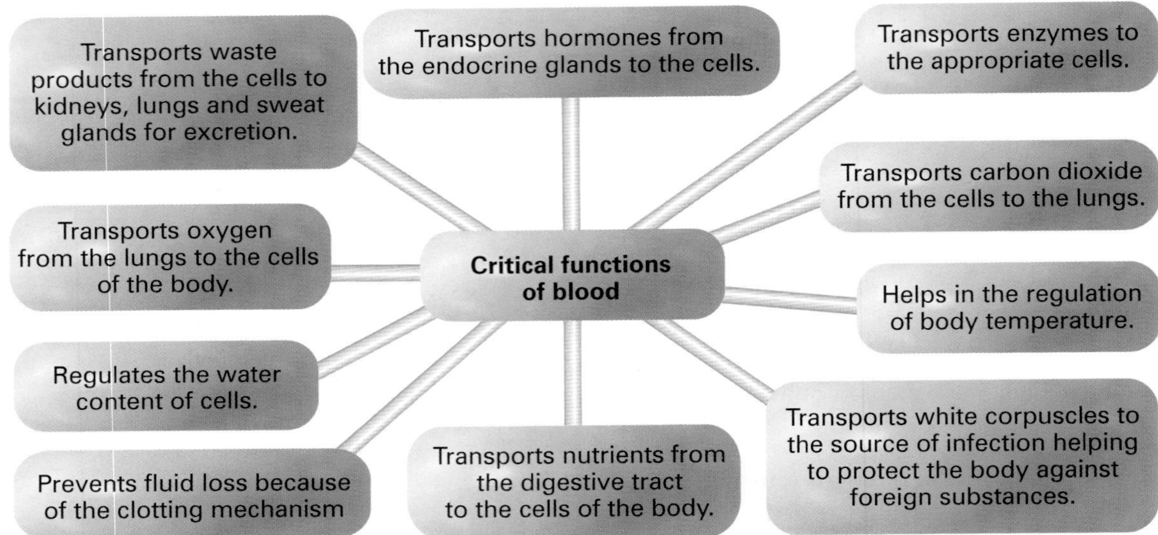

Figure 14.4 The blood is critical to the body in various ways

Constituents of blood

Blood consists of plasma and corpuscles. Plasma is the liquid portion and accounts for about 55% of the volume. It contains:

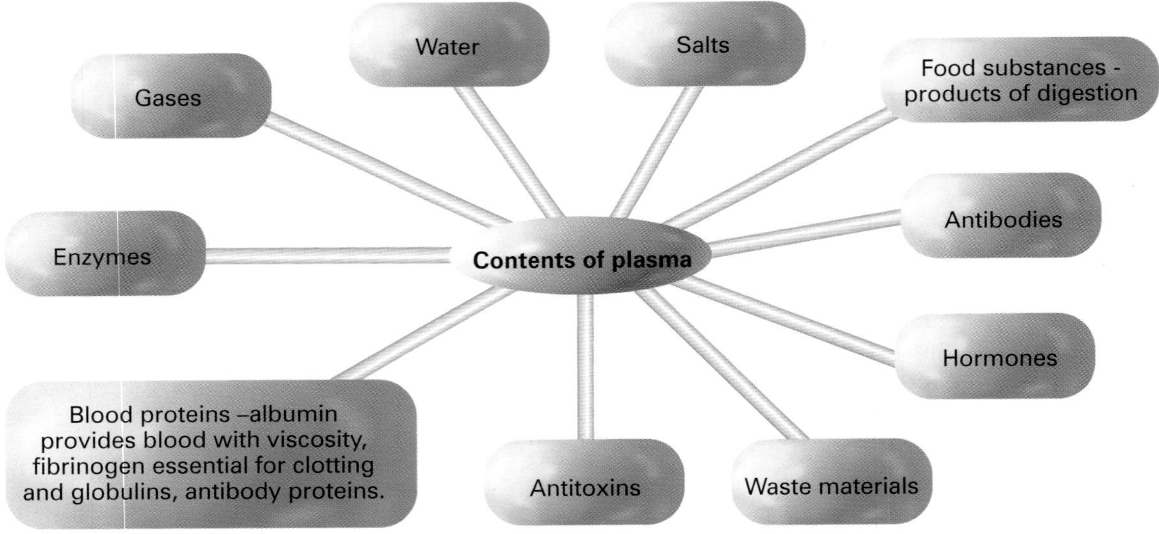

Figure 14.5 Contents of plasma

The corpuscles in the blood are **erythrocytes** (or red blood cells) which contain haemoglobin and transport oxygen around the body, **leucocytes** (or white blood cells) and **platelets**. The white blood cells are divided into two groups:

- Granular – developed from red bone marrow and called **neutrophils**, **eosinophils**, **basophils**.
- Agranular – developed from lymphoid and myeloid tissue and called **lymphocytes** and **monocytes**.

Neutrophils and monocytes	Basophils
These are phagocytic – they ingest bacteria and dead matter.	These are also involved in fighting irritants, releasing **histamine** to aid vasodilation and increase permeability of blood vessels, **heparin** a quick acting anticoagulant which helps to prevent clotting and **serotonin** which also aids vasodilation.
Eosinophils	**Lymphocytes**
These produce **antihistamine** which helps to fight an allergic reaction caused by an irritant.	These help to produce antibodies, which will deactivate antigens.

Blood vessels

These are the vessels along which the blood flows.

Arteries

These are thick walled blood vessels which convey blood from the heart to the capillaries. They help to maintain blood pressure. The thick elastic walls are important in that most of the force of each heartbeat is taken up in the elastic walls of the large arteries, and they continue pushing the blood forward in the pause between each heartbeat.

Arterioles

These are small arteries which convey blood to the capillaries.

Capillaries

These are microscopic blood vessels composed of a single layer of cells, which connect arterioles and venules. Their main function is to allow the passage of nutrients and waste products between the blood cells and the tissue cells.

In addition to the change of substances they have an important function in helping to regulate body temperature. The capillaries widen when the body heats up and this allows more blood to reach the surface of the skin where it is cooled.

Veins

These have much thinner walls than the arteries and they convey blood back to the heart from the capillaries. They contain valves to prevent back flow, allowing blood to move towards the heart.

The arteries and veins are similarly distributed throughout the body and those associated with a particular organ or tissue often run together.

Venules

These are found when groups of capillaries join together. They collect blood from the capillaries and drain it into veins.

Circulation of blood around the body

Arteries carry blood from the heart to all parts of the body. They branch out and become smaller arterioles, which in turn carry blood to the capillaries, the microscopic blood vessels in the tissues.

Interchange of tissue fluids (interstitial fluid) takes place. This is when oxygen and nutrients are received by the tissues and carbon dioxide and other waste products (the result of cell metabolism) are removed.

The capillaries then drain into venules which form veins to carry the deoxygenated blood back to the heart.

Blood pressure

Blood pressure is the force exerted by the blood on the walls of any blood vessels, in particular arteries. The factors which affect blood pressure are:

- The force of the heartbeat.
- The volume of blood in the cardiovascular system.
- The resistance to the flow of blood in the arteries.

A decrease in volume due to blood loss causes blood pressure to drop. An increase in blood volume, for example excessive salt intake leading to water retention, will cause blood pressure to increase. The blood pressure also varies depending on the activity of the body.

Measuring blood pressure

Blood pressure is measured using a **sphygmomanometer**. The two measurements are:

- **Systolic blood pressure** is the force exerted by the blood on the arterial walls during ventricular contraction. It is the highest pressure measured in the arteries.
- **Diastolic blood pressure** is the force exerted on the arterial walls during ventricular relaxation. It is the lowest blood pressure measured in the arteries.

The difference between the systolic and diastolic pressure is called pulse pressure.

What is normal blood pressure?

The average healthy adult male will have a blood pressure of 120 over 80. This would be a systolic pressure of 120 mm Hg (millimetres of mercury) and a diastolic pressure of 80 mm Hg. Strenuous exercise, stress, fear or excitement can all raise the systolic blood pressure, which is normally at its lowest when asleep. Blood pressure may become raised as a result of some illnesses, with increasing age, or when overweight and unfit.

Disorders of the cardiovascular system

Angina pectoris

This literally means chest pain and it occurs when circulation is reduced for some reason and insufficient oxygen is being carried in the blood to the muscles of the heart. This may occur when stressed or after eating a large meal and then taking strenuous exercise. It is a fairly common condition in men over 50 but it can start as young as 30; in women it usually starts after the menopause. It is a result of coronary artery disease when a narrowing of the arteries restricts the blood flow and there is an increased risk if the sufferer smokes, has high blood pressure, a family history of coronary artery disease or is obese. Other symptoms include a feeling of pressure in the chest, extreme anxiety, dizziness, sweating and difficulty in breathing.

Atherosclerosis

This is a condition also known as hardening of the arteries. It is caused by fatty substances such as cholesterol, cellular waste, calcium and fibrin (clotting material) being deposited in the walls of the arteries. This build up, called plaque, may partially or totally block the blood flow through the artery and this can cause a heart attack or stroke. It is a slow progressive disease which may progress rapidly in the third decade for some people or not until the fifties or sixties for others.

Deep vein thrombosis (DVT)

This is a blood clot within a deep vein, most commonly in the calf or thigh and it may partially or completely block the flow of blood in the vein. It occurs when the flow of blood is restricted in a vein and a clot forms. It can be caused by poor circulation because of other problems such as a recent heart attack or stroke, varicose veins, inactivity, or it may develop during a long haul flight.

The symptoms include tenderness in the area, a reddening of the skin, pain, swelling, fever, rapid heartbeat, joint pain and soreness.

DVT may also be caused by an injury to the vein following surgery, during pregnancy, or as a result of severe infection, liver disease and some cancers.

Hypertension

This is a condition where the blood pressure is consistently higher than normal, even when relaxing. It puts extra strain on the heart and the circulatory system and increases the risk of coronary artery disease, heart attack, stroke and kidney disease. It can be a natural consequence of getting older and there is some evidence that this is genetically linked.

As the arteries harden and become narrower as a result of age or a diet high in fat, the circulation is restricted and this puts added pressure on the heart as it works harder to keep the blood flowing. There are a number of factors which contribute to this condition; these are lack of exercise, smoking, obesity, stress and excessive alcohol consumption.

There can be specific causes which can occur any time; these include kidney problems, complications during pregnancy, certain hormone imbalances, some heart conditions and side-effects of drugs such as steroids. Symptoms of severe hypertension are breathlessness, headaches and dizziness.

When suffering from hypertension it is advisable to adopt a healthy lifestyle: give up smoking, lose weight if necessary, increase exercise, follow a healthy diet, cut down on fatty foods, learn to relax and avoid stressors. Reflexology, yoga, tai chi or other complementary therapies may also help to produce a sense of well-being, thus reducing stress which exacerbates high blood pressure.

Hypotension

This is a condition in which the arterial blood pressure is abnormally low. It may occur after excessive fluid loss or blood loss. Other causes include pulmonary embolism (an obstruction of the pulmonary artery or one of its branches), severe infection, allergic reactions, Addison's disease and drugs. Some people suffer temporary hypotension when they faint.

Stroke

This is damage to part of the brain caused by a reduced blood supply as a result of blockage in a blood vessel or a blood vessel rupturing. Those most at risk from a stroke are those who suffer with high blood pressure, heart disease, diabetes, smoke, drink excessive amounts of alcohol or are obese. The results of a stroke can vary depending on which part of the brain was affected, paralysis and loss of sensation may occur in varying degrees.

PRACTICE IN CONTEXT

Research the effects of age on the cardiovascular system and practise working the reflex points of this system.

ASSESSMENT OF KNOWLEDGE

1. What does the cardiovascular system consist of?
2. Where is the heart located?
3. What are the two lower chambers of the heart called?
4. Where does the blood transport waste products to and why?
5. How does the blood contribute to protecting the body?
6. How is fluid loss prevented?
7. Give two differences between arteries and veins.
8. What is the blood pressure of an average healthy adult?
9. What are the classic symptoms of deep vein thrombosis?
10. What are the factors that contribute to hypertension?

15 The lymphatic system

This is a subsidiary circulatory system which is composed of lymph, lymph vessels, nodes and ducts as well as highly specialised lymphoid organs and tissues, including the thymus, spleen and tonsils. Lymph vessels are found in all parts of the body except the central nervous system, bone, cartilage and teeth.

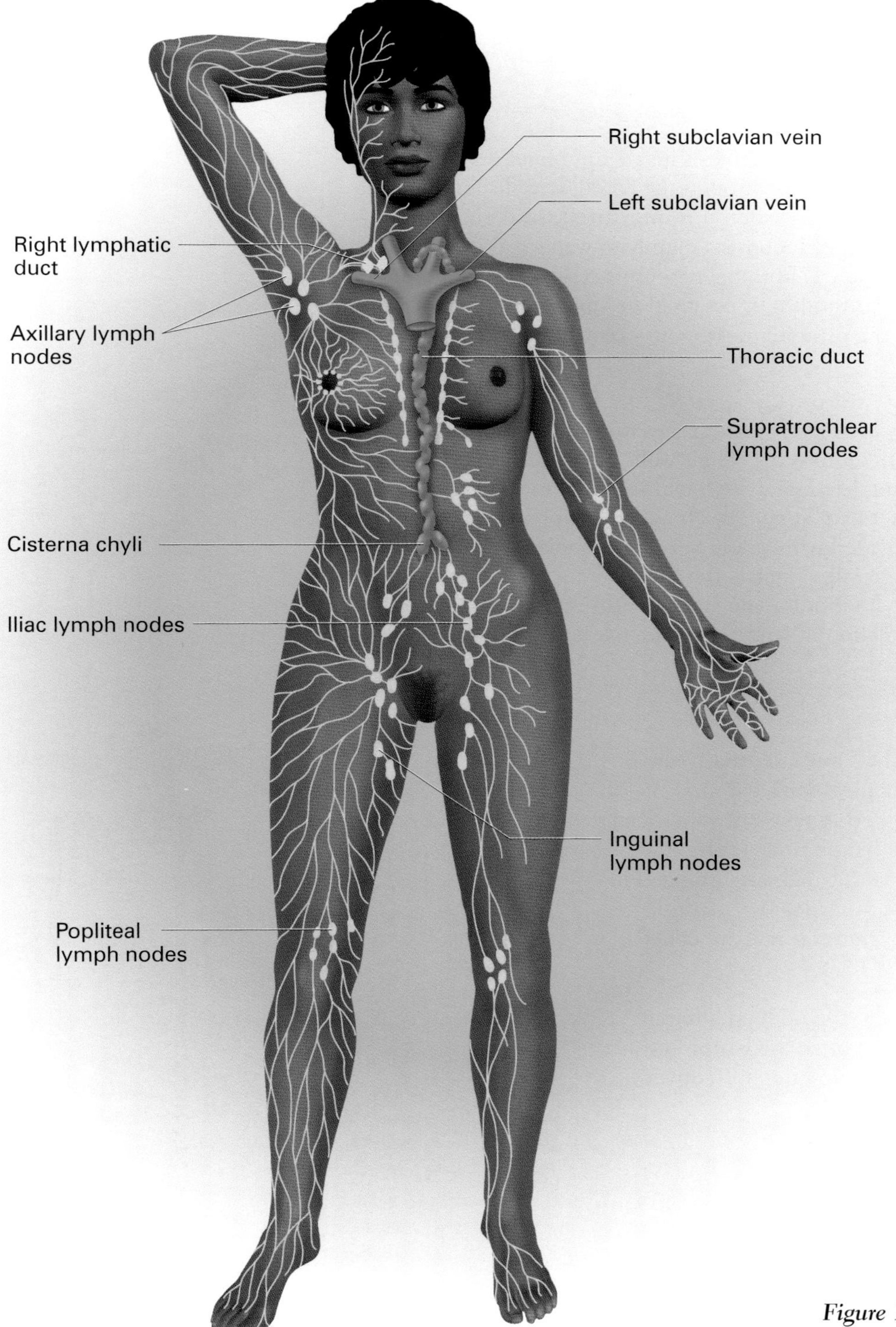

Figure 15.1 *The lymphatic system*

Functions of the lymphatic system

The lymphatic system conveys excess fluid, foreign particles and other materials from the body's tissues and cells. It also transports fats from the digestive tract to the blood. Lymphocytes are produced which deal with waste products and toxins that build up in the tissues. The development of antibodies occurs in the lymphatic system and this helps to protect the body against disease and provide immunity against further attack. Antibodies are proteins produced by the body to protect it against invasion by antigens, which may prove dangerous or irritating. The primary functions of the lymphatic system therefore are to protect the body from disease, clean it of waste and toxins and maintain fluid balance.

Lymph

Blood itself does not flow into the tissues but remains inside the blood vessels. Certain parts of the blood however permeate through the capillary walls and into the tissue spaces, this is called interstitial fluid. When this **interstitial fluid** enters the lymphatic vessels it is then called lymph. It consists mainly of water and important substances found in blood plasma such as fibrinogen, a protein which, when converted to fibrin by the action of thrombin, is essential in blood clotting and serum albumin, which helps to regulate the osmotic pressure of plasma.

Lymph vessels

There are lymph capillaries into which tissue fluid passes from the tissue spaces running alongside the body's arteries and veins. Their walls are thin and permeable, allowing larger molecules including bacteria, which cannot enter the blood capillaries, to be carried away. There are larger vessels called lymphatics, which are the size of small veins and are provided with valves to prevent backflow. The larger vessels eventually converge into two large ducts – the thoracic duct and the right lymphatic duct, which drain into the innominate veins, returning the lymph into the blood. So there is a constant circulation of lymph into the tissues via the capillaries and back again into the bloodstream.

Lymph nodes

These are situated around the body. They are usually small groups of oval or bean shaped structures found around major arteries and these groups are arranged in two sets; superficial and deep. The outer region of the lymph node (cortex) contains densely packed lymphocytes, which are arranged in masses called lymph nodules. The inner region (medulla) contains lymphocytes arranged in strands, these are called medullary cords.

The lymphatic vessels carry lymph to the node in afferent (convey towards a centre) vessels and once the lymph has been filtered it is taken from the node in efferent (convey away from a centre) vessels.

Lymph ducts

From the lymph nodes the lymphatic vessels combine to form lymph trunks and they empty into the two main ducts:

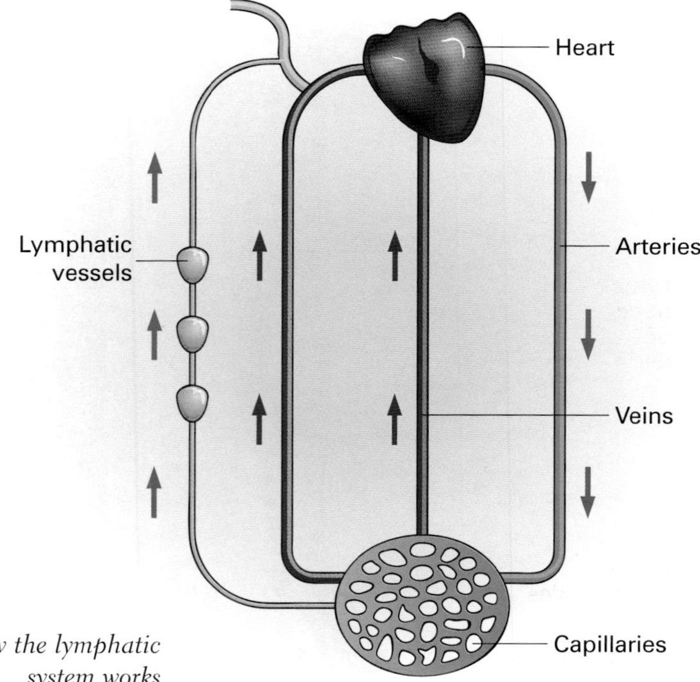

Figure 15.2 How the lymphatic system works

- The **thoracic duct** – the main collecting duct of the lymphatic system beginning as a dilation called the cisterna chylli and receiving lymph from the left side of the head, neck, chest, the left upper extremity and the entire body below the ribs.
- The **right lymphatic duct** – receives lymph from the right side of the head and neck, the thorax and the right arm.

From these two ducts the lymph returns to the blood circulation via the subclavian veins and the cycle repeats itself continuously.

Lymph organs

The lymph organs are the:

- Tonsils
- Thymus gland
- Spleen

The tonsils

These are part of a ring of lymphoid tissue, which encircles the entrance to the food and air passages in the throat. They play a part in the body's defence against disease, reacting to ingested material that poses a threat to health. This immunity is provided by the lymphocytes that are processed in the tonsils and the production of antibodies in the tonsils, which deal with local infection. Infected tonsils are enlarged and inflamed with spots of pus exuding from the surface.

The adenoid is situated at the back of the nose and any infection breathed in is filtered and destroyed. Adenoids are present at birth but usually disappear by puberty.

Thymus gland

This is a mass of lymphatic tissue situated in the upper thoracic cavity. Its function is to produce antibodies to destroy foreign particles. It is large in children and by puberty it reaches maximum size, becoming involuted and most of it being replaced by fat and connective tissue.

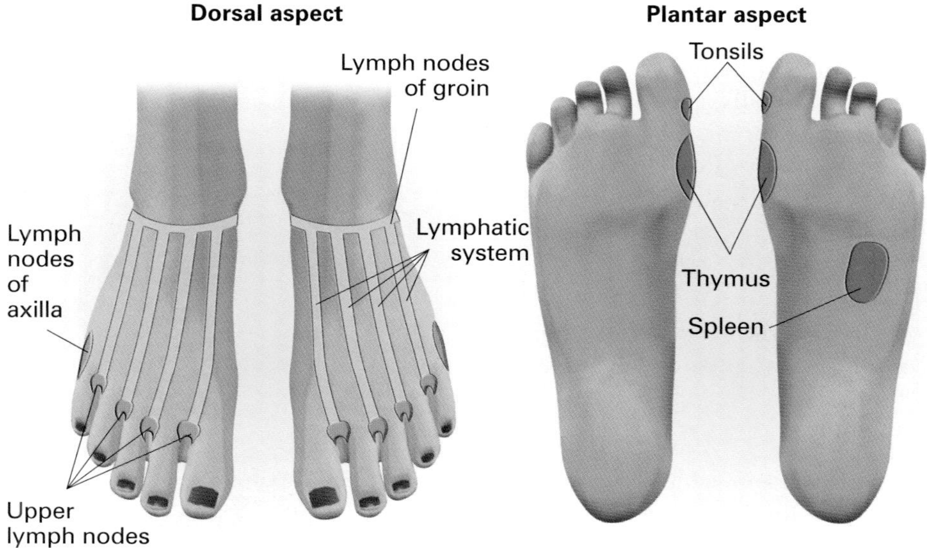

Figure 15.3 Foot map – lymphatic system

Spleen

This is the largest mass of lymphatic tissue in the body and is situated between the fundus of the stomach and diaphragm. It is one of the main filters of blood, removing worn out red blood cells and abnormal cells, with white cells and platelets filtered selectively. It makes antibodies, which immobilise foreign particles, stores blood and releases it into the circulatory system in times of need, for example when there is a heavy blood loss during haemorrhage.

Immunity

Immunity is a specific resistance to disease and it requires the production by the body of a specific antibody to destroy a specific antigen.

Definition of terms

- **Immunity** is when the body is resistant to injury, particularly by poison, foreign bodies and parasites due to the presence of antibodies.
- An **antigen** is a chemical substance which when introduced into the body causes the production of specific antibodies to neutralise the effects.
- An **antibody** is a protein the body produces in response to the exposure to a specific antigen in the body.

Disorders of the lymphatic system

The normal antigen–antibody response which provides immunity sometimes goes wrong. This leads to three problems:

- Allergy
- Autoimmunity
- Tissue rejection

Allergy

Allergic reaction to a substance can occur at any time, even when the body has been exposed to it for some time. The antigens which cause an allergic reaction are called allergens. Some common causes of allergic reaction are milk, eggs, strawberries, nuts, penicillin, cosmetics, plants or even house dust. Immediate reactions may be localised: reddening of the skin, oedema, watery eyes, runny nose, bronchial asthma, dermatitis or hives. The most severe reaction is anaphylactic shock, which may produce life-threatening effects such as asphyxia.

Autoimmune disease

Occasionally the immune response of the body breaks down and an abnormal immune response occurs against the body's own tissues which are seen as foreign. Autoimmune diseases include rheumatoid arthritis, lupus, rheumatic fever, glomerulonephritis, pernicious anaemia and multiple sclerosis.

Acquired **I**mmune **D**eficiency **S**yndrome (AIDS) is a disease which lowers the body's immune system. Those suffering from this disease are then susceptible to many different illnesses. These may include a general malaise, fever, cough, sore throat, shortness of breath, muscular aches, weight loss, skin cancer and pneumonia.

Lymphatic disease

Some common illnesses and diseases such as cancer, heart, digestive and kidney diseases are directly affected by the proper health and functioning of the lymphatic system. When this system malfunctions a significant number of diseases and related conditions may occur.

Oedema

This is an excessive build up of fluid in the tissues. It may be caused by an excessive amount of lymph being formed and an increase in the permeability of the capillary walls, a blockage in the system between the lymph capillaries and the subclavian veins, or an increase in blood pressure, when interstitial fluid is formed faster than it passes into the lymphatics. It may be localised in the area of an injury or it may be general as a result of heart or kidney conditions. Subcutaneous oedema commonly occurs in the legs and ankles due to the influence of gravity, and in women it may occur before menstruation.

Tissue rejection

After transplant the body recognises the new tissues as foreign and produces antibodies against them. This is often treated with immunosuppressive drugs.

PRACTICE IN CONTEXT

Discuss with your tutor and colleagues the different ways in which the immune system can be weakened and what steps you can take to prevent this occurring. Practise working the reflex points of the lymphatic system.

ASSESSMENT OF KNOWLEDGE

1. What is the main function of lymphocytes?
2. What is the name of the lymph nodes in the groin?
3. What are antigens?
4. What does interstitial fluid consist of?
5. What are the names of the two large ducts which drain lymph into the innominate veins?
6. Which lymph organ stores blood?
7. What is an antibody?
8. What is anaphylactic shock?
9. What is oedema?
10. Give two examples of autoimmune disease.

16 The respiratory system

What is the respiratory system?

Respiration is the process by which oxygen is taken into the body and used for the oxidation of food materials; this liberates the energy necessary to support life, and carbon dioxide and water are released as waste. The respiratory system comprises organs that exchange the gases oxygen and carbon dioxide between the blood and the atmosphere. Oxygen is essential for cells to survive and it is brought into the body every time we inhale, and carbon dioxide is released when we exhale; this process is called respiration. The cardiovascular system and the respiratory system together are responsible for supplying oxygen to the tissues and eliminating carbon dioxide.

Definition of terms

External respiration

The physical means by which the oxygen is obtained and the carbon dioxide is removed from the body.

Internal respiration

A chain of chemical processes which takes place in every living cell. Oxygen is released to the tissues and carbon dioxide is absorbed by the blood ready for removal.

The respiratory system consists of the following:

- The nose
- Pharynx
- Larynx
- Trachea
- Lungs
- Bronchi
- Bronchioles
- Intercostal muscles
- Diaphragm

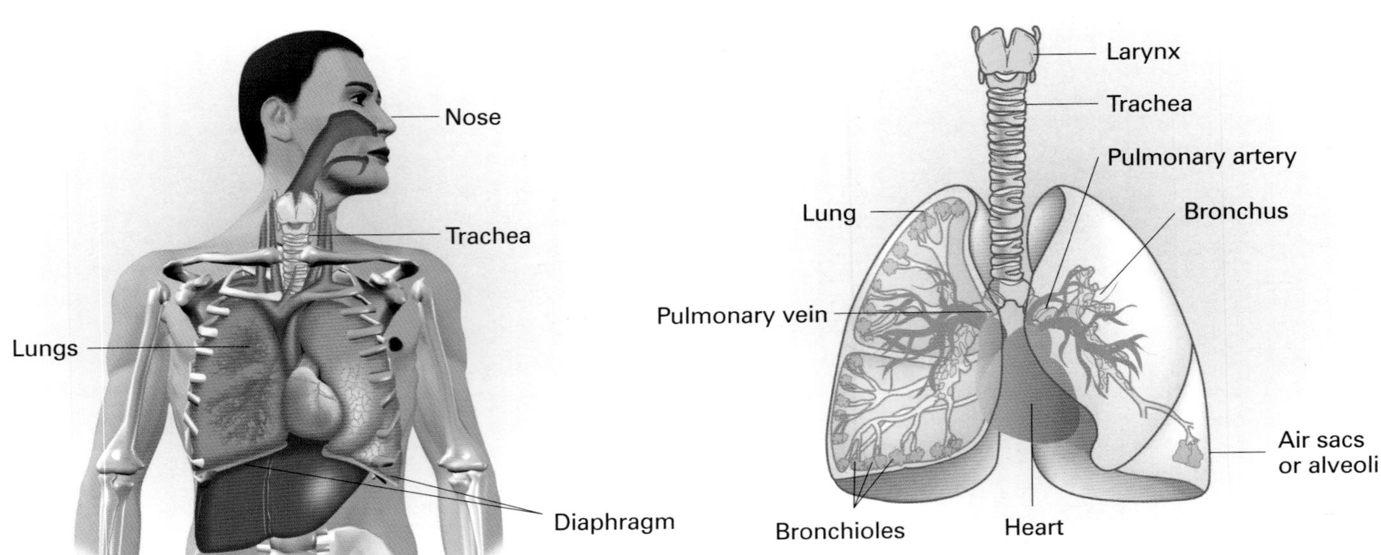

Figure 16.1 The respiratory system

The nose

The nose is the natural pathway for air entering the body and it also acts as protection against irritants such as dust, which the nose will expel by sneezing so that foreign bodies do not enter the lungs.

The nostrils are lined with coarse hairs, which protect the entrance to the nose. Air entering the nose is warmed to body temperature and moistened by contact with the mucous membrane and then filtered by the tiny hairs or cilia and the mucous from the mucous membrane. The cilia then moves the mucous gradually into the pharynx where it is swallowed. In the upper part of the nasal cavities the olfactory nerve endings detect smells in the air.

Pharynx and larynx

The throat is the area which leads into the respiratory and digestive tracts from the oral and nasal cavities to the oesophagus and trachea. It is made up of the pharynx which, together with the trachea, nose and mouth, form the **upper respiratory tract**. The pharynx (throat) and larynx (voice box) have two main functions:

1. To channel food and liquid into the digestive tract.
2. To transport air into the lungs.

The pharynx is made up of:

- The **nasopharynx** which lies above the soft palate and forms the back of the nose.
- The **oropharynx** at the back of the mouth is part of the airway between the mouth and the lungs.
- The **laryngopharynx** is the lowest part of the pharynx and is involved entirely with swallowing.

The movements of the pharynx are carefully co-ordinated to ensure that respiratory gases end up in the lungs and food ends up in the oesophagus.

The larynx is situated between the pharynx and the trachea and it is the body's voice box, containing the vocal cords which vibrate to produce speech.

The function of the larynx in respiration is its secondary function. The opening from the pharynx into the larynx is called the glottis and is closed by the epiglottis. When we breathe in or out the epiglottis opens to allow air into the lungs.

Trachea

The trachea or windpipe, as it is more commonly known, is a tubular passageway for air approximately 12 cm in length and 2.5 cm in diameter. It extends from the larynx to the right and left bronchi. The wall of the trachea is made up of smooth muscle and elastic connective tissue with hoops of cartilage that hold open the elastic tissue. It is lined with mucous membrane and cilia, which waft invading germs and foreign particles back up into the throat to be swallowed.

Lungs

The two lungs fill most of the thorax and each one is divided into lobes containing a dense network of tubes. The right lung is larger and is divided into three lobes. The left lung is slightly smaller, as the heart takes up more room on the left side of the thorax, and it is divided into two lobes. The largest of the tubes in the lungs are the bronchi and the smallest are the bronchioles, which terminate in air sacs called alveoli where the exchange of oxygen and carbon dioxide takes place. The second system of tubes is formed by the pulmonary arteries, which enter the lungs alongside the right and left bronchi. These tubes branch into smaller blood vessels running alongside the bronchioles and at the alveoli they form small capillaries.

The pleural membrane encloses and protects each lung and they are held open by the surface tension created by the fluid produced by the pleural membrane.

Bronchi and bronchioles

Where the trachea terminates in the chest it divides into the right bronchus which enters the right lung and the left bronchus which enters the left lung. Inside the lungs the bronchi further divide into secondary and tertiary (third) bronchi which become smaller tubes called bronchioles. These bronchioles terminate in air sacs called alveoli.

Intercostal muscles

The internal and external intercostal muscles are situated between the ribs. When the external muscles are contracted they move the ribcage upwards, helping to increase lung volume during inspiration (breathing in). When the internal muscles are contracted they force air out of the lungs during expiration (breathing out).

Diaphragm

This is a sheet of muscle which forms the floor of the thoracic cavity. When it contracts it flattens, increasing the vertical space in the thoracic cavity, allowing the lungs to expand and fill with air during inspiration. When this muscle is relaxed it increases in size becoming dome shaped. This reduces the space in the thoracic cavity and this helps to squeeze air out of the lungs during expiration.

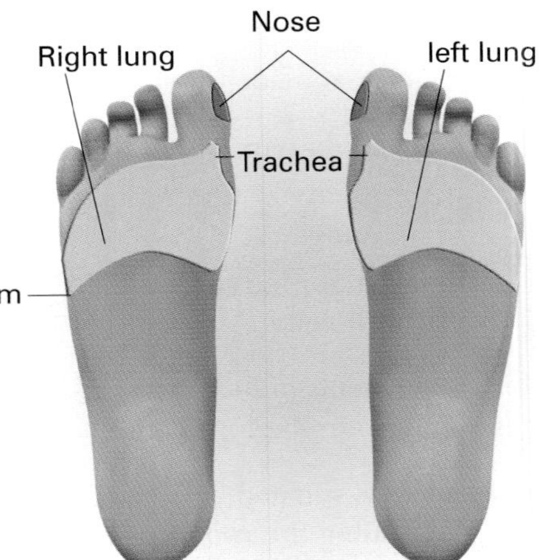

Figure 16.2 Foot map – reflex areas of respiratory system

Breathing

We breathe on average twelve times per minute. This rate will increase considerably during physical exercise up to eighty times per minute. In a 24-hour period we breathe in and breathe out more than 8000 litres of air. Oxygen in the air we breathe is carried to the body's tissues to produce the energy required for life via the lungs, the heart and the blood vessels. Oxygen enters through the mouth, nose and trachea into the lungs where it travels to the alveoli, via the bronchioles, and the exchange of oxygen and carbon dioxide takes place. Oxygen is taken up by the haemoglobin in the blood and the red blood cells discharge carbon dioxide back into the lungs to be exhaled.

Disorders of the respiratory system

Allergic rhinitis

This is an inflammation of the nasal passages resulting in a runny, itchy and inflamed nose. Caused by an allergy, the most common being hay fever, it is prevalent in families with eczema and asthma as there is probably an inherited factor that affects the way the immune system reacts to allergens.

Asthma

This condition affects the lungs and causes the walls of the bronchioles to swell and produce mucous resulting in wheezing and difficulty with breathing. The bands of muscle around the outside of the bronchioles tighten, further blocking the flow of air. The cause is often an allergic reaction to pollens, house dust, animal hair, fur or feathers, tobacco smoke, pollutants, a change in the weather and respiratory infections.

Emphysema

This condition occurs when the alveolar walls lose their elasticity and remain filled with air during expiration. Damage occurs, which then reduces the surface area for normal exchange of oxygen and carbon dioxide. In severe cases there is extreme breathlessness and in most cases it is caused by long-term irritation.

Lung cancer

This is a common form of malignancy usually developing in the main bronchus; as the tumour grows it may erode a blood vessel. A major cause is long-term exposure to an irritant such as inhaled smoke.

Pulmonary embolism

This is a condition where a blood clot causes a blockage in the lungs and restricts blood flow, which prevents adequate amounts of oxygen being absorbed into the lungs. Symptoms may be shortness of breath, a cough which may bring up blood, chest pain when breathing, elevated heart rate and sweating.

PRACTICE IN CONTEXT

Practise working the reflex points of the respiratory system. Choose one disorder of the respiratory system and discuss with your tutor and colleagues the main reflex points to be worked during a reflexology treatment.

ASSESSMENT OF KNOWLEDGE

1. Why does the body need oxygen?
2. What is respiration?
3. Where is the trachea situated?
4. How many lobes does the right lung have?
5. What are the tiny air sacs in the lungs called?
6. What is the function of the pleural membrane?
7. What is the function of the intercostal muscle?
8. What is the main cause of asthma?
9. What is allergic rhinitis?
10. What effect does emphysema have on the lungs?

17 The skin

What is the skin?

The skin is the largest organ of the body. It provides a protective outer covering to the underlying structures and prevents the invasion of bacteria.

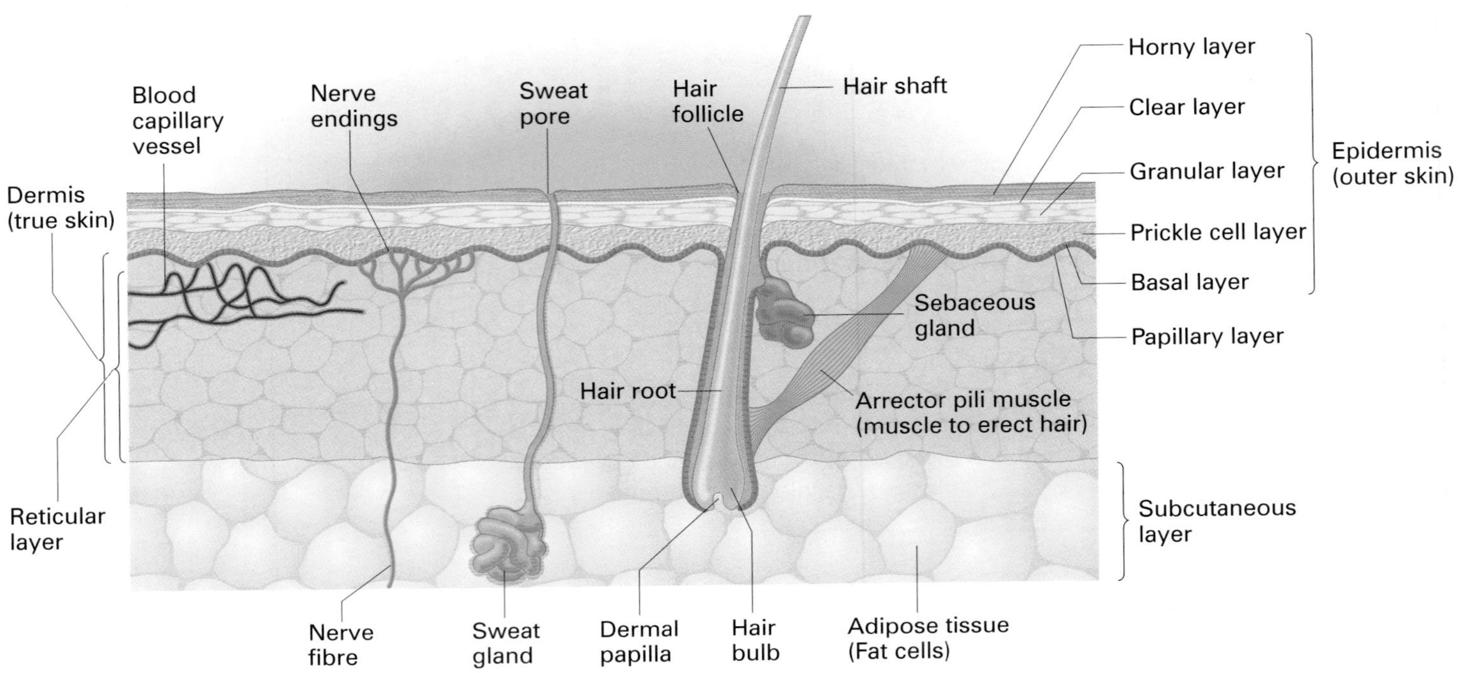

Figure 17.1 The skin

The skin has three main layers:

1 The **epidermis**, the surface of the skin, thinnest on the eyelids and thickest on the soles of the feet and palms of the hands. It is extremely sensitive to touch.

2 The **dermis**, which supports the epidermis and provides contour and elasticity, is composed of dense connective tissue.

3 The **hypodermis**, or subcutaneous layer, is made up of adipose tissue containing fat cells, muscles and veins.

The epidermis

The layers of the epidermis are:

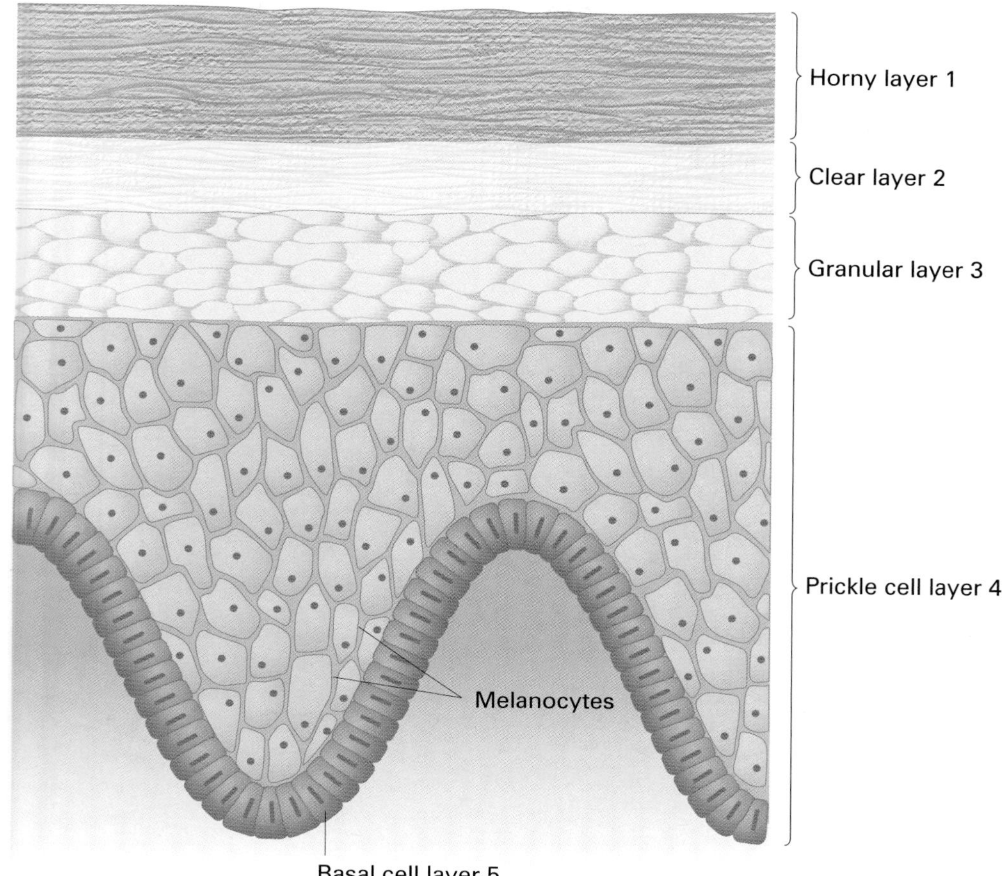

Figure 17.2 The layers of the epidermis

Note: Cell renewal is the change of living cells containing a nucleus (the vital body in a cell, essential for its growth and reproduction) into dead, horny flat cells with no nucleus which are constantly shed from the surface of the skin.

Stratum germinativum – basal layer

This is the deepest layer of the epidermis and it receives nutrient fluid from the blood vessels of the dermis. It is in this layer that the development of new cells (mitosis) occurs.

Melanin forming cells called **melanocytes** are formed in this layer. Melanin is the skin's natural protection against the harmful effects of ultraviolet light and is responsible for the change in skin colour when exposed to the sun.

Stratum spinosum – prickle cell layer

Towards the upper part of this layer, chemical changes take place and the keratinisation process has begun. Keratinisation is the change of living cells containing a nucleus into layers of flat cells composed of the hard durable protein keratin.

Stratum granulosum – granular layer

The cells of this layer become flattened and the nucleus begins to disintegrate, there is a loss of fluids which contributes to the transformation of cells into keratin, a tough fibrous protein.

Stratum lucidum – transparent layer

This is made up of small, tightly packed transparent cells with no nucleus. This layer is thought to be the barrier zone controlling the transmission of water through the skin. It is more evident in the thickest areas of the skin, the soles of the feet and the palms of the hands.

Stratum corneum – horny layer

This consists of several layers of skin that are very tough and with no nucleus. The superficial layers are constantly being shed and the cells beneath contain an epidermal fatty substance resembling beeswax which keeps them waterproof and helps prevent the skin from cracking and becoming open to bacterial infection.

The dermis

This is the chief supportive section of the visible surface skin, or epidermis. It is composed of dense connective tissue which is tough, highly elastic and flexible and creates the strength, contour, elasticity and smoothness of the skin.

The tissue is highly sensitive and fibrous and comprises:

- Collagen – a protein that is the main constituent of connective tissue.
- Elastin – a protein that is a constituent of connective tissue.
- Fibroblast cells that form collagen and elastin fibres and the ground substance of loose connective tissue.
- Blood and lymph vessels to transport blood and its constituents and waste products.
- Sensory nerve endings to receive messages.
- Hair follicles.
- Sudoriferous glands which excrete sweat.
- Sebaceous or oil glands.
- Papillary muscles to move the hair in the follicle.

The hypodermis, or subcutaneous layer

This layer is an area for the formation and storage of fat. It is a combination of adipose tissue containing fat cells and areolar tissue containing elastic fibres which makes this layer elastic and flexible.

Functions of the skin

Protection

Skin provides a protective covering for underlying internal organs and is a barrier to bacterial invasion. Sebum is produced to keep the skin supple and prevent it drying out. The basal layer contains melanocytes, which produce melanin to protect the skin against ultraviolet radiation, and langerhans cells, which initiate an immune response to invading foreign bodies.

The sensory nerve endings in the skin serve as a warning system to protect the body from injury as they instigate a reflex action to any painful stimulus.

The skin is also waterproof and therefore prevents the absorption of water and the loss of essential body fluids.

Temperature control

Skin plays an important part in the process of maintaining a constant body temperature of 36.8 °C. The loss of heat from the body is controlled by the blood supply and the sweat glands of the skin.

When the body temperature rises the capillaries in the skin dilate allowing heat from the extra blood brought to the surface to be lost by radiation, convection and conduction.

When the body temperature lowers the capillaries in the skin constrict and this conserves the heat within the body.

Evaporation of sweat from the skin's surface also helps to regulate body temperature because when the temperature rises the sweat glands are sent a message by the brain and they are then stimulated to produce sweat which then evaporates on the surface of the skin and cools the body.

Sensation

The skin contains sensory nerve endings which when stimulated by external stimuli send messages to the brain which in turn responds via the motor nerves.

The nerve receptors are located at different levels in the skin and some messages are interpreted before reaching the brain when reflex action occurs.

The sensory nerve endings in the skin react to heat, cold, pain, touch, and pressure.

Motor nerves supply the arrector pili muscle, which is attached to the hair follicle and causes it to stand on end. Secretory nerve fibres innervate the sweat and oil glands of the skin.

Absorption

Since the skin acts as a waterproof barrier very little absorption takes place. The very superficial layers of the stratum corneum are capable of absorbing small amounts of moisturising or conditioning products. There is a passage via the hair follicles to some fatty substances and minute amounts of water may be absorbed over a large surface area.

Excretion

Perspiration is excreted by the sweat glands, removing waste from the skin.

Secretion

Sebum is secreted by the sebaceous glands and this is the skin's natural moisturiser, which helps to keep it soft, supple and intact.

Vitamin production

The skin synthesises vitamin D, which is essential for the formation and maintenance of healthy bones. The fatty substance present in the skin, 7-dehydrocholesterol, is converted to vitamin D when exposed to ultra violet light from the sun.

Disorders of the skin

Acne vulgaris

This affects adolescents between the ages of 14 and 20 and is an inflammatory condition of the sebaceous glands. Its characteristics are greasy shiny skin with enlarged pores, inflammation in and around the sebaceous glands, comedones, papules, pustules, nodules, cysts and sometimes scarring. At puberty the increase in androgens causes the sebaceous glands to enlarge and increase sebum production; the sebaceous follicles then become an environment that allows the bacteria to thrive which contributes to the acne condition.

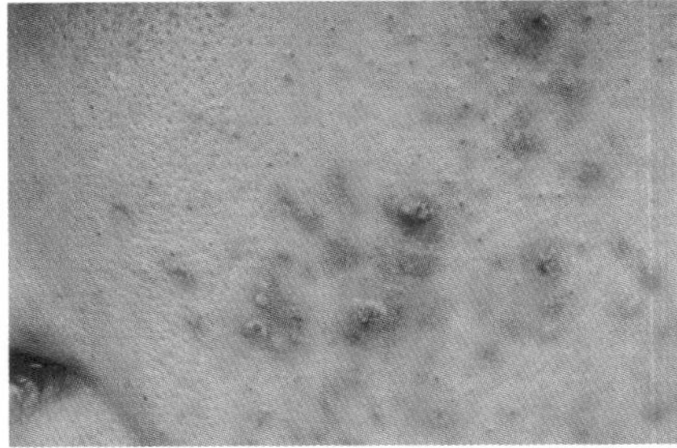

Acne

Eczema

This is a skin condition caused by a sequence of inflammatory changes triggered by the skin's intolerance to a sensitiser. The characteristics are redness, itchiness, scaling, blisters, weeping and cracking of the skin. The appearance of eczema may include one or more of these features and therefore one person's eczema may vary greatly from the next.

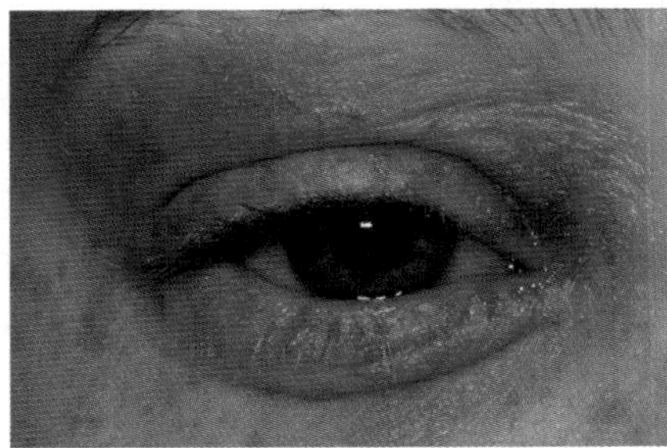

Eczema

Eczema may be:

- **endogenous** – caused by an internal stimulus via the bloodstream

or

- **exogenous** – caused by external contact with a primary irritant to which the skin is allergic. Some common irritants are cosmetics, perfumes, detergents, dyes, rubber and soap.

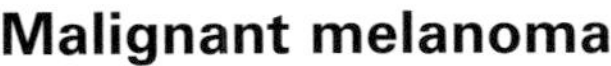

Malignant melanoma

This is a skin cancer due to cancerous changes in skin pigment cells – the cancerous cells divide without control or order. The main cause is intermittent intense exposure to sunlight. It may occur on any skin surface and can affect any age group. Often the first sign of melanoma is the change in size, shape, colour or feel of an existing mole. The signs to look for are asymmetry (when the shape of one half does not match the other), irregular shaped border, uneven or mixed colour, or a change in size.

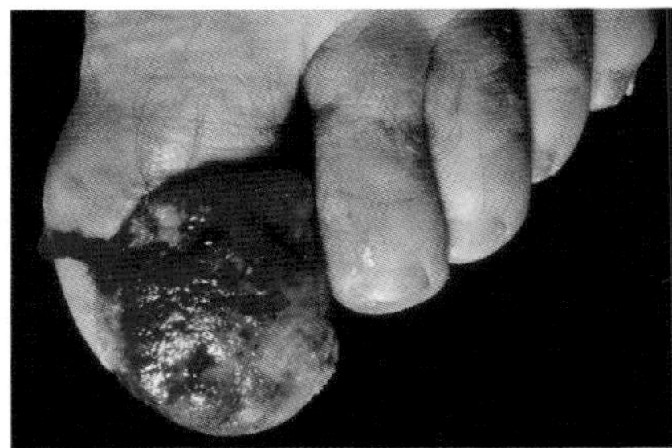

Malignant melanoma

Psoriasis

This is a fairly common skin disorder, which affects about 2% of caucasians at some time during their lives. It may appear at any time but the most common age at which it develops is between the ages of 15 and 30, and is more likely to occur in someone who has one or both parents with the disorder. Psoriasis is characterised by red, slightly raised plaques or papules covered in white scaly skin. Its exact cause is unknown but it may be triggered by trauma, infection, emotional stress or hormone changes.

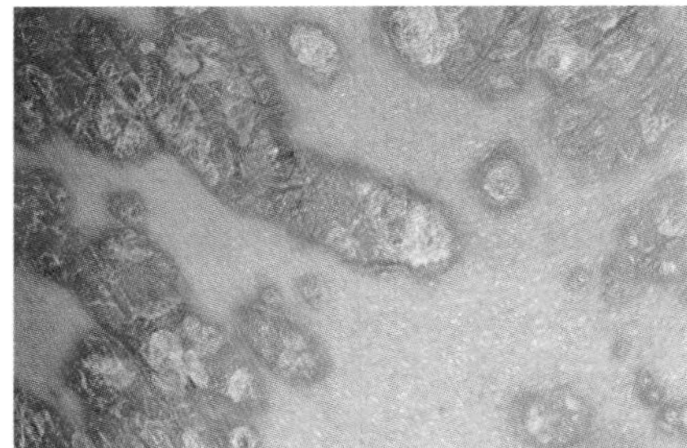

Psoriasis

Rosacea

This is a chronic hypersensitivity of the face normally affecting the nose and cheeks. The characteristics are excessive oiliness, redness (which sometimes takes on a butterfly shape across the cheeks and nose), papules and pustules, and a lumpy appearance. It usually appears in middle age and is more common in women than men, but more severe for a man when rhinophyma occurs (a large bulbous purple veined nose).

This condition is aggravated by eating hot, highly spiced foods, alcohol, very hot tea and coffee, exposure to sunlight, emotional stress and digestive disorders. They cause the already weakened and congested blood vessels to dilate even more and the sensitive skin to become more inflamed.

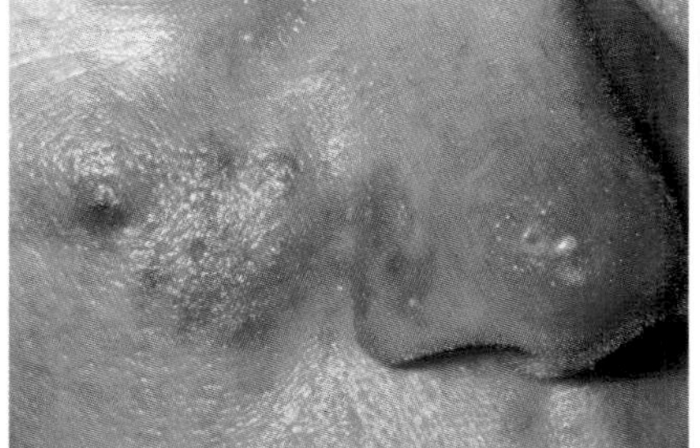

Rosacea

PRACTICE IN CONTEXT

Research the different skin types there are. Discuss with your tutor and colleagues the significance of the sebaceous glands and sudoriferous glands in maintaining a healthy skin.

ASSESSMENT OF KNOWLEDGE

1. Which two layers of the epidermis make up the active area of cell renewal?
2. What is a nucleus?
3. Where are melanocytes found?
4. What is melanin?
5. What is keratinisation?
6. Which layer of the epidermis is more evident on the soles of the feet?
7. How do the sensory nerve endings in the skin help to protect the body?
8. How does the skin help to control body temperature?
9. What causes eczema?
10. What are the physical characteristics of acne?

18 The digestive system

The digestive system depends on a number of different organs, glands and the enzymes they produce working together to change the food we eat into a digestible form that is absorbed from the small intestine and carried by the blood for immediate use or storage. Digestion is the process by which the system breaks down the food into molecules small enough to be absorbed by the cells. The organs and glands which assist the digestive system are the liver, gall bladder and the pancreas.

The digestive system includes:

- The mouth
- The pharynx
- The oesophagus
- The stomach
- The small intestine
- The large intestine
- The rectum and anal canal

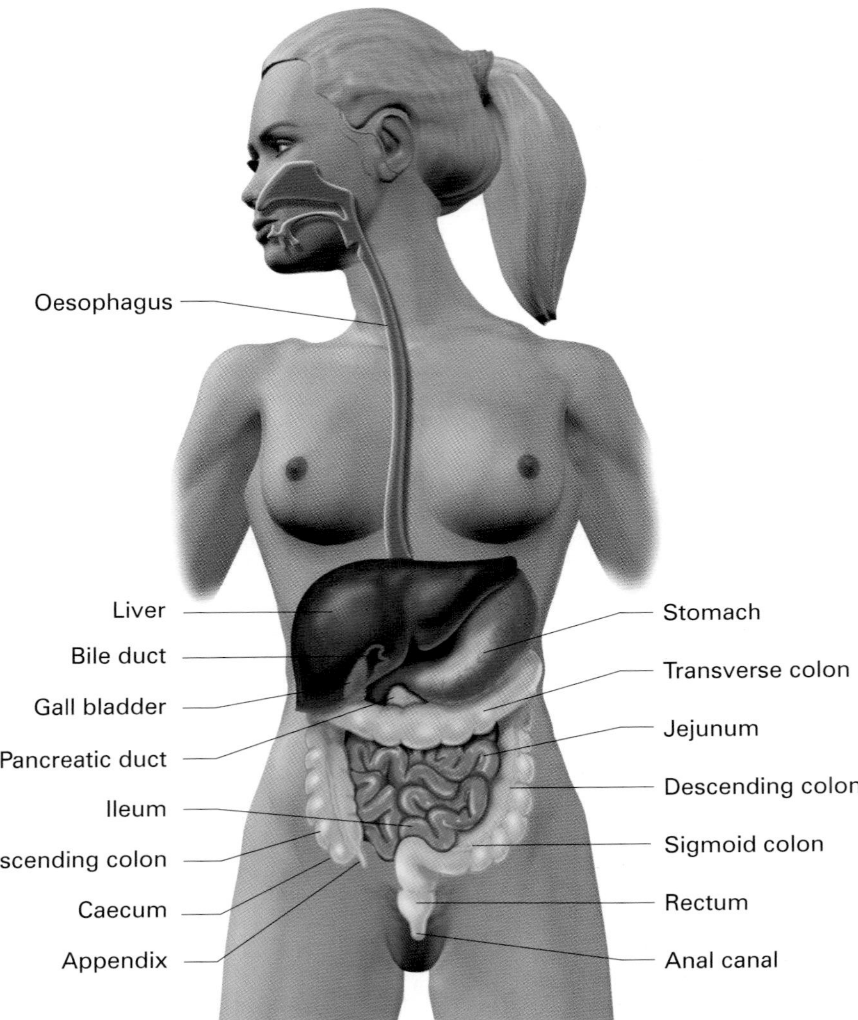

Figure 18.1 *The digestive system*

What is digestion?

Digestion occurs in several stages:

1. **Ingestion** is the taking in of food through the mouth.
2. **Digestion** is the breakdown of food by chemical and mechanical means.
   - *Chemical digestion* occurs when enzymes present in the secretions from the glands of the digestive system react with the food swallowed, breaking it up into small molecules which may pass through the walls of the digestive organs to be utilised by the body's cells.
   - *Mechanical digestion* is a combination of voluntary and involuntary movements that aid the chemical process.

   Digestion starts in the mouth but takes place mainly in the stomach and small intestine. The secretions from the glands of the digestive system are:
   - saliva from the salivary glands
   - gastric juice from the stomach
   - intestinal juice from the small intestine
   - pancreatic juice from the pancreas
   - bile from the liver.
3. **Absorption** This is the uptake of fluids or other substances by the tissues of the body. Digested food is absorbed into the blood and lymph from the alimentary canal and transported to the cells to provide energy. The stomach also plays a very small part in absorption as it does allow some water, electrolytes, certain drugs and alcohol to permeate through the walls into the bloodstream.
4. **Excretion** is the final stage of digestion when the indigestible food substances, i.e. those which have no value to the body, are eliminated.

The process of digestion

1. Digestion begins in the mouth where the food is mechanically broken down by the teeth and chemically broken down when mixed with saliva produced by the salivary glands. This makes the food easier to swallow, as it is formed into a rounded mass of food called a **bolus**.
2. After swallowing the food, by contraction of the muscles in the walls of the pharynx, digestion occurs automatically as there is now no control over its movement. The food is carried down the oesophagus by involuntary muscular contractions. This process is termed **peristalsis**.
3. When the food reaches the stomach it is acted upon chemically by the digestive juices, secreted from the glands of the mucous membrane and mechanically by the muscles of the stomach wall. The food is broken down into a semi-fluid called **chyme**. It then passes into the **duodenum**, the first and smallest part of the small intestine, via the **pyloric sphincter** muscle, which relaxes to allow the chyme to pass through.
4. **Pancreatic juice** from the pancreas and **bile** from the liver neutralises the acid chyme, the enzymes from the pancreas process the proteins, carbohydrates and fats further, and bile helps in the emulsification of fats. The bile is stored in the gall bladder until it is required in the small intestine.
5. The digested food then travels along the **jejunum** where the useful nutrients from the food are absorbed. The **ileum**, which is the final part of the small intestine, absorbs

any remaining nutrients into the bloodstream and the material which is of no use to the body enters the large intestine through the **iliocaecal valve** to be eliminated.

6 The remaining food material accumulates in the ascending colon and then by means of peristalsis moves through the transverse and descending colon to the rectum via the **sigmoid colon**. These solid faeces are stored in the rectum before being released through the anus.

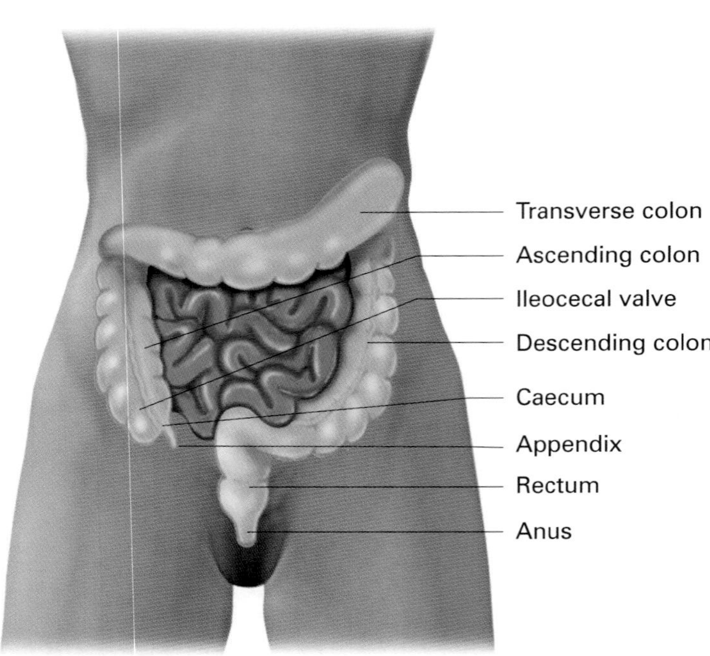

Figure 18.2 *The large intestine*

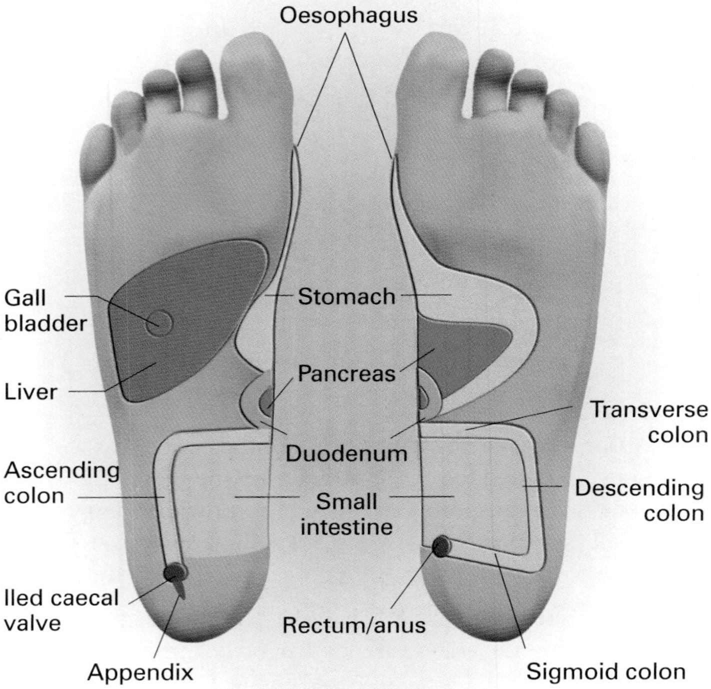

Oesophagus
Gall bladder
Stomach
Liver
Pancreas
Transverse colon
Duodenum
Ascending colon
Small intestine
Descending colon
Iled caecal valve
Rectum/anus
Appendix
Sigmoid colon

Figure 18.3 *Foot map – reflex areas of digestive system*

Disorders of the digestive system

Appendicitis

An inflammation of the appendix causing abdominal pain and tenderness. Vomiting and diarrhoea sometimes occurs.

Constipation

A condition when bowel evacuation occurs infrequently or when passage of faeces causes pain or difficulty.

Diarrhoea

Frequent bowel evacuation or passage of abnormally soft or liquid faeces. It may be caused by intestinal infection or inflammation, irritable bowel syndrome or anxiety.

Diverticulitis

This is inflammation of the diverticula (small pouches formed at weak points) in the colon. It is caused by infection and results in abdominal pain, constipation and diarrhoea.

Gallstones

These are solid lumps or stones that collect in the bile ducts or gall bladder, causing pain, nausea and vomiting. They develop when the chemical composition of bile is upset.

Hepatitis

This is an inflammation of the liver which may be acute or chronic (a prolonged illness). Both types are most commonly caused by hepatitis viruses, or excessive intake of alcohol. The most common are hepatitis A, B and C.

- Hepatitis A is caused by ingesting the virus through contaminated food and water or using contaminated cutlery and it does not usually cause permanent damage to the liver.
- Hepatitis B is more serious and often causes extensive liver damage. It is spread through body fluids and the most common methods of cross-infection are sexual contact with an infected person and contaminated needles. Much less frequently it may be contracted through needles used for tattooing, acupuncture or ear piercing.
- Hepatitis C spreads in the same way as the B virus. It almost always leads to chronic hepatitis and liver damage although initially the effects are less severe than those of the A and B virus.

Hepatitis caused by excessive alcohol can be acute or chronic and contribute to cirrhosis of the liver. Hepatitis may also occur as a result of some rare genetic disorders or autoimmune diseases. There are a range of symptoms: fatigue, headaches, loss of appetite, nausea, vomiting and fever. As the disease progresses other symptoms include jaundice, brown urine and abdominal pain.

Hernia

This is a protrusion of an organ or tissue from the body cavity in which it lies.

Irritable bowel syndrome

This is recurring abdominal pain caused by abnormal muscular contractions in the intestine with either diarrhoea or constipation. The cause is unknown but is often stress related and may follow a severe infection of the intestine. It may also be aggravated by certain foods.

Peritonitis

Acute inflammation of the membrane lining the abdominal cavity, caused by bacteria spread as a result of an accident, surgical wounds or rupture of the appendix.

Ulcerative colitis and Crohn's disease

These are conditions in which there is a long-term inflammation of the digestive tract. Crohn's may affect any part of the digestive tract from the mouth to the anus and ulcerative colitis affects only the colon and rectum. These conditions are sometimes classified as autoimmune disease and often run in families.

PRACTICE IN CONTEXT

Practise working the reflex points of the digestive system and discuss with your tutor and colleagues what foods should be included in the diet to maintain the health of the digestive system.

ASSESSMENT OF KNOWLEDGE

1. Name three organs and glands which assist the digestive system.
2. What is meant by the term 'chemical digestion?'
3. Name five secretions from the glands of the digestive system.
4. What is a bolus?
5. What is peristalsis?
6. Which is the first and smallest part of the small intestine?
7. What is the function of pancreatic juice and bile?
8. What is appendictis?
9. Which organ of the body does hepatitis affect?
10. What are the characteristics of irritable bowel syndrome?

19 The urinary system

What is the urinary system?

The body is continuously producing by-products and waste as a result of the metabolism of nutrients, which must be removed to prevent the body poisoning itself. It has several methods of ridding itself of these waste products through the excretory systems in the body. **Excretion** is the name given to the process by which the body eliminates waste. The urinary system is one of the main systems responsible for excretion and it consists of:

- Two kidneys
- Two ureters
- The bladder
- The urethra

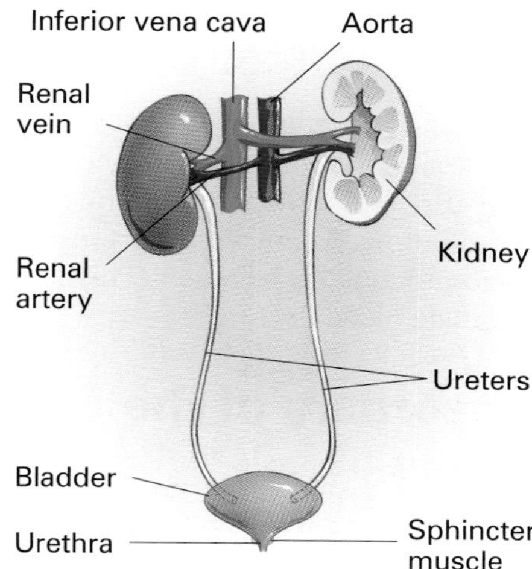

Figure 19.1 *The urinary system*

The kidneys

The kidneys are found just above the waist on the back wall of the abdomen. They contain thousands of tiny filtering units called **nephrons** and each nephron is divided into two parts:

- The **glomerulus**, or filtering part.
- The **tubule**, where water and essential nutrients are extracted from the blood.

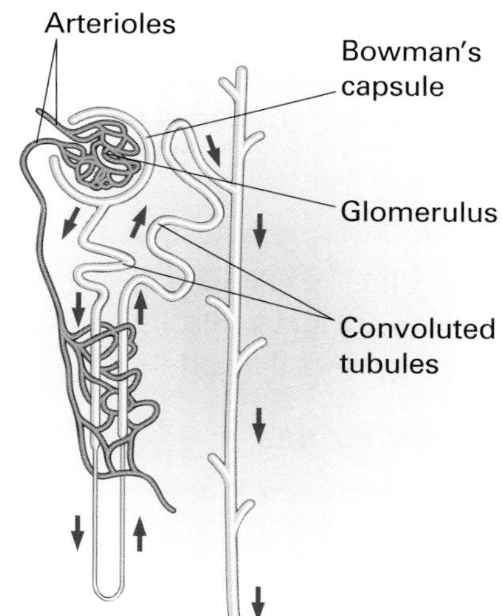

Figure 19.2 *A nephron*

The glomerulus contains a knot of tiny blood capillaries which have very thin walls. Water and waste pass easily across these walls into the collecting system of tubules on the other side. The tubules run between the glomeruli to a collecting system, which drains into the bladder. Each glomerulus is surrounded by a **Bowman's capsule** and it is here that most of the filtered water and salt is reabsorbed.

The kidneys are responsible for filtering nitrogen containing waste, the most common compound of which is urea, out of the bloodstream and regulating the amount of water passed out of the body, maintaining the correct balance of salt in the body.

The kidneys receive about one litre of blood every minute through a renal artery. This is then filtered, separating the watery element (plasma) of blood which passes into the tubule from the rest – water, salt and other valuable substances (glucose, amino acids, minerals and vitamins) which are absorbed back into the bloodstream. Some water, urea and other waste substances are then passed in the form of urine, down two tubes (**ureters**), to the bladder for excretion.

The ureters and urethra

The ureters are two tubes through which urine passes from the kidneys to the bladder. They have one-way valves in the opening to the bladder to prevent urine from flowing back to the kidneys when the bladder is full. The urine passes out of the bladder through the urethra which is situated at the lowest point in the bladder, the opening of which is kept closed by a sphincter, a circular muscle which contracts to seal the passageway. During urination this sphincter muscle relaxes at the same time as the bladder wall contracts to expel the urine.

The bladder

This is a hollow, thick walled, muscular organ lying in the lower part of the pelvic basin between the pubic bones and the rectum. It is a reservoir for urine. The bladder walls are composed of a number of muscular layers, which stretch when the bladder is filling and then contract when it is emptying. There is an almost continuous trickle of urine from the kidneys to the bladder and when the bladder starts to resist, the need to pass urine is felt.

Functions of the urinary system

The main function is to help keep the body in homeostasis (the body's internal environment remaining balanced) by controlling the composition and volume of blood. Waste is filtered from the blood and excreted from the body in the form of liquid urine. There are three processes involved in the formation of urine: filtration, reabsorption and secretion. This system also helps to control the pH of the blood and regulate blood pressure.

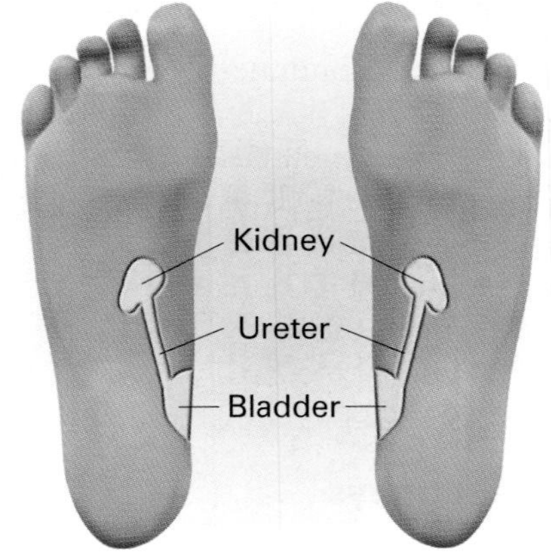

Figure 19.3 Foot map – reflex areas of the urinary system

Disorders of the urinary system

Cystitis

This is an inflammation of the urinary bladder, often caused by infection. The characteristics are a desire to pass urine frequently and a burning sensation; it is sometimes accompanied by cramp-like pain in the abdomen.

Glomerulonephritis

This is an inflammation of the kidney, which may result in damage to the glomeruli, the network of blood capillaries. It may be caused by an allergic reaction to a streptococcal infection of the throat. There are many forms of this disease and it will affect each individual in a different way.

Gout

A hereditary condition associated with an excessively high level of uric acid in the bloodstream and joints. It is caused by an overproduction of uric acid or trouble excreting normal amounts.

Kidney stones

These may be small or large and form in the kidneys or bladder. They can pass straight through or increase in size, causing an obstruction to the flow of urine. They can be extremely painful when passing through and blockage may occur, causing infection and in extreme cases kidney damage.

PRACTICE IN CONTEXT

Practise working the reflex points of the urinary system and investigate the effect on the system of excess salt in the diet.

ASSESSMENT OF KNOWLEDGE

1. What does the urinary system consist of?
2. Where are the kidneys positioned in the body?
3. What is the function of the glomerulus?
4. What is the chief regulating function of the kidneys?
5. Where is the urethra found?
6. What is the function of the bladder?
7. What are the three processes involved in the formation of urine?
8. What are the causes of gout?
9. What are the characteristics of cystitis?
10. In extreme cases, what affect will kidney stones have on the kidneys?

20 The endocrine system

What is the endocrine system?

The endocrine system is responsible for controlling many of the body's functions, providing the driving force behind the mental and physical activity, growth and reproduction of humans. It works in conjunction with the nervous system. The nervous system controls muscular contraction and secretion from glands whilst the endocrine system initiates changes in the metabolic activities of tissues. It consists of endocrine or ductless glands, which are also referred to as organs of internal secretion as they secrete chemical substances called hormones directly into the bloodstream.

The endocrine glands are composed of millions of cells, each of which makes hormones or chemical messengers, which are then transported by the blood to the target cells in the body. The glands of the endocrine system are:

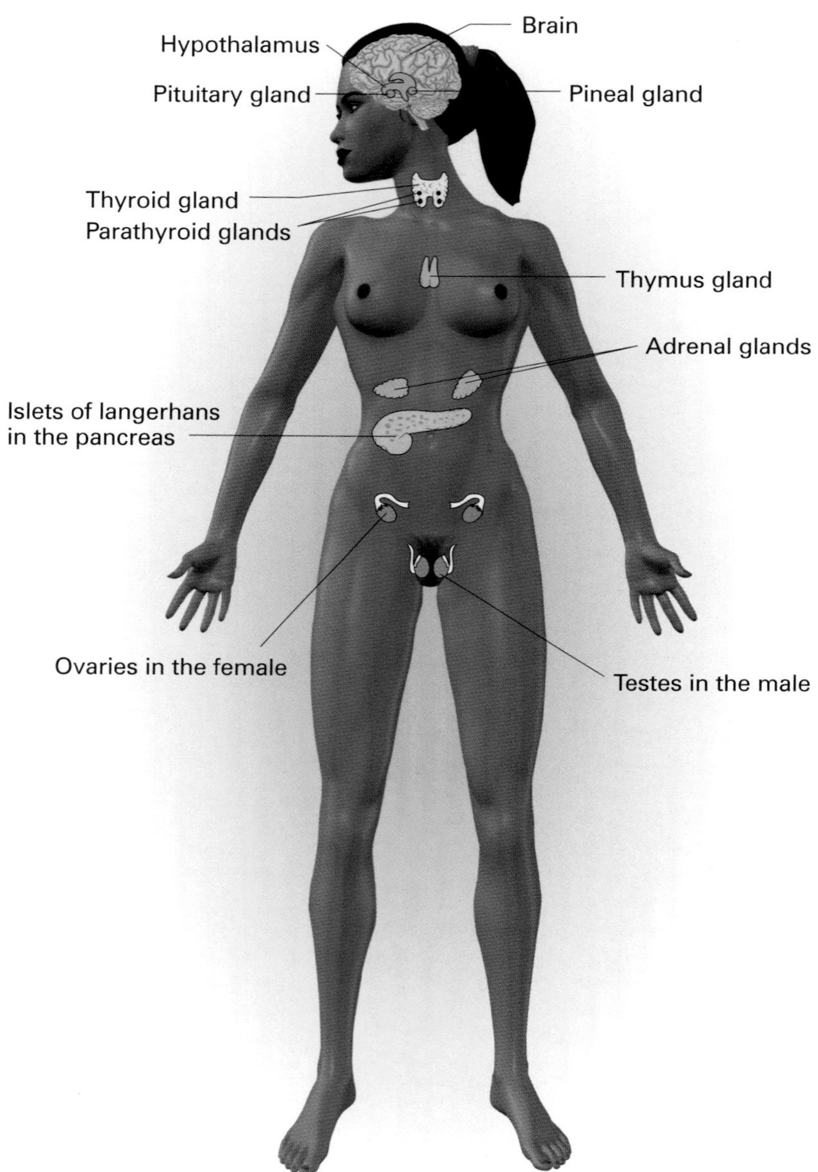

Figure 20.1 The endocrine system

Hormones

Hormones are chemical substances produced by one gland or organ and carried to other organs and tissues where they influence growth, activity and nutrition, helping to maintain homeostasis. When this balance is upset and hormone levels become either excessive or deficient disorders will occur. For example, an excessive amount of sex hormones, in particular androgens, causes cessation of menstruation and hair growth on the face. An undersecretion of corticosteroids from the adrenal glands causes a condition known as Addison's disease. The symptoms include weakness, loss of energy, low blood pressure and dark pigmentation of the skin.

Some hormones affect most parts of the body and increase the rate of chemical reaction in all of the body's cells, for example the growth hormone.

Some hormones only affect certain tissues, called 'target tissues', and only these tissues respond to the hormone. This is because these tissues have specific receptors which receive a hormone and so initiate a response.

The endocrine glands

Pineal gland

This is situated in front of the cerebellum and is thought to produce a hormone called melatonin (in darkness not bright light), which informs the brain when it is day and night. It inhibits the growth and maturation of the gonads (sex glands) until puberty.

Pituitary gland

This gland is situated at the base of the brain and is often called the master gland because its hormones help to control so many of the other endocrine glands in the body. However, it is known that the **hypothalamus** produces secretions which regulate the pituitary gland.

The gland has two parts, the anterior and the posterior lobes.

The anterior lobe produces the following hormones:

Hormone	Action/effect
• Thyroid stimulating hormone (TSH)	Controls the thyroid gland
• Adrenocorticotrophic hormone (ACTH)	Stimulates the adrenal cortex
• Somatotrophin or growth hormone (GH)	Controls general body growth
• Follicle stimulating hormone (FSH)	Stimulates the production of eggs in the ovaries and sperm in the testes
• Luteinising hormone (LH)	Prepares the uterus for implantation of the egg and prepares the mammary glands for milk production in the female. In the male it stimulates the testes to develop and secrete testosterone.
• Prolactin (PRL)	Initiates and maintains milk secretion

The posterior lobe stores the following hormones produced by the hypothalamus:

Hormone	Action/effect
• Vasopressin antdiuretic hormone (ADH)	Decreases urine volume
• Oxytocin	Stimulates the uterus to contract and the mammary glands to produce milk

Hypothalamus

This is an area of the brain near the pituitary gland and is the link between the nervous system and the endocrine glands. It has special nerve cells which make releasing factors, which act on cells of the anterior pituitary before they can send out their hormones.

Thyroid gland

The thyroid gland has two lobes situated on either side of the trachea and by a narrow strip of tissue. The thyroid gland is responsible for regulating the body's metabolic rate and influencing the growth of the body. It secretes thyroxine which if over-secreted (hypersecretion) causes **hyperthyroidism** or **exophthalmic goitre**. This causes an enlarged thyroid, bulging eyes, rapid pulse, excessive sweating and restlessness.

If there is an under-secretion (hyposecretion) it causes cretinism, poor mental and physical development in children, or **myxoedema** in middle age. The characteristics of the latter condition are a slowing down of metabolism, puffy tissues and a slowness of speech and movement.

Parathyroid glands

There are two pairs of parathyroid glands situated on the posterior surface of the thyroid gland. These glands together with the thyroid gland regulate the levels of calcium in the blood. The thyroid lowers the amount of calcium and the parathyroid controls calcium metabolism.

When blood calcium levels are high calcitonin is released by the thyroid gland and excess calcium is then deposited in the bones.

When blood calcium levels become too low, parathormone is released by the parathyroids and calcium is reabsorbed.

Thymus gland

This is a lymph organ. The thymus gland lies behind the sternum in front of the heart. It is thought to be important in helping the process of cellular immunity by processing T cells and B cells, lymphocytes that help with cellular immunity.

Adrenal glands (suprarenals)

These glands are situated immediately above the kidneys. Each gland consists of two distinct parts, the outer part, or **cortex**, and the inner core, or **medulla**.

Adrenal cortex

The adrenal cortex secretes hormones called **steroids**. The most important fall into three main groups:

1. **Mineralocorticoids** – the most important of these is aldosterone. Its functions are sodium and chloride retention and potassium excretion. The water and electrolyte balance in the body are maintained by these functions.
2. **Glucocorticoids** – cortisone and hydrocortisone (cortisol). These assist in the conversion of carbohydrate into glycogen. They increase the blood sugar level, help utilise fat and suppress the natural reaction to inflammation. A deficiency in cortisone production can cause the pituitary to stimulate an overproduction of adrenal androgens, thereby creating hypertrichosis.

3 **Sex hormones** – a small number of both **androgens** (male hormones) and **oestrogens** (female hormones) are secreted. They are influential in sexual development and growth but are not as important as the sex hormones produced by the gonads. In females, however, the adrenals are the principal sources of androgens, which are capable of stimulating facial and body hair. Under-secretion of adrenal cortex hormones causes Addison's disease, the characteristics of which are low blood pressure, an excessive loss of salt, dehydration, muscle weakness, increased pigmentation of the skin, menstrual disturbances and loss of body hair.

Adrenal medulla

The adrenal medulla secretes **adrenalin** and **noradrenalin**. They are known as the 'fight or flight' (see page 80) hormones because they prepare the body to cope with danger or stress. A surge of adrenalin when the body faces danger or excitement causes the heart to beat faster and more strongly, which then raises the blood pressure. At the same time the blood vessels constrict and blood is diverted to the muscles and heart where it is most needed. The liver is stimulated to convert glycogen into glucose, supplying the muscles with the necessary fuel to provide extra energy.

Pancreas

This gland is situated in the abdomen and is attached to the duodenum by the pancreatic duct. It is an endocrine gland secreting **insulin** and also an exocrine gland (secreting onto a free surface or into ducts) as the pancreatic juice is secreted directly into the intestine to aid digestion and not into the bloodstream. The **Islets of langerhans** are cells in the pancreas which secrete insulin necessary for controlling the sugar level in the body. A deficiency of insulin results in diabetes mellitus.

Ovaries and testes (gonads)

The male gonads or testes secrete **androgens**, the most important one being **testosterone** and **oestrogen** in small amounts. Testosterone is the hormone responsible for the development of the secondary sexual characteristics of the male, such as the distribution of hair, deepening of the voice and enlargement of the genitalia.

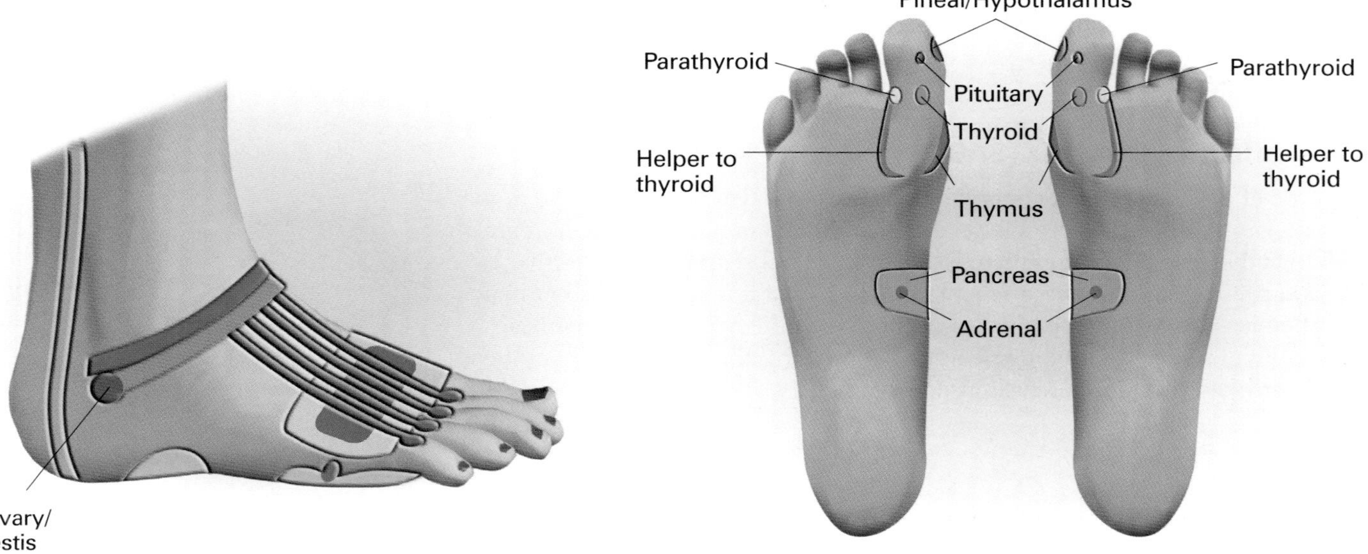

Figure 20.2 Foot map – reflex areas of the endocrine system

The female gonads or ovaries produce ova and secrete the hormones **oestrogen** and **progesterone** and small amounts of **androgens**. They regulate menstruation and play an important part in the development of secondary sexual characteristics.

Progesterone's principal function is to initiate changes in the endometrium (the lining of the womb) in preparation for pregnancy. The ovaries also produce a hormone called **relaxin**, which helps dilate the cervix towards the end of pregnancy.

Disorders of the endocrine system

Cushing's syndrome

This condition is a combination of symptoms caused by adrenal overactivity as a response to excessive cell development of the adrenal cortex, a tumour of the adrenal cortex or anterior pituitary gland, administration of steroids, cortisone or hydrocortisone. The effects of this condition may include:

- Obesity of the face, neck and trunk.
- Muscle weakness and wasting of the legs.
- Osteoporosis resulting in fractures.
- Reduction in protein synthesis, thinning of the skin with stretch marks particularly in the abdominal and thigh areas.
- Poor wound healing and bruising of the skin.

Diabetes

This is a metabolic disorder caused by a deficiency or absence of insulin or an interference with insulin activity, thus reducing the ability of the body to convert food into energy and control the amount of glucose in the blood. There are two types of diabetes:

- **Insulin dependent** – the body stops producing insulin and injections of insulin must be given regularly.
- **Non-insulin dependent** – when a small amount of insulin is produced but not enough to control glucose levels. Sufferers may control this condition with exercise and a healthy well-balanced diet to control weight and burn off excess glucose in the blood. In some cases oral medication is required to increase the release of insulin from the pancreas and increase its effect on body cells.

Seasonal affective disorder (SAD)

This is a type of depression that occurs at particular times, symptoms get worse in the autumn and winter when days are shorter and the amount of natural daylight is greatly reduced. In addition to depression there is a slowing of mind and body, excessive sleeping and over eating. There is a school of thought that it is caused by abnormal levels of chemicals, such as serotonin and dopamine, in the brain, these chemicals play an important role in controlling sleep patterns, eating and moods. Another theory is that sufferers may have a lower eye sensitivity to light.

Thyroid disease

This includes hypothyroidism and hyperthyroidism.

- **Hypothyroidism** is underactivity of the thyroid gland and is more common in women than men. It can cause lethargy, memory loss, heavy periods, hoarse voice, increased weight and intolerance to cold. The eyes may become swollen, the skin dry and the hair dull and lifeless.
- **Hyperthyroidism** is overactivity of the thyroid gland. It can cause a racing pulse, tremor in the hands, weight loss in spite of increased appetite, diarrhoea and an intolerance of heat. The sufferer requires less sleep, may become emotional and suffer anxiety attacks, and the most striking feature is protrusion of the eyes.

PRACTICE IN CONTEXT

Practise working the reflex points of the endocrine system and investigate the effect of hormones on the body systems.

ASSESSMENT OF KNOWLEDGE

1 Which other system of the body does the endocrine system work closely with?
2 What is the common name for 'organs of internal secretion'?
3 What are 'target tissues'?
4 Where is the pituitary gland situated?
5 Name three hormones produced by the anterior lobe of the pituitary gland.
6 What is the function of vasopressin antidiuretic hormone?
7 Which gland is responsible for regulating the body's metabolic rate?
8 Which hormone is released into the body when blood calcium levels are too low?
9 What does insulin control?
10 What are the effects on the body of Cushing's syndrome?

21 The nervous system

What is the nervous system?

This is the control centre and communication network of the body and it works in conjunction with the endocrine system. The functions of the nervous system are: to sense change within the body, to sense change in the environment outside the body, and to interpret and respond to the changes to maintain homeostasis. These responses are in the form of muscular contraction or glandular secretion, and the response from the nervous system is much faster than the response from the endocrine system but they are equally effective in their roles.

The nervous system is divided into the central nervous system, consisting of the brain and spinal cord, and the peripheral nervous system, consisting of the spinal and cranial nerves.

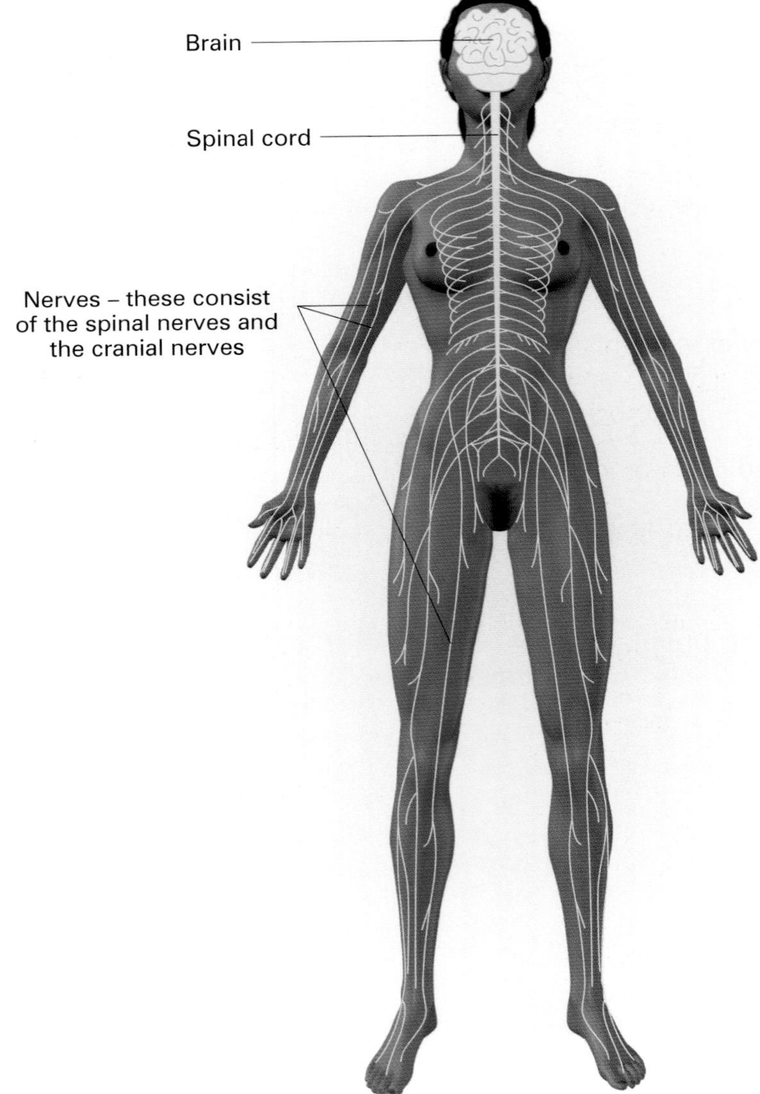

Figure 21.1 The nervous system

Organisation of the nervous system

The following shows how the nervous system is organised.

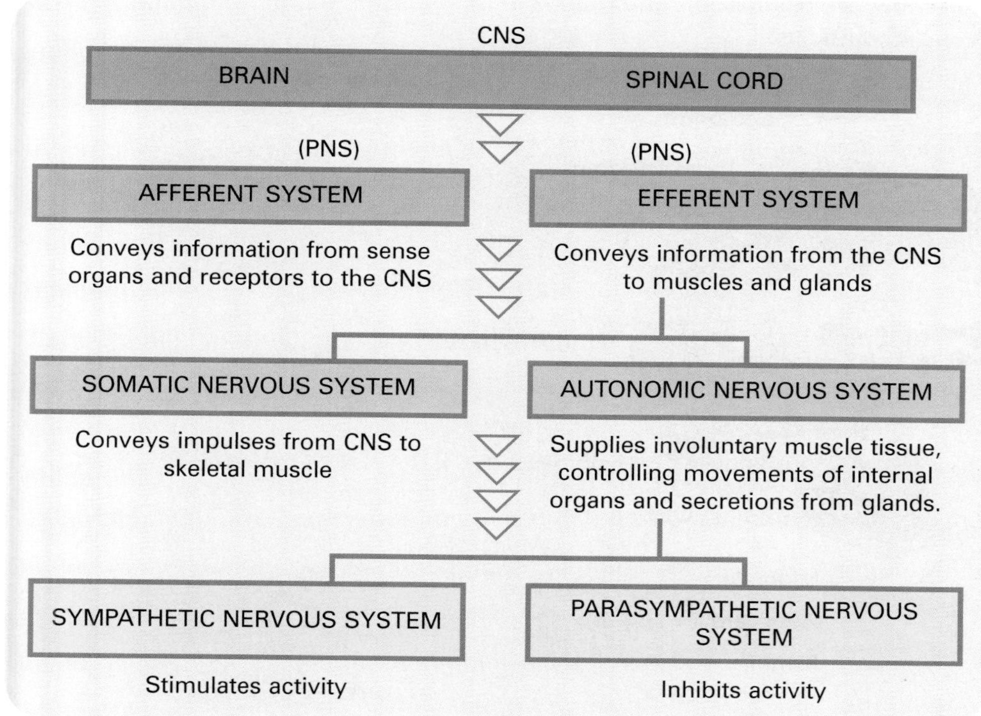

Autonomic nervous system

The two parts of this system have opposing effects on the body in stressful situations. The sympathetic nerves speed up body activity, the parasympathetic nerves slow down body activity. The sympathetic impulses become stronger as a reaction to stress. The heart beats faster, blood vessels dilate, the liver produces more glucose, the pupils of the eyes dilate, hair stands on end, sweat glands produce more sweat and blood pressure rises due to the constriction of small arterioles in the skin. This prepares the body to cope. When the stressful situation passes the parasympathetic nerves take over and help the function of the organs to return to normal.

The cells, which make up the nervous system are called **neurones** and they come in various shapes and sizes. Each neurone is a nerve cell of grey matter with projections called **dendrites** and **axons**. The long fibrous axon has a delicate covering called a **neurilemma** and most axons have a **myelin sheath** which acts as an insulator protecting the axon from injury and speeding the flow of nerve impulses along its length. These impulses are then carried to the nerve cell via the dendrites.

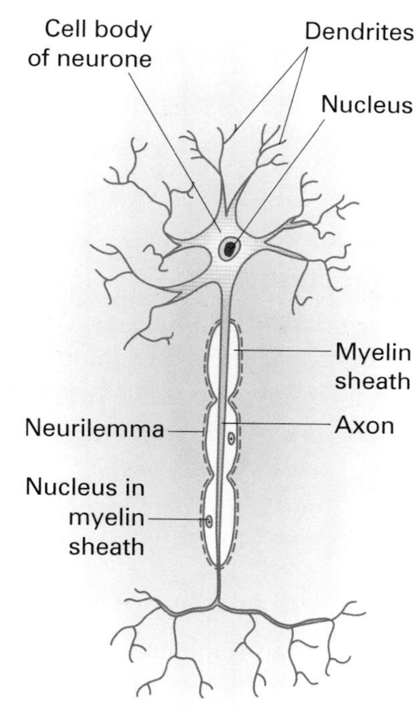

Figure 21.2 *A neurone*

The brain

The brain is one of the largest organs in the body and it consists of:

- The **brain stem** – which comprises the medulla oblongata, pons varolii and the midbrain.
- The **cerebrum** – which makes up about seven-eigths of the weight of the brain and occupies most of the cranium.
- The **thalamus** and **hypothalamus** above the brain stem.
- The **cerebellum** – which lies below the cerebrum and behind the brain stem.

The brain is protected, by the cranial bones and the cranial meninges which is composed of dense fibrous connective tissue. The cerebrospinal fluid also acts as a protection against injury, circulating around the brain and through the ventricles in the brain serving as a shock absorber for the central nervous system. It has a good supply of blood vessels, which provide oxygen and nutrients.

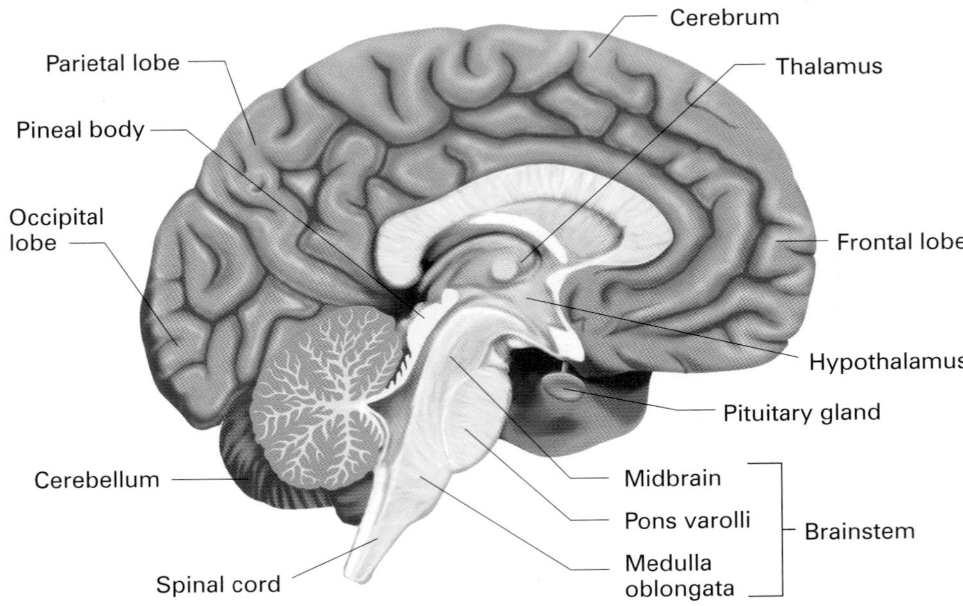

Figure 21.3 The brain

Brain stem

- The **medulla oblongata** contains centres which help to control the heart rate, the depth and rate of breathing and other non-vital autonomic reflexes such as swallowing, sneezing and coughing.
- The **pons varolii** is a bridge connecting the spinal cord with the brain and parts of the brain with each other.
- The **midbrain** is the highest part of the brain stem and is situated centrally under the cerebrum just below the hypothalamus.

Thalamus and hypothalamus

The thalamus is the main relay station for sensory impulses and it interprets sensory messages to the brain. It is also concerned with memory and certain emotions. The hypothalamus is an important area just above the pituitary gland. It is responsible for controlling many body activities and most of them are related to homeostasis:

- It helps to control the autonomic nervous system, regulating the heartbeat, controlling the secretion of many glands, the movement of food through the digestive tract and contraction of the urinary bladder.
- It receives sensory impulses.
- It is the principal intermediary between the nervous system and the endocrine system. When it detects certain changes occurring in the body it releases chemicals that stimulate or inhibit the anterior pituitary gland.
- It controls normal body temperature.
- It stimulates hunger and inhibits food intake when full.

- It produces a sensation of thirst when fluid is reduced in the body.
- It helps to maintain sleeping and waking patterns.

Cerebrum

Often referred to as the cerebral cortex, the cerebrum is divided into four lobes, each of which takes its name from the bone under which it lies.

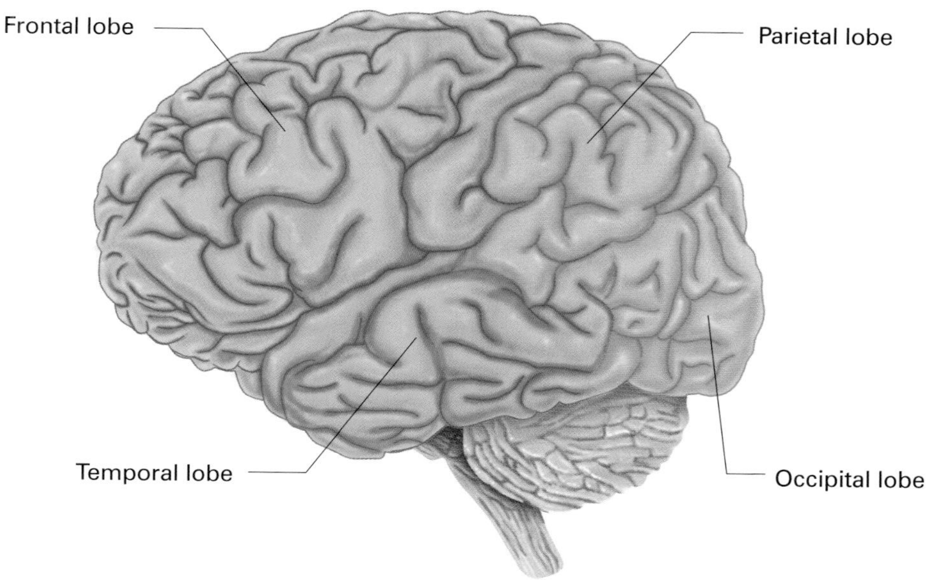

Figure 21.4 *The cerebrum*

The functions of the cerebrum are:

- Mental activities involving memory, intelligence, sense of responsibility, thinking and reasoning.
- Sensory perception of pain, temperature, touch, sight, hearing, taste and smell.
- Initiation and control of voluntary muscle contraction.

Cerebellum

This is a motor area of the brain controlling subconscious movements of the skeletal muscles, movements required for posture, co-ordination, balance and delicate movements, for example playing the piano or typing a letter. Messages are transmitted from the inner ear to the cerebellum, which responds by sending impulses to the muscles necessary for maintaining balance.

Cranial nerves

There are twelve pairs of cranial nerves, ten of which originate from the brain stem. Each pair has a number denoting the order in which they arise from the brain and a name indicating their distribution or function. Some cranial nerves are sensory only, others have both functions and are referred to as mixed. They are shown in the table overleaf.

Name	Classification	Function
I. Olfactory	sensory	smell
II. Optic	sensory	vision
III. Oculomotor	mixed	motor – movement of the eyelid and of eyeball, constriction of the pupil sensory – muscle sense
IV. Trochlear	mixed	motor – movement of the eyeball sensory – muscle sense
V. Trigeminal	mixed	motor – chewing sensory – touch, pain, temperature from the upper eyelid down to the jaw
VI. Abducent	mixed	motor – movement of the eyeball sensory – muscle sense
VII. Facial	mixed	motor – facial expressions, secretion of saliva and tears sensory – taste and muscle sense
VIII. Vestibulocochlear	sensory	conveys impulses associated with hearing and equilibrium
IX. Glossopharyngeal	mixed	motor – swallowing and secretion of saliva sensory – taste and regulation of blood pressure and muscle sense
X. Vagus	mixed	motor – swallowing and visceral muscle movement sensory – sensations from, pharynx, larynx, respiratory passageways, lungs, oesophagus, heart, stomach, small intestine, part of large intestine and gall bladder
XI. Accessory	mixed	motor – swallowing and movement of the head sensory – muscle sense
XII. Hypoglossal	mixed	motor – movement of tongue during speech and swallowing sensory – muscle sense

The spinal cord

The spinal cord begins as a continuation of the medulla oblongata extending down the vertebral column. Its main function is conveying impulses to and from the brain and the peripheral nervous system. Its second function is to provide reflexes which are fast responses to internal or external stimuli, helping to maintain the body's internal balance or homeostasis.

There are 31 spinal nerves, which are named according to the region from which they emerge. They are as follows:

- Eight pairs of cervical nerves
- Twelve pairs of thoracic
- Five pairs of lumbar
- Five pairs of sacral
- One pair of coccygeal

Each spinal nerve splits into branches which in turn split into smaller branches to form a network which radiates all over the body.

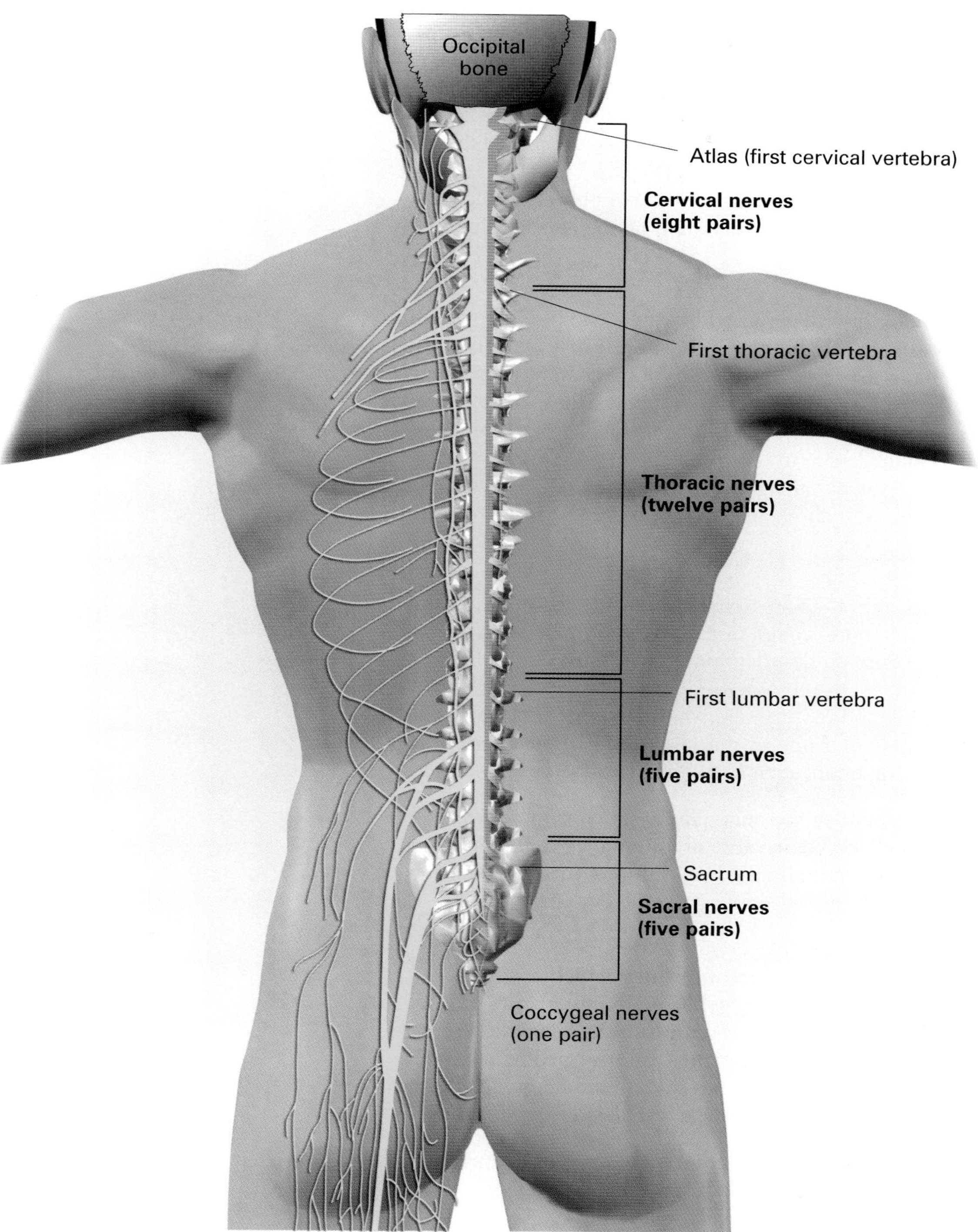

Figure 21.5 *The spinal nerves*

Disorders of the nervous system

Bell's palsy

This is a condition which results in weakness or total physical paralysis of one half of the face; however it usually recovers spontaneously. It is caused by a swelling of the facial nerve which activates the muscles. This results in a loss of the covering layers or damage to the nerve fibres themselves. The symptoms start with pain behind the ear and weakness of the face that usually appears after two to five days. The condition may affect the eye and mouth which may begin to droop. Other symptoms may include loss of taste, intolerance of loud noise and altered sensation on the affected side.

Cerebral palsy

This term refers to a group of motor disorders caused by damage to the brain cells in the motor area of the brain, before, during birth or in infancy. It may be caused when the mother is exposed to rubella in the first three months of pregnancy, if the baby is starved of oxygen during the birth or hydrocephalus in infancy. This is not a progressive disease but once the damage is done it is irreversible. Most people with cerebral palsy have damage to some degree in the cortex, basal ganglia and cerebellum. The location and severity of damage will determine the symptoms. It may cause deafness, partial blindness, inability to speak, or mental retardation.

Epilepsy

This is a condition marked by recurrent seizures, sometimes called fits. This occurs when nerve cells in the brain temporarily go out of control and fire off excessive and random signals. It is a relatively common disorder and it often starts in childhood or teenage years, abating after adolescence and sometimes disappearing altogether in adulthood. It often runs in families and most sufferers have no symptoms between seizures, leading relatively normal lives. Epilepsy may also occur when a person has a progressive condition that affects the brain, such as Alzheimer's disease.

It is thought that a chemical imbalance in the brain causes sufferers to be susceptible to epileptic seizures or there may be a specific cause of disturbance in the brain which instigates a fit. These could include strokes, head injuries, meningitis, damage from alcohol or drug abuse or other brain infections. In some circumstances the condition may develop for no obvious reason.

The most common symptom of epilepsy is recurrent seizures, which occur spontaneously and may be preceded by a strange feeling and unusual taste or smell. There may also be a sensory disturbance, known as an 'aura'. Occasionally, a seizure may be triggered by rhythmical flashing lights. A seizure can vary greatly in severity. Major seizures (tonic) occur when brain cells on both sides of the brain are affected at the same time. Tiny seizures (petit mal) cause only a brief loss of responsiveness.

The seizure often follows a pattern. The person becomes unconscious and may become rigid and arch the back, make rapid twitching or jerking movements, have a rigid jaw or froth at the mouth, breathe noisily and with difficulty.

Minor epileptic seizures are not always noticed as the person may just be staring blankly, appear to be daydreaming, complain of a pins and needles sensation, be twitching their mouth, eyelids, head or limb or just be making strange noises.

Multiple sclerosis (MS)

This is a progressive condition and is the result of the destruction of the protective tissue around the nerves in any part of the brain or spinal cord. It is often classified as an autoimmune disease when the body's own immune system attacks its own tissues. Some people are genetically susceptible to this condition, but it is thought that a viral infection may be responsible for triggering the condition.

There are a considerable number of symptoms: a tingling sensation and general weakness or numbness in the arms and legs may be felt if the spine is affected, there may also be a more frequent passing of urine or incontinence. Blurred vision, a loss of colour vision or pain in or around the eye, may be a result of 'optic neuritis' inflammation of the nerves carrying impulses from the eyes. MS that affects the brain can result in an unsteadiness when walking, slurring of speech and twitching of facial muscles. In more advanced stages, stiffness and spasms may affect the legs and the arms become clumsy and tremor may affect them.

Parkinson's disease

This is a progressive disorder of the nervous system when the nerve cells in the part of the brain that control movement stop functioning properly. The cause is unknown and the symptoms do not appear until about 80% of the chemical dopamine in the brain has been lost and there are, tremors, rigidity and slowness of movement which causes stooped posture, problems with swallowing, drooling and a shuffling gait. Other signs are soft, mumbling speech, problems with handwriting, difficulty with everyday activities and depression.

PRACTICE IN CONTEXT

Investigate the way in which the nervous system affects all the other systems in the body.

ASSESSMENT OF KNOWLEDGE

1 What are the functions of the nervous system?
2 Which system conveys information from the central nervous system to the muscles and glands?
3 What is the action on the body of the parasympathetic nerves?
4 What is a neurone?
5 What are the names given to the projections on each neurone?
6 Which area of the brain contains the control centre for the vital reflex of swallowing?
7 Give three functions of the cerebrum.
8 How many spinal nerves are there?
9 Name five characteristics of Parkinson's disease.
10 What is the effect of multiple sclerosis on the nerves?

22 The reproductive system

What is the reproductive system?

Reproduction is the means by which life is sustained and genetic material is passed from generation to generation maintaining the continuation of human life.

The reproductive organs of the male and female are different both anatomically and physiologically. The function of the male reproductive system is to produce numerous, minute spermatazoa (reproductive cells), store them and transfer them to the female reproductive system. The functions of the female reproductive system are to produce ova (reproductive cells), provide a place for the fertilised ovum to grow, nourishment to sustain it and provide milk to feed it after birth.

Male reproductive system

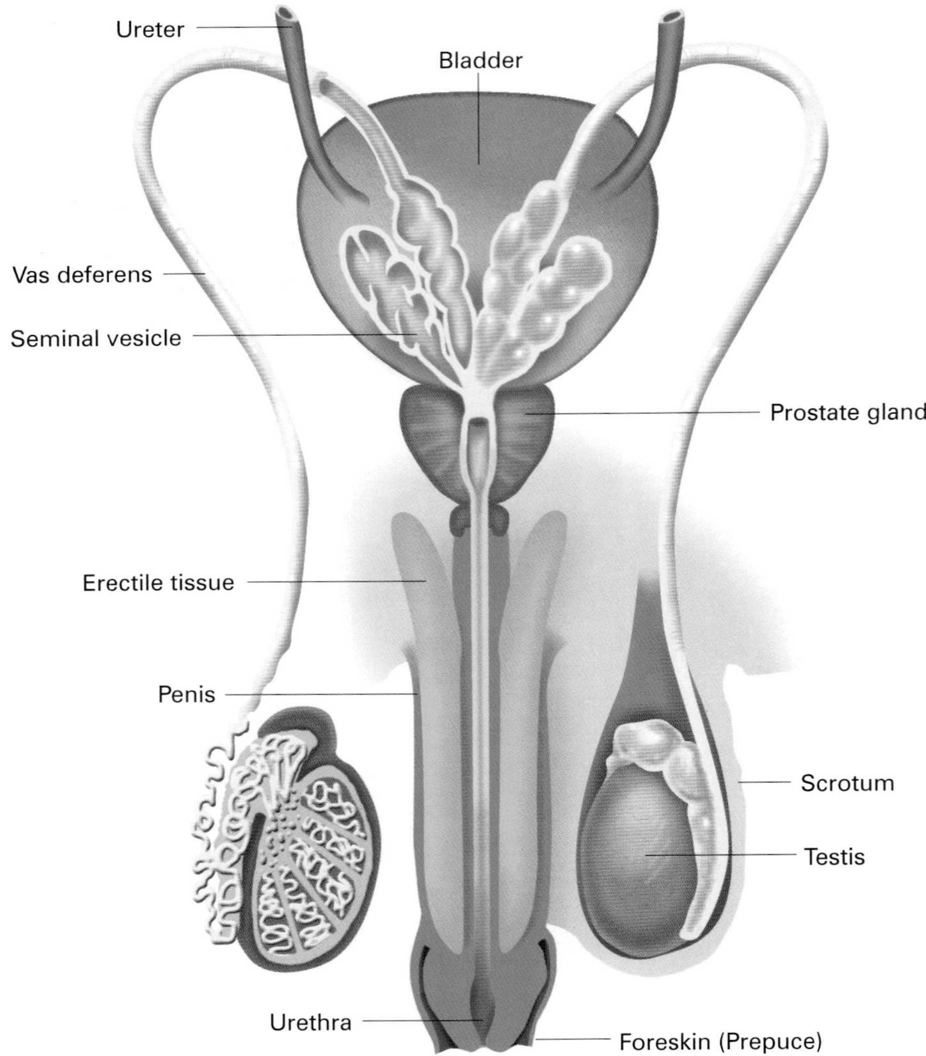

Figure 22.1 The male reproductive system

The organs of the male reproductive system are:

- The **testes** (part of the endocrine system), which produce sperm and testosterone. Testosterone controls the development, growth and maintenance of the male sex organs.
- **Ducts** and **glands** that store or transport sperm.
- **Accessory glands** to add secretions, seminal fluid, to aid motility and viability of spermatozoa.
- The **penis**, erectile tissue, dilates with blood under the influence of sexual stimulation, to ejaculate spermatozoa into the vagina of the female.

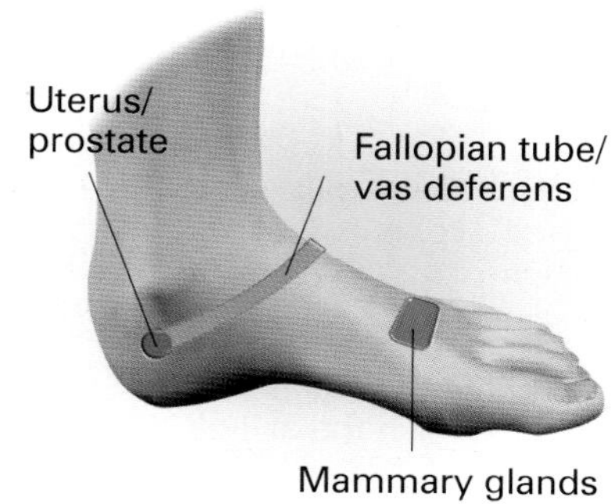

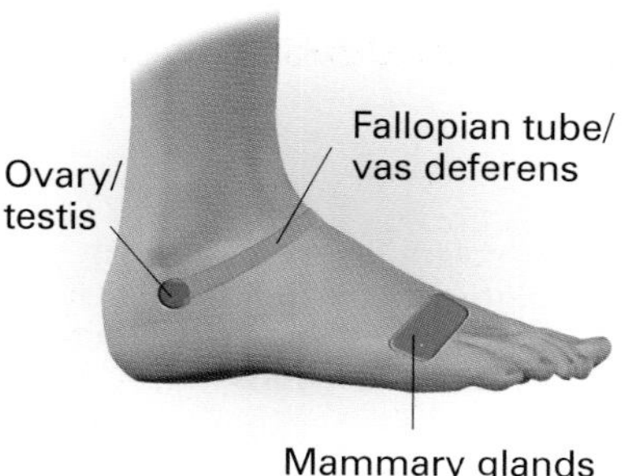

Figure 22.2 Foot map – male and female reproductive areas

Female reproductive system

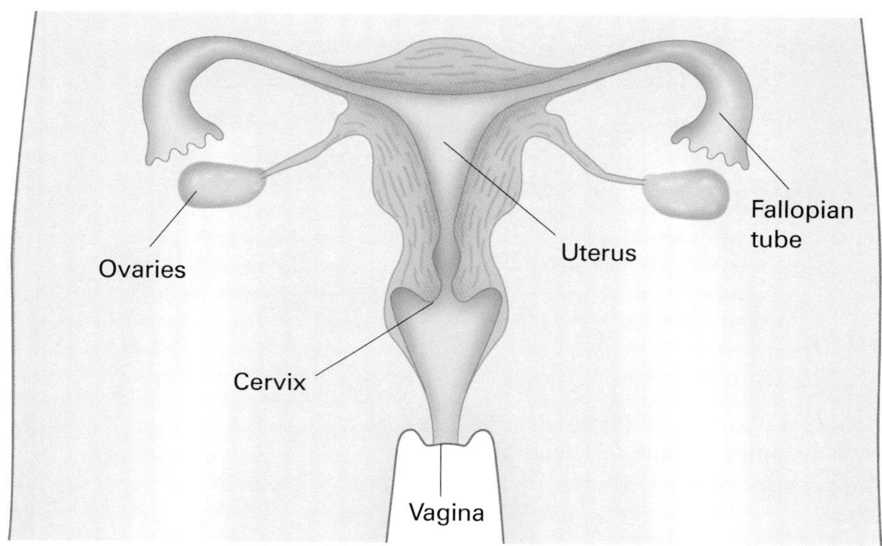

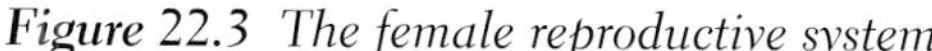

Figure 22.3 The female reproductive system

The organs of the female reproductive system are:

- The **ovaries** which produce ova and secrete female sex hormones: progesterone, oestrogens and relaxin.
- The **fallopian tubes** which transport the ova to the uterus where it develops into an embryo. An unfertilised ovum disintegrates and is removed during menstruation.
- The **uterus** or **womb** – the site of menstruation and the environment for the developing embryo.
- The **vagina** – a passageway for menstrual flow and where the penis is inserted during sexual intercourse. It is also the lower part of the birth canal through which the baby is delivered.
- The **mammary glands**.

Mammary glands

The breasts or mammary glands are accessory glands of the female reproductive system. Each gland consists of 15–20 lobes separated by adipose tissue. The size of the female breasts is determined by the amount of adipose tissue present.

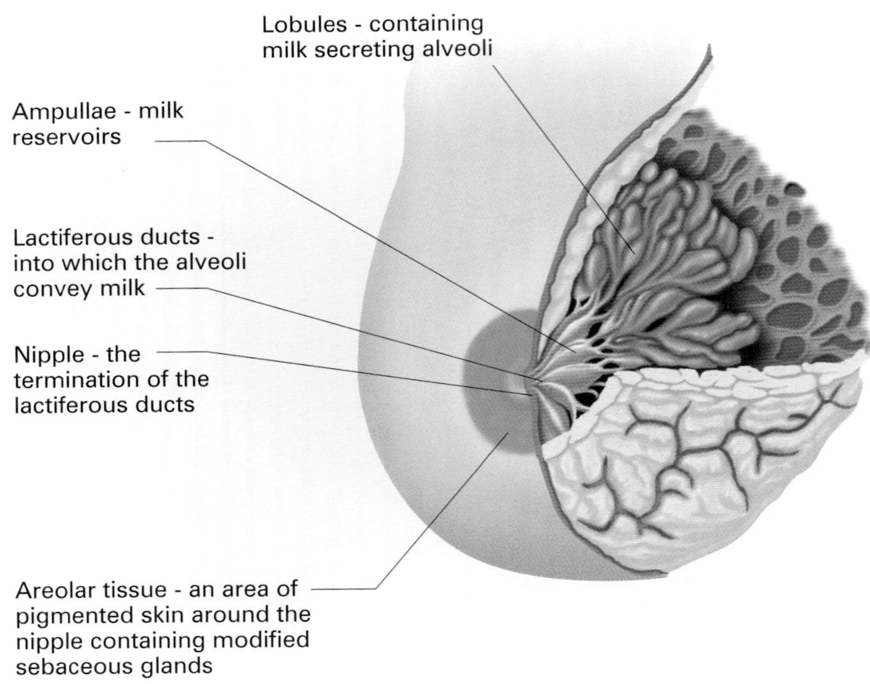

Figure 22.4 The breast

The function of the female breasts is the secretion and ejection of milk, commonly called lactation. The secretion of milk is controlled by the hormone prolactin with some help from progesterone and oestrogen. Oxytocin stimulates the release of milk in response to the stimulation of the nipple by the baby sucking.

Menstrual cycle

This occurs regularly in females throughout their childbearing years, which lasts approximately 35 years. It is a series of changes in the endometrium (the mucous membrane lining of the uterus) of a non-pregnant female and these changes are controlled by the hypothalamus, which acts as a menstrual clock.

An egg is released from an ovary and travels to the womb. If it is fertilised it will be nourished by secretions from the cells lining the womb, until it burrows into the wall itself and receives nourishment from the mother's own blood supply.

When the egg is not fertilised, the lining of the womb breaks up and is shed during the menstrual flow, a new lining then forms for the next egg to be released.

Reproduction

Fertilisation is accomplished when the spermatozoa penetrates the surface of the egg and they fuse together to form a single nucleus, which then begins to divide and within 72 hours travels into the uterus where it burrows into the lining to be nourished. The placenta then forms and by the twelfth week it is a separate organ which allows substances to pass from the mother to the foetus ensuring its development. The placenta is attached to the foetus via the umbilical cord and waste products pass back to the mother after nutrients and oxygen have been received from her. The foetus continues to develop until it reaches the end of the gestation period when the mother goes into labour and the baby is delivered.

Disorders of the male reproductive system

Benign prostatic hypertrophy

An enlargement of the prostate gland is a common condition in men over 50. It is thought to be linked to hormonal changes that occur with age. The cells of the prostate grow and multiply, which then compresses the urethra causing an obstruction to the flow of urine, making it difficult to empty the bladder completely. The bladder may then become distended causing swelling and pain in the abdomen and eventually incontinence may result, requiring surgical repair.

Impotence

This occurs when a man cannot achieve or maintain an erection. It is a common problem which affects most men at some time in their lives, and the causes may be systemic, neurological, psychological or physical. Psychological problems include mental fatigue, anxiety or stress, depression or relationship problems. Physically an erection depends on nerve signals, which are triggered by sexual arousal, and these may be blocked by taking medication to treat depression and high blood pressure or diuretic drugs. It also may occur in those suffering from diabetes, multiple sclerosis, Parkinson's disease, or after surgery or injury to the genitals, spine or pelvic area. For those suffering from hardening of the arteries – more common amongst heavy smokers, diabetics, sufferers of high blood cholesterol and high blood pressure – blood flow may be restricted to the penis.

This condition may also occur if damage has been caused to the blood vessels through injury, radiotherapy to the pelvic area or surgery to the prostate gland and bladder. As men get older the reduction in testosterone levels may contribute to this problem; other physical causes are excessive alcohol consumption and drug abuse.

Infertility

This is an inability to fertilise the ovum. This may be caused by an insufficient number of spermatozoa being produced, an obstruction in the seminal tract to the transportation of sperm or degenerative changes to the male reproductive system which have caused sterility. Some steroid treatment given at puberty may also have an adverse effect on fertility in the male.

Prostate cancer

Tumours of the male reproductive system often involve the prostate gland. It is usually slow to grow and can be treated effectively but this relies heavily on early detection and diagnosis. It is more common in older men. Sometimes there are no obvious symptoms, however pressure may be exerted on the urethra as the tumour grows and this constricts the flow of urine from the bladder making urination painful and difficult. Symptoms may include frequent urination, difficulty urinating, a strong urge to urinate but little flow, waking constantly during the night or dribbling urine before or after urination. In the more advanced condition there may be abdominal pain and problems with the nerves that supply the legs.

Testicular cancer

This is a disease which is caused by an abnormal growth of the cells of the testicles. Causes are unknown but it is thought that those men who were born with an undescended testicle are more susceptible. It most often affects men aged between 15 and 35. If caught early it can usually be treated and cured. Characteristics may include a lump, irregularity or enlargement in either testicle, a dull ache in the groin or lower abdomen, a feeling of heaviness, pain or discomfort in the scrotum or a sudden collection of fluid.

Disorders of the female reproductive system

Amenorrhoea

This is the absence of menstruation. Primary amenorrhoea is when a woman has never menstruated. It can be caused by endocrine disorders in the pituitary or hypothalamus or through genetic abnormalities of the ovaries or uterus. Secondary amenorrhoea occurs to most women at some time and it is when one or more periods are missed. Causes may include changes in body weight, for example, obesity can affect ovarian function, and the extreme loss of weight, which characterises anorexia nervosa, can halt menstrual flow.

Dysmenorrhoea

This is painful menstruation caused by contraction of the uterus during menstruation. In some cases it may be accompanied by nausea, vomiting, headache, fatigue and nervousness. An underlying gynaecological disorder may cause the pain, conditions such as endometriosis, a backward tilting uterus, fibroids, inflammation of the fallopian tubes or abnormal adhesions. The pain may sometimes extend into the back or thighs and can resemble a constant dull ache or cramps that come and go.

Endometriosis

This occurs when endometrial tissue normally only found in the lining of the uterus grows outside attaching itself to various sites such as the ovaries, cervix, abdominal wall, bowel, ureters, bladder or the vagina. This misplaced tissue still responds to the hormonal changes of the menstrual cycle and therefore it may bleed during menstruation, causing irritation, pain and sometimes cramps. In time scar tissue develops and this can cause adhesions which bind structures together that are normally separate and this may interfere with their normal function.

Infertility

This is an inability to conceive. It may be due to failure to ovulate, obstruction of the fallopian tubes or disease in the uterus.

Mastitis

This is inflammation of the breast caused by bacterial infection via damaged nipples.

Ovarian cancer

This is cancer of the female reproductive system affecting about 1 in 70 women and usually develops between the ages of 50 and 70. This condition may grow to a large size before it exhibits symptoms, which may be a vague dragging sensation in the lower abdomen. Occasionally bleeding may occur in women who have been through the menopause. There may be an accumulation of fluid in the abdomen which causes swelling, as does a very large growth.

Pelvic inflammatory disease

This is an infection of the female reproductive organs usually affecting the uterus and fallopian tubes, but it may spread to the ovaries and pelvic cavity. It normally starts with a sexually transmitted infection such as gonorrhoea or chlamydia. Much less often it may be caused when the neck of the womb is open. When an intrauterine contraceptive device is fitted, during miscarriage, abortion or after childbirth, the risk is greater if the woman already has an untreated infection.

Symptoms are severe abdominal and lower back pain, high temperature, nausea, vomiting or abnormal vaginal discharge. The worst outcome of PID is infertility and an increased risk of ectopic pregnancy.

Uterine fibroids

These are swellings in the muscular walls of the uterus. They are extremely common, are benign and in most women cause no problems. The fibroids seem to depend on oestrogen for their growth, growing during pregnancy but shrinking spontaneously after the menopause. They are more common in women over 40 and in women of African-Caribbean and Asian origin. The most common symptom is heavy periods but if the fibroid grows to a large size there may be a swelling in the abdomen and if it presses on the bladder will cause frequent urination, or incontinence. Fibroids grow rapidly during pregnancy and if it outgrows its blood supply and degenerates it can be very painful.

PRACTICE IN CONTEXT

Practise working the reflex points for the male and female reproductive system (see page 151).

ASSESSMENT OF KNOWLEDGE

1. What is the function of the male reproductive system?
2. What is the function of the female reproductive system?
3. What hormones do the ovaries secrete?
4. In which part of the mammary gland is milk stored?
5. What happens to an unfertilised egg?
6. What is the function of the placenta during pregnancy?
7. Which psychological problems contribute to impotence in men?
8. What are the characteristics of testicular cancer?
9. What is meant by the term ‘secondary amenorrhoea’?
10. When does the condition endometriosis occur?

23 The special senses

The special senses include smell, taste, sight, hearing and balance, and they allow us to detect changes in the environment.

The sense of smell

The nose has two functions – respiration (see Chapter 16) and sense of smell, which has a connection with the part of the brain that has grown to be the sorting house for emotional responses. Our sense of smell provides us with a warning system giving us valuable information about the environment and it is closely linked with our sense of taste.

Structure and function of the olfactory system

The sensory receptors for smell are found in the roof of the nasal cavity just below the frontal lobes of the brain. This is known as the **olfactory area** and it contains millions of **olfactory cells**. Each of these cells has about a dozen fine hairs called cilia which are surrounded by mucous to keep the cilia moist and trap odorous substances. These cilia help to increase our sensitivity to smell.

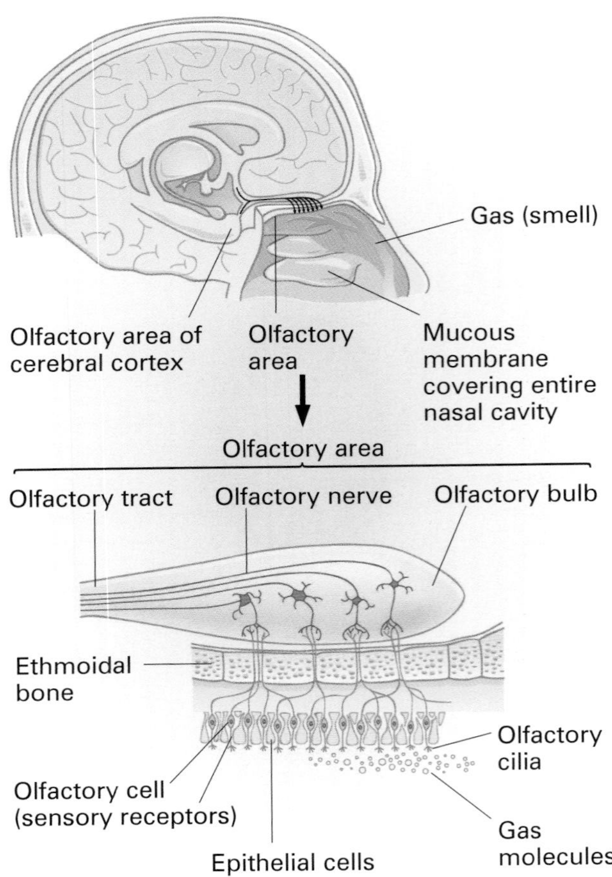

Figure 23.1 *The olfactory system*

The process of smelling

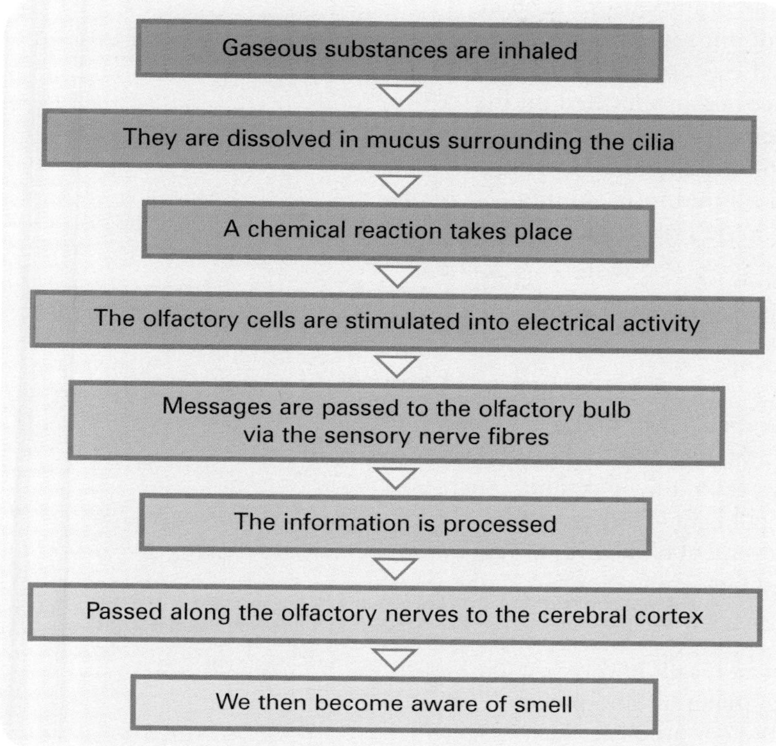

Gaseous substances are inhaled
They are dissolved in mucus surrounding the cilia
A chemical reaction takes place
The olfactory cells are stimulated into electrical activity
Messages are passed to the olfactory bulb via the sensory nerve fibres
The information is processed
Passed along the olfactory nerves to the cerebral cortex
We then become aware of smell

The limbic system

This is the part of the brain which deals with emotions, moods, our motivation, memory and creativity. It is sometimes referred to as the primitive brain. It is closely connected with the part of the brain, which receives the messages from the olfactory cells in the nose.

This connection explains why smells evoke particular memories and feelings and smells are so richly endowed with emotional significance. The smell of a mother's scent can provide instant comfort to a child. A perfume may remind us instantly of a place where we may have first worn the fragrance. The smell of freshly baked bread may make us feel instantly hungry and the smell of a new-born baby can stimulate maternal feelings long after the children have left home.

Some smells will bring back memories of special occasions. This is because we remember those things which have emotional significance. The areas of the brain which process memories and recall events are closely linked to the limbic system and this in turn is linked to the centres in the brain for the sense of smell.

Odour stimulates the release of neurotransmitters, which in turn have a beneficial effect on the body, for example:

- **Encephaline** and **endorphins** help to reduce pain and create a feeling of well being.
- **Serotonin** helps us to relax and have a calming effect.
- **Noradrenaline** helps to stimulate and wake us up.

The sense of taste

The sense of taste provides us with less information than the other senses. Its chief role is to select and appreciate food and drink, but much of our sense of taste is in fact linked with our sense of smell. The receptors for sensations of taste are located in our taste buds, which are most numerous on the tongue, but also located on the soft palate and in the throat. We have four primary taste sensations: sour, salt, bitter and sweet. Most tastes are combinations of these four and modified by the sense of smell. In order to taste food it must be dissolved in liquid form, so the saliva plays an important part in dissolving the substances to be tasted. The nerve cells then pass messages to the brain and together with the sense of smell perception of taste occurs.

Sight

The eye is the organ of the sense of sight. It is situated in the orbital cavity and is supplied by the optic nerve. Clear vision depends on the co-ordination of two processes, the refraction of the light rays and the accommodation of the eyes to the light. The pupils of the eyes dilate in poor light and they constrict in bright light. The size of the pupil is controlled by the autonomic nervous system. The movement of the eyes to view an object is caused by the muscular activity of six muscles and the oculomotor, trochlear and abducent cranial nerves.

The lacrimal glands secrete tears which are composed of water, salts and lysozyme (a protective bactericidal enzyme) that wash away irritating materials and prevent microbial infection. It also helps to prevent drying out of the conjunctiva, the membrane lining the eyelids.

Disorders of the eye

Blepharitis

This is an allergic inflammation of the eyelid caused by staphylococcal infection or allergy to dandruff or cosmetics used on the eye.

Cataract

This is an opacity in the lens of the eye that results in blurred vision. It may be congenital or as a result of metabolic disease such as diabetes, through injury or prolonged exposure to infra-red rays.

Conjunctivitis

This is inflammation of the conjunctiva or membrane inside the eyelid and covering the cornea. It becomes red and swollen and is caused by infection. Allergic conjunctivitis may be caused by a variety of antigens such as pollen, dust, spores, animal dander or cosmetics.

Glaucoma

A condition in which loss of vision occurs because of abnormally high pressure in the eye. It can be acute, occurring rapidly with accompanying pain and blurred vision, or chronic, when the pressure gradually increases over a period of time. It is the second-most common cause of blindness in the elderly.

Hearing and balance

The ear is the organ of hearing and is supplied by the vestibulocochlear cranial nerve. It contains receptors for sound waves and receptors for balance, and is divided into three parts: the external, middle and inner ears.

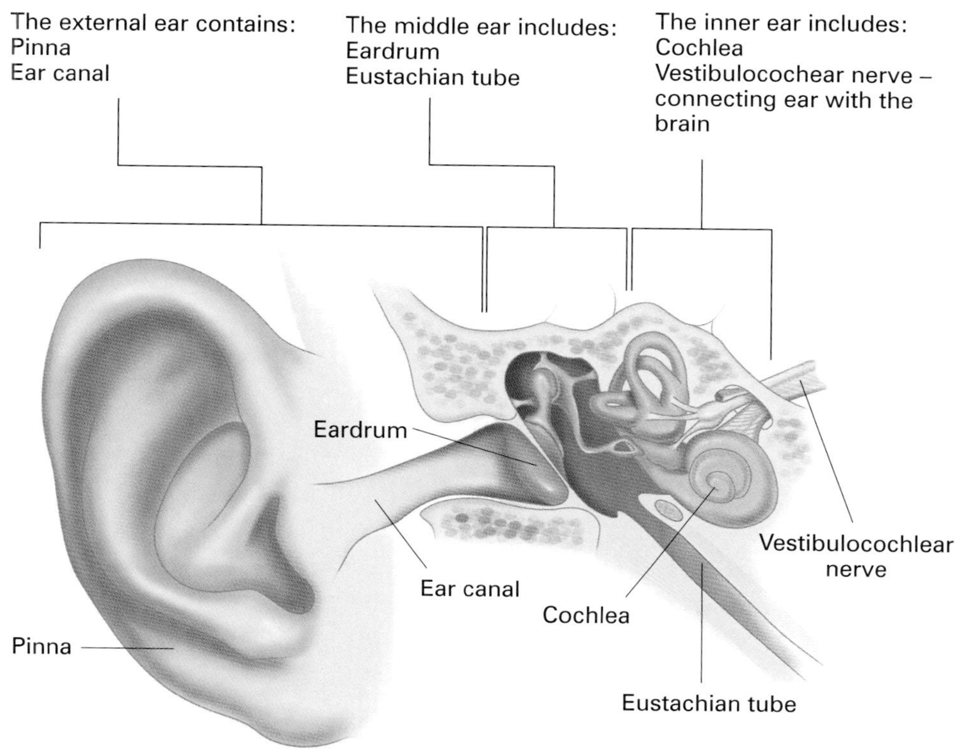

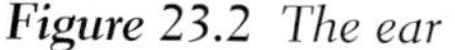
Figure 23.2 *The ear*

The external ear collects the sound waves and directs them inwards to the middle ear or tympanic cavity, which is a small air-filled cavity separated from the external ear by the eardrum. There is an auditory tube in this part of the ear which is responsible for equalising air pressure.

The inner ear contains the organs of hearing and balance. Sound waves pass from the middle to the inner ear in a series of vibrations, which ultimately lead to the generation of nerve impulses, which reach the brain and sound is perceived.

The ear is also responsible for the monitoring of the position of the body and movements of the head. The inner ear in particular contains a maze of tubes filled with fluid, all at different levels and angles, working together to maintain balance. Together with the brain, eyes and muscles, the body remains balanced and in an upright position as long as nothing disturbs the equilibrium.

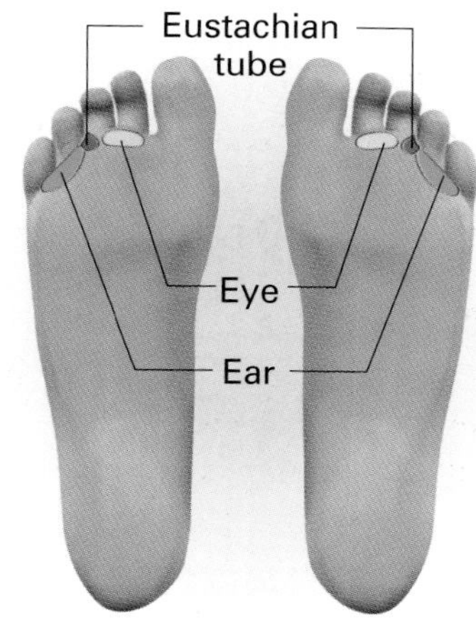

Foot map – Eye, ear and eustachian tube reflexes.

Disorders of the ear

Méniere's syndrome

This is a disorder of the inner ear and has several characteristics, which include fluctuating hearing loss, vertigo, vomiting and tinnitus (ringing in the ears). This can be progressive, lasting for years, and result in total loss of hearing.

Motion sickness

This is a functional disorder of perpetual movement characterised by nausea and vomiting. The more common varieties are car and sea sickness. Emotional and visual factors can affect this condition.

Otitis

This is inflammation of the ear, affecting the outer ear. Acute **otitis media** affects the middle ear usually due to viral or bacterial infection, and symptoms include pain and high fever. The condition, **secretory otitis media**, or glue ear, is an accumulation of fluid in the middle ear, which can cause hearing loss and often affects children. Inflammation of the inner ear causes vertigo, vomiting, loss of balance and deafness.

PRACTICE IN CONTEXT

Practise working the reflex points of the ears and eyes and investigate the effects on the body of an inner ear disorder.

ASSESSMENT OF KNOWLEDGE

1. How does the sense of smell protect the body?
2. Where are the sensory receptors for smell found?
3. Which neurotransmitters when stimulated by odour have a relaxing and calming effect?
4. What is the chief role of our sense of taste?
5. What two processes does clear vision depend upon?
6. What is the function of the lacrimal glands?
7. What is conjunctivitis?
8. What is the second most common cause of blindness in the elderly?
9. What are the two main functions of the ear?
10. What is tinnitus?

- Maintaining standards in business
- Research for setting up a business
- The business plan

Setting up in **Business**

24 Maintaining standards in business

Setting up in business or working for someone else will require the reflexologist to comply with current legislation and local bylaws. To maintain professional standards it is also necessary to follow the industry codes of practice, as well as establishing or following their own personal policies, practices and procedures. This is equally important whether they own their own business, employ other people, work alone providing a mobile service, work for an employer or work away from their employer's premises.

Legal requirements in health and safety

The working environment must be maintained to a high level of health and safety as this will help in the prevention of accidents and cross-infection. It also indicates a high level of commitment to the client in providing a professional and safe sanctuary for the therapeutic treatment and an atmosphere conducive to relaxation.

There are several Acts of Parliament and EU (European Union) directives, implemented in the United Kingdom, relating to health and safety in the workplace which are relevant to the reflexologist. European law has had an impact on health and safety legislation in recent years and it is enforced by means of directives. A directive sets out the standards that each member state must achieve and the UK implements these directives by formulating regulations.

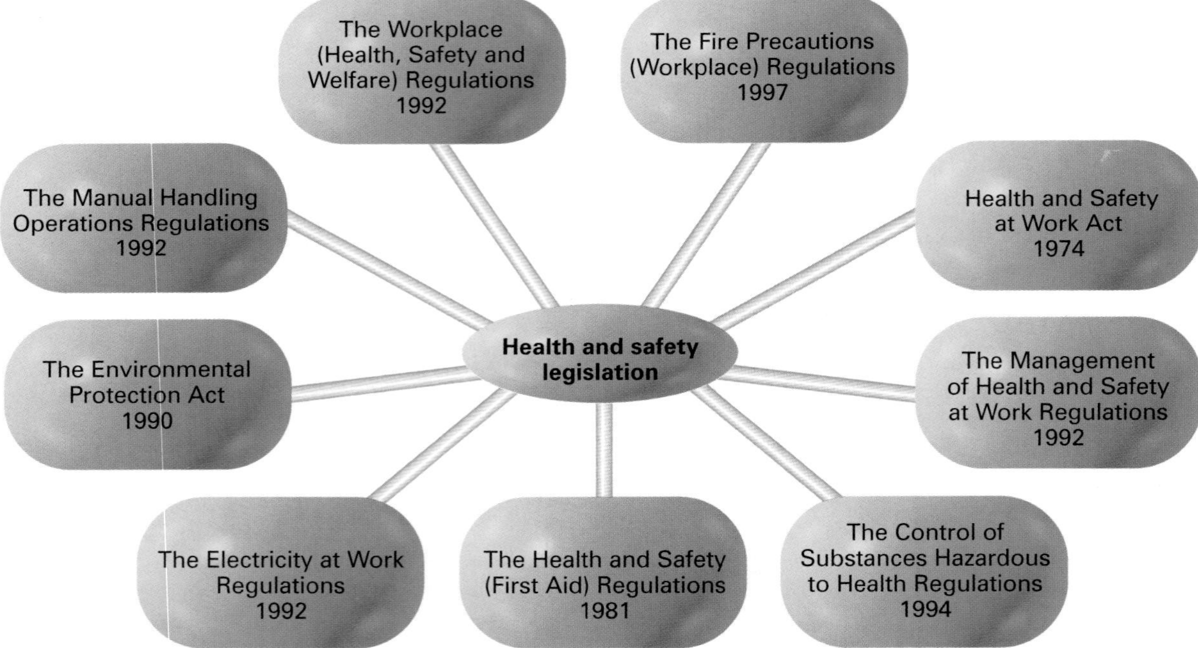
Health and safety legislation
The Workplace (Health, Safety and Welfare) Regulations 1992
The Fire Precautions (Workplace) Regulations 1997
The Manual Handling Operations Regulations 1992
Health and Safety at Work Act 1974
The Environmental Protection Act 1990
The Management of Health and Safety at Work Regulations 1992
The Electricity at Work Regulations 1992
The Health and Safety (First Aid) Regulations 1981
The Control of Substances Hazardous to Health Regulations 1994

Figure 24.1 *There are several Health and Safety Acts to be taken into account when starting a business*

The Health and Safety at Work Act 1974

This Act imposes general obligations and duties on all those concerned with health, safety and welfare in the workplace, and it still forms the basis of health and safety regulations in the UK. New regulations have come into effect in response to the EU directives stating how these obligations and duties must be fulfilled.

The duties of the employer are to ensure, as far as is reasonably practicable, the health, safety and welfare of all employees by providing and maintaining safe systems of work, ensuring safety in the handling, storing and using of equipment and substances. They must also provide information, instruction, training and supervision to ensure health and safety. The environment must be well maintained and access to and exit from the premises should be without risk. When there are a number of employees working in a business the employer must also provide adequate facilities for their welfare whilst at work.

This Act also requires the employee to take reasonable care of themselves and anyone for whom they are responsible. They have to comply with statutory duties and requirements and they must not intentionally or recklessly misuse anything provided in the interest of health, safety or welfare. To prevent cross-infection certain rules of hygiene should be followed.

- Sanitise equipment using an appropriate method.
- Clean floors daily.
- Wash curtains regularly.
- Wipe over work surfaces with disinfectant.
- Clean sinks after use.
- Use clean bedlinen or a disposable cover for each client.
- Use clean towels for each client.
- Place soiled towels in a laundry basket after use.
- Wash your hands before touching the client.

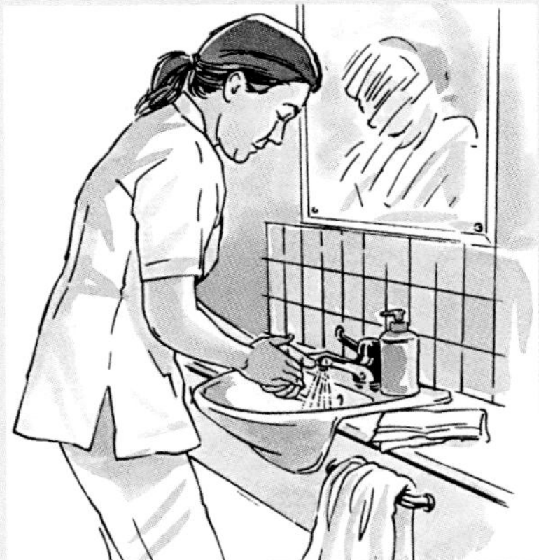

Figure 24.2 Washing hands before and after treatment helps prevent cross-infection

- Cover cuts or abrasions in the skin.
- Clean all equipment after use.
- Replace tops and lids on bottles and containers to prevent contamination.
- Use disposable spatulas to remove products from containers.
- Put waste in a closed waterproof container.
- Sharps box must be used to dispose of sharp objects and broken glass.
- Check client for contraindications.
- Clean all spillages immediately.

The Management of Health and Safety at Work Regulations 1992

The principal duties of an employer according to these regulations are:

- To assess health and safety risks to employees, clients and any others who may visit the business premises.
- To implement, monitor and review any preventative measures that have been put in place.
- To complete health and safety records.
- To appoint the necessary number of competent people, to implement evacuation procedures and to provide training.
- To provide employees with comprehensive and relevant information regarding health and safety.
- To consult with an elected health and safety representative on health and safety issues.

Monitoring health and safety is important and regular health and safety checks must be made to ensure the business is complying with legislation. Random checks can also be made to ensure that all staff members are fulfilling their obligations in maintaining the standards laid down by the management.

The Workplace (Health, Safety and Welfare) Regulations 1992

These regulations ensure that all places of work meet the health, safety and welfare needs of the employees.

- The workplace must be well maintained and everything kept in good working order with repairs carried out to a safe standard and in good time. Ventilation must be effective and the working temperature, sanitary and rest facilities should provide reasonable comfort. The lighting must be suitable and floor, ceilings, walls, fixtures, fittings and soft furnishings must be kept clean. The floor covering should be suitable for the workplace, with no uneven or slippery surfaces, and it should be kept clear of obstruction. If there is a staircase on the premises it should have a substantial and secure handrail.
- Waste products must be disposed of in a covered receptacle, which must be emptied regularly. Cleaning must be carried out using suitable materials that will not expose anyone to a health and safety risk.
- The working area of the reflexologist should provide sufficient room to work safely and the seating provided should give adequate support to the lower back.
- A changing room with provision for outdoor clothes must be supplied when special workwear is required and there should be secure facilities provided for clothes. There should be suitable provision for eating and rest facilities arranged in such a way that non-smokers will not experience discomfort from tobacco smoke.
- The sanitary conveniences must be adequately ventilated, lit, clean, easily accessible and in sufficient numbers. For 1–5 people 1 WC and 1 wash station, and for 6–25 people 2 WCs and 2 wash stations. There must be suitable means provided for the disposal of sanitary items in a convenience used by women. Washing facilities must be provided in the immediate vicinity of each sanitary convenience or changing room and they must be clean, well lit and ventilated with a clean supply of hot and cold running water, soap to wash with and the means to dry the hands.
- An adequate supply of drinking water should be supplied which is easily accessible with sufficient drinking vessels or a water fountain.

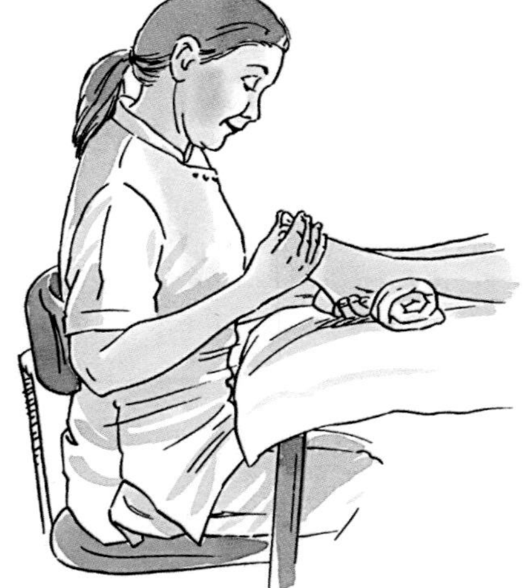

Figure 24.3 *Good back support prevents backache and maintains the correct position*

The Manual Handling Operations Regulations 1992

Manual handling operations is the transporting or supporting of a load either by hand or bodily force. It includes lifting, putting down, pushing, pulling, carrying or moving. A 'load' is any item or object that is being supported or transported.

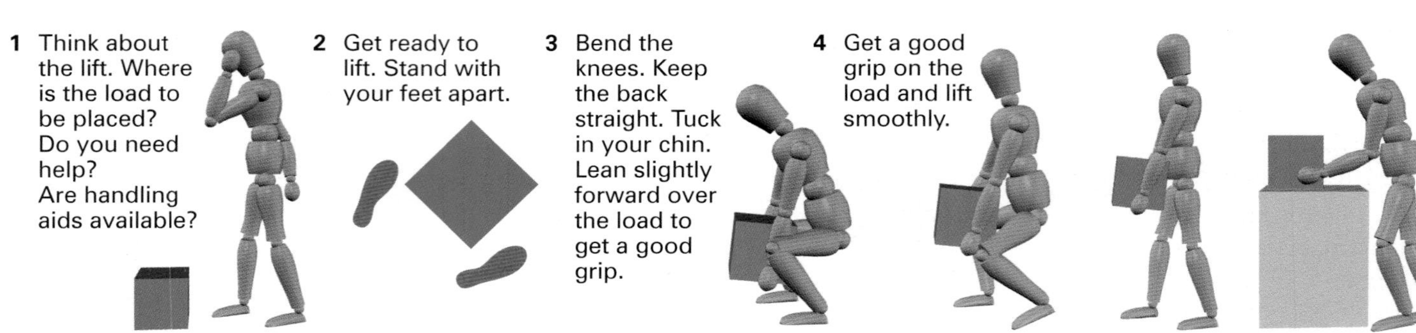

1 Think about the lift. Where is the load to be placed? Do you need help? Are handling aids available?
2 Get ready to lift. Stand with your feet apart.
3 Bend the knees. Keep the back straight. Tuck in your chin. Lean slightly forward over the load to get a good grip.
4 Get a good grip on the load and lift smoothly.

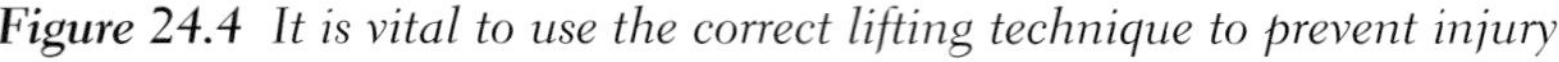

Figure 24.4 *It is vital to use the correct lifting technique to prevent injury*

The reflexologist may be expected to receive, transport and use portable equipment which may be classed as a load. These regulations implement a European directive on the manual handling of loads to prevent injuries such as strains, sprains, back injuries or cumulative damage which causes incapacity. Never lift an elderly or disabled person; instead use steps to allow them access to a high couch or use a low portable couch or chair that they may sit or lie on easily.

It is the duty of an employer, when a task is unavoidable, to assess any risks involved and then avoid them or reduce them as much as possible. This may be achieved by:

- delivering goods to the point of use
- carrying out a task *in situ* without transporting anything heavy
- using trolleys to transport anything large or heavy
- splitting loads to make them smaller or lighter
- asking for assistance to distribute the load.

When moving something heavy, think carefully about the task and plan ahead:

- Choose the flattest straightest route.
- Remove any obstacle you may trip over.
- Look for a place en route to stop and rest.
- Make sure the area you are placing the load is clear.
- Check the load has an even distribution of weight.
- Make sure there is nothing sharp protruding from the load.
- Ask for assistance in lifting and carrying.

The Control of Substances Hazardous to Health Regulations (COSHH) 1994

More commonly referred to as the COSHH regulations, these state that every employer has a legal obligation to assess the risks associated with hazardous substances used in the workplace and to take steps to eliminate or control these risks. The regulations apply to all substances which have an adverse effect on health if they are not handled, stored or used correctly.

There are several steps to be taken by a competent person within the business or organisation, and these are:

- Inspect the workplace and make a list of all hazardous substances.
- Assess the potential risk to health, evaluate the measures in place and devise new measures to be taken in the safe storage, handling, transportation, use and disposal of hazardous substances.
- All staff will require training in the use of these substances and the effectiveness of the measures taken must then be monitored.
- Keep detailed records of measures taken and safety checks made to comply with the legislation.

The reflexologist does not require the use of any substances that are hazardous to health as part of the treatment; however, to maintain standards in health and safety and prevent cross-infection, there are cleaning substances which may be used and pose a risk to health. The place of work may be part of a larger establishment and this may necessitate the reflexologist coming into contact with hazardous substances relevant to other businesses or practices.

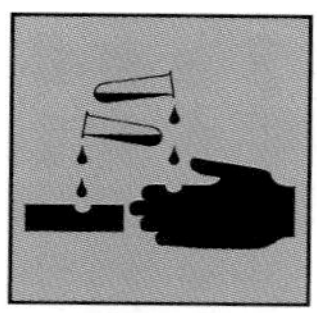
(a) Corrosive

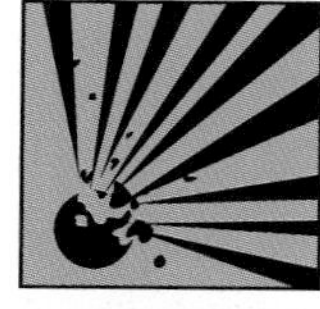
(b) Explosive

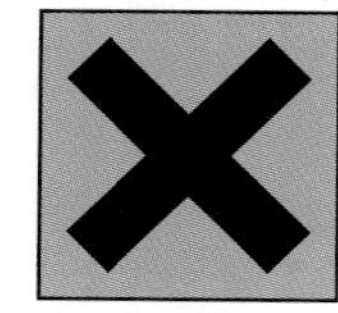
(c) Harmful

(d) Highly flammable

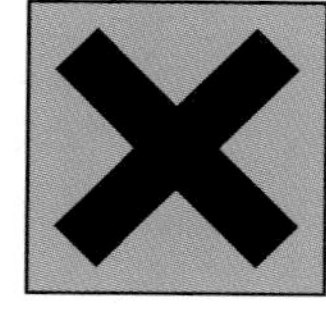
(e) Irritant

(f) Oxidizing

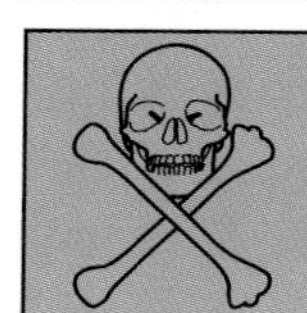
(g) Toxic

Figure 24.5 *COSHH classification*

The effects of hazardous substances may cause different problems. They may:

- cause irritation when exposed to the skin or eyes
- burn the skin when making direct contact
- give off fumes, which may irritate the eyes or lungs
- cause breathing difficulties, irritating or restricting the air passages
- cause allergies sensitising the skin immediately or after repeated exposure.

Any product which has been identified as hazardous must be stored in the following way – in a cool dry place, well ventilated, out of direct sunlight, in a metal cupboard, in the correct container, away from naked flames or heat and out of reach of children.

The Health and Safety (First Aid) Regulations 1981

According to these regulations, the employer is obliged to ensure that there is adequate first aid provision for their employees. The requirements vary depending on the number of employees and the type of work which is carried out. In a small clinic with five members of staff comprising of a receptionist, two reflexologists and two other therapists, there is a minimum requirement.

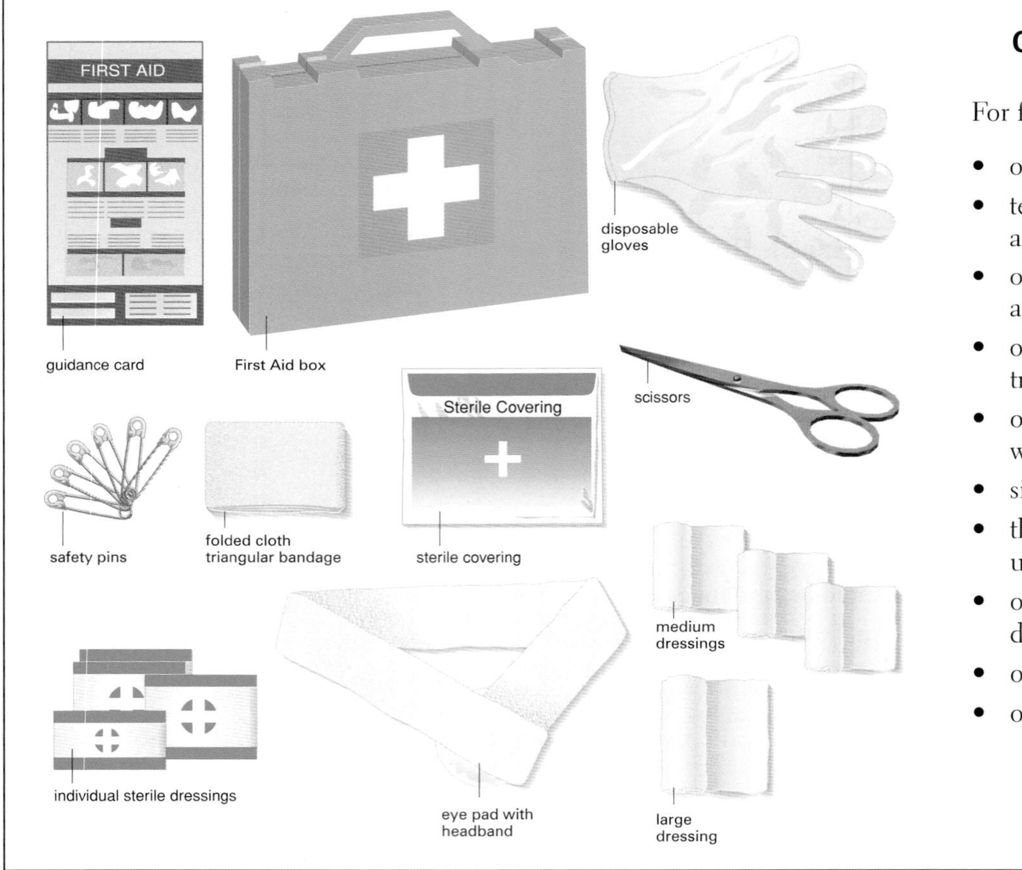

Contents of first aid box

For five employees:

- one guidance card
- ten individually wrapped sterile adhesive dressings, assorted sizes
- one sterile eye pad with attachment
- one individually wrapped triangular bandage
- one sterile covering for serious wounds
- six safety pins
- three medium sized sterile unmedicated dressings
- one large sterile unmedicated dressing
- one pair of disposable gloves
- one pair of scissors.

Most minor accidents and injuries which occur may be treated by the appointed person, who will hold a current first aid certificate. Any person qualified to administer first aid would also be in a position to help with the more serious problems while the injured party is waiting to be seen by a doctor.

For guidance on the responsibilities of the first aid representative, see page 215.

Accidents, no matter how minor, must be recorded in an accident book, which should be kept for a minimum of three years from the date of the last entry.

The following is an example of an accident report form.

The Complementary Therapy Clinic
Hardwicke Crescent Sheffield SH5 10A

Date : 20th September 2001

Time : 11.30 am

Name : Jayne Salt Signed ....

Address : 7 Burton Avenue

Tel. No. : 0789 653421

Status : Client

Description of accident :

Miss Salt had been resting for ten minutes in the relaxation area having a herbal tea after her reflexology treatment. She slipped and fell when the heel of her shoe broke as she was walking to reception to make her next appointment. As she slipped she banged her arm on a shelf, grazing her elbow. The injury was superficial but first aid was applied.

Location of accident : In the reception area next to the product display.

Nature of injuries : Slight graze to the elbow, superficial bleeding.

Action taken : The first aid representative was called. He provided the necessary treatment by cleaning the graze and covering it with a waterproof dressing.

Witness 1 : Kathleen Fitzgerald Status : Therapist Signed ....

Witness 2 : Faye Ramjaun Status : Manageress Signed ....

First aid rep : Jason Clarke Status : Sports therapist Signed ....

The Fire Precautions (Workplace) (Amendment) Regulations 1999

These regulations update the Fire Precautions Acts of 1971 and 1999 and provide for the minimum safety standards in the workplace. To comply with these regulations the risk of fire in the workplace must be assessed. When five or more people are employed in the business, a formal record must be kept of the risk assessments and the measures proposed to deal with those risks.

All members of staff must be informed of the results of risk assessment and written reports must be made available on request. Training in fire and evacuation procedures must be given and smoke alarms or automatic fire detectors should be provided. Any means of escape must be clear of obstruction and doors must be unlocked and in good working order. The correct fire fighting equipment must be provided and maintained in good working order. A fire certificate is required when more than 20 people work in the business or where more than 10 people work other than on the ground floor.

To reduce the risk of fire and to ensure safe evacuation in the case of fire there are certain precautions to be taken.

FIRE PRECAUTIONS
➢ COSHH assessment of all substances should cover fire risks and suitable control measures put in place. ➢ Combustible material must be removed from areas it is not required. ➢ Candles should not be left burning. ➢ Rubbish must be disposed of regularly. ➢ Flammable materials must be used and stored safely. ➢ Electrical equipment must be regularly checked. ➢ Plug sockets must not be overloaded. ➢ Portable heaters must be placed in a safe position. ➢ Smoking should only be allowed in designated safe areas. ➢ Ashtrays must be used rather than waste bins and floors. ➢ Fire exits and the passageway to them must be kept clear. ➢ Fire extinguishers must be kept in an easily accessible place. ➢ Fire exits must be kept unlocked during working hours. ➢ Fire doors must not be wedged open. ➢ Fire drills should be carried out to check evacuation procedures.

In the case of a very small fire breaking out, which may be easily controlled, the fire extinguishers may be used. Two people should always be present to put out the fire, as long as it does not endanger their safety. It is essential to use the correct fire extinguisher for the type of fire. In accordance with regulations, all fire extinguishers should be red in colour with a coloured panel indicating their contents.

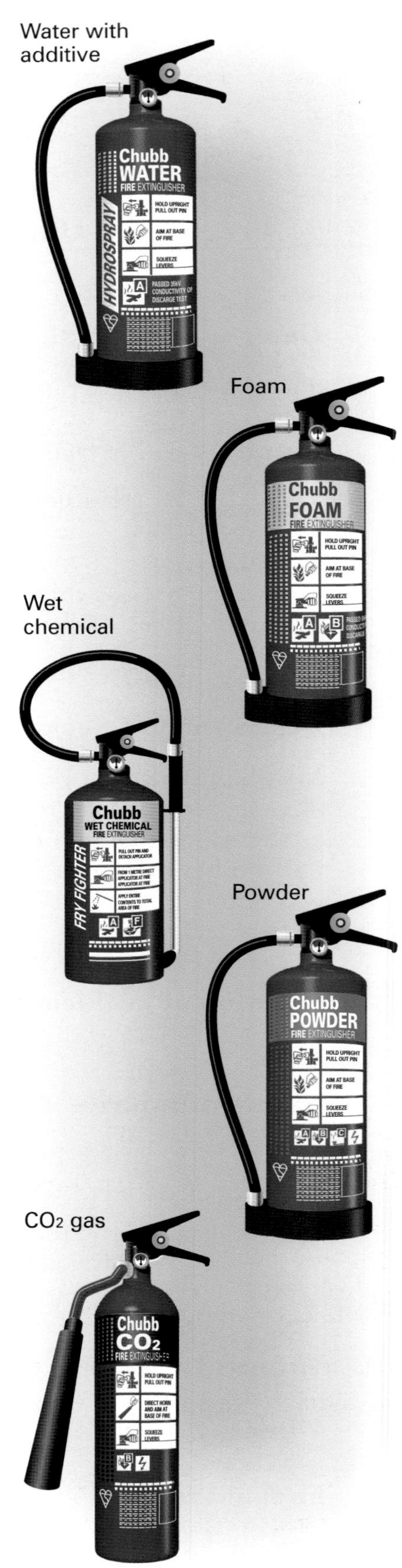

Fire extinguishers

The following table shows the contents of fire extinguishers.

COLOUR	CONTENTS	USE
RED	Water	Paper, fabric, wood, textiles
BLUE	Powder	Paper, textiles, wood, burning liquid, electrical
BLACK	Carbon dioxide	Burning liquid and electrical
CREAM	Foam	Burning liquid

Fire evacuation procedure

This is the procedure to follow when there is a fire.

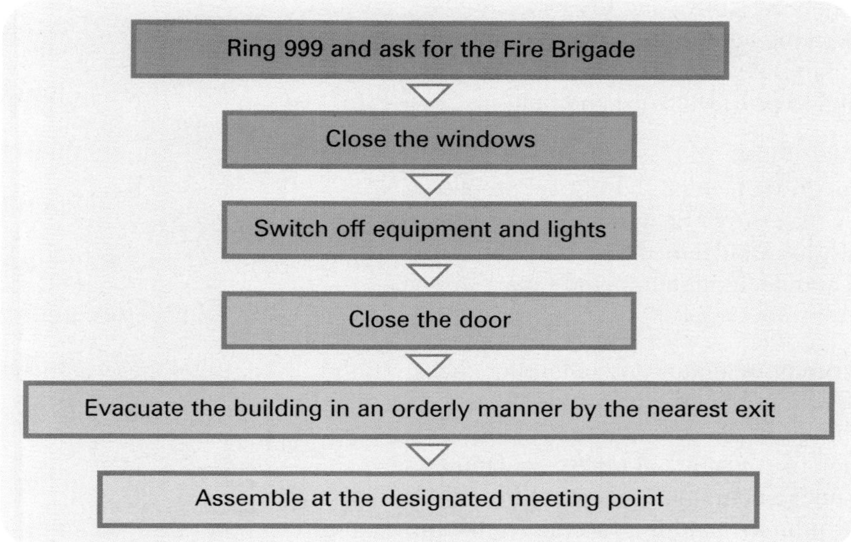

For maximum safety the following points must be considered.

- Never use a lift – always use the staircase or fire escape when above ground level.
- Never stop to collect personal belongings and only re-enter the building when the all clear has been given.
- All employees must be aware of their role and responsibilities in the event of fire and special arrangements must be made for disabled employees, clients or visitors.

The Electricity at Work Regulations 1992

These regulations govern electrical safety in the workplace, where all electrical equipment and systems must be suitable for the work involved and safe to use. Care must be taken to buy, install and maintain equipment taking into account manufacturers' instructions and recommendations.

Regular tests must be carried out at least once a year on all electrical appliances and by a qualified electrician. A written record of each test must be made with the date and name of the person carrying out the tests.

The Environmental Protection Act 1990

When disposing of waste chemicals in the course of work it is important to comply with this Act. Any person has the duty to dispose of waste safely in such a way that it does not cause harm to the environment or any individual. To comply with this Act you must ask the supplier for information about the safe use and disposal of their products, and training must be provided for all employees in the safe use and disposal of chemicals. It is important that chemical substances are not disposed of where they may be found by an unauthorised person, in particular children.

Enforcing health and safety law

All legislation establishes that each individual member of the workforce, from the owner down to the most junior member of staff, is responsible for maintaining health and safety within the workplace. It is important to understand the implications of incorrect action or ignoring health and safety legislation. Insurance cover is provided only if the rules and regulations laid down by law are being followed.

The enforcing authorities are the Health and Safety Executive and the local authority, council or borough. Both of these enforcing authorities are responsible for appointing suitably qualified inspectors whose main roles are to ensure that law relating to health and safety is complied with and to provide advice and help in matters of health and safety.

The powers of the health and safety inspector are to visit, enter and inspect premises at any time. If there is a suspected problem they may carry out an investigation and take any samples, photographs or measurements that are deemed necessary. They should have unlimited access to records, books and documentation and may interview anyone they consider appropriate.

The occasions when an inspector may visit the premises are to carry out a spot check, if there has been a complaint from a member of the public or if an accident has occurred on the premises. The visit may result in an improvement notice being served if they believe that there is a contravention of a health and safety regulation and that it may be continued or repeated. The notice contains a statement from the inspector detailing their belief that a law has been broken and the specific regulation, with reasons to support their findings. A specific period of time will be given to put the situation right and this should not be less than 21 days.

If the inspector believes that there is a risk of serious injury because of a work activity, a prohibition notice may be served. This contains the inspector's belief that there is a risk of personal injury, the problems that create the specific risk, supporting evidence and a statement directing the unsafe activity to cease. This notice can take effect immediately, causing the hazardous activity to stop.

The worst outcome of an inspector's visit is prosecution and the circumstances which may cause this are:

- when there is a failure to comply with an improvement or prohibition notice
- when the inspectors have been obstructed in the course of their duties
- breaching any health and safety regulations
- making false statements in documentation required to be kept by law
- failing to carry out any of the general duties of the HASWA 1974 or other relevant statutes.

Prosecution may result in a fine or a term of imprisonment and any person involved in an offence will be prosecuted. It is the responsibility of every member of staff to ensure that health and safety documentation is accurate and up to date and that all breaches of health and safety are reported immediately to their line manager.

Consumer protection

The reflexologist must be aware of the responsibilities to his or her client in relation to selling goods and services. There are three Acts that are important and these are:

The Supply of Goods and Services Act 1982

This act helps to protect any consumer from faulty goods and poor service. It applies to the supply of a service, goods supplied as part of a service, free gifts supplied with promotional products, hire goods and goods supplied in part exchange. In supplying goods, this Act requires them to be of reasonable quality, fit for the purpose they were sold, and they must fit their description. When providing a service you must work within a reasonable time, work with reasonable care and charge a reasonable price.

The Consumer Protection Act 1987

This Act safeguards the consumer from products used or sold that are not safe. It is the responsibility of the supplier of goods to provide clear instructions for use and safe handling and to ensure that goods conform to the approved standards. This Act also makes it an offence to give misleading price information about goods and services.

Trade Descriptions Act 1968

This Act provides protection for the consumer who has been misled or given inaccurate descriptions of the goods or services offered. The retailer must not make false claims about goods or services; this includes information in an advertisement, a brochure, provided verbally, or in a price list.

25 Research for setting up a business

The nature of reflexology treatment provides great flexibility when setting up in business. As a service, it can work successfully as a stand alone business as well as alongside other businesses or within other professional practices. There are many health service workers training in reflexology to gain additional skills that will help their patients, and doctors are becoming more aware of the benefits of reflexology, particularly as an antidote to stress, and are providing locations within a medical practice or health centre. There are also many physiotherapists and chiropodists providing reflexology as an additional service, which complements their existing practice.

More recently, as complementary and alternative therapies increase in popularity, complementary therapy centres are becoming more widely available and a number of different therapies are offered under the same roof; existing beauty salons are also adding holistic therapies to their range of treatments.

Whatever the location or reason to start a business, it is important for the individual to research the prospective market thoroughly and identify the need for the proposed business. The success of any business is in supplying a service or product that the consumer needs or wants.

The reception area of a health and beauty salon within a hotel

The research plan

To establish the viability of the proposed business a research plan will help. This should include:

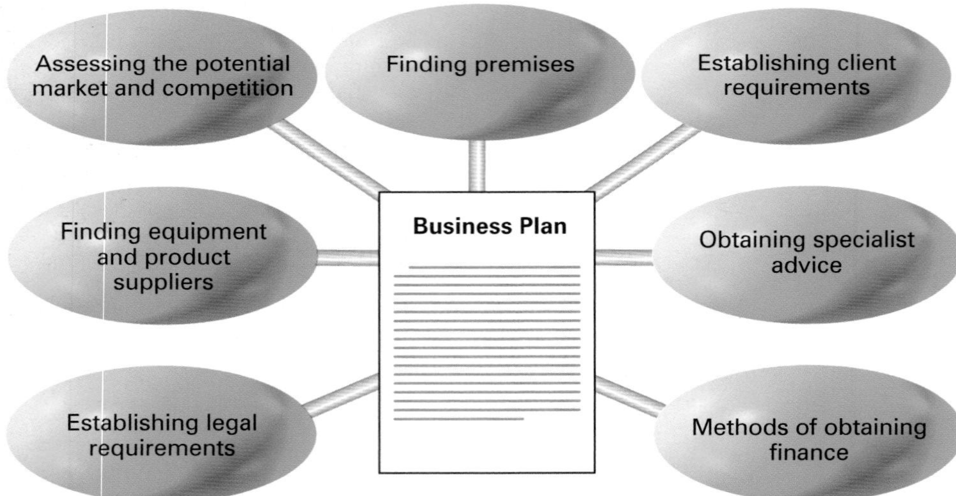

Figure 25.1 *A research plan will help to establish the viability of a business*

Assessing the potential market and competition

Market research is collecting, collating and analysing data relevant to the business to help establish its viability.

- You will need to assess how many people are likely to want your service and if the numbers will be sufficient to make your business viable, whether it is a growing or static market and what share in that market do you think you will achieve.

- Look at your competitors, in particular, how well established they are, how your services or prices compare with theirs and what will you provide that they don't. One of the easiest ways in which to achieve this is to visit your competitor/s as a client and gain reliable first-hand knowledge.
- Market research allows you to establish if there is a market segment on which to concentrate. Market segmentation is dividing an existing market into a number of smaller submarkets, and identifying groups of customers with similar requirements, e.g. the housebound, patients in hospital, the elderly, sports people, health and fitness fans or pregnant mums. Look for a gap in the market that you could fill.

The more information you acquire about potential clients and the current market, the better the chance of minimising risk and maximising success.

Establishing client requirements

Your clients will come from all walks of life and different age groups; they will have varying lifestyles and may have particular health problems or disabilities. It is important to be able to cater for the clients individual requirements and these could include some or all of the following:

- Providing a mobile service for those people who are housebound or find it difficult to travel.
- Providing flexible opening hours for those people who work 9–5, Monday to Friday. Most clients appreciate a late or weekend appointment.
- Providing your services *in situ*, possibly working from a room within another business or a large building servicing many businesses. These businesses could be high-powered and stressful and may appreciate the services of a reflexologist to be available as an antidote to the stresses and strains of the job. Some large organisations provide hair, beauty and massage services for their staff as a perk of the job.
- Providing other services which complement reflexology.
- Providing easy access to your premises for disabled clients.
- Providing a professional and relaxing environment in which to have the treatment, using quality equipment and products.

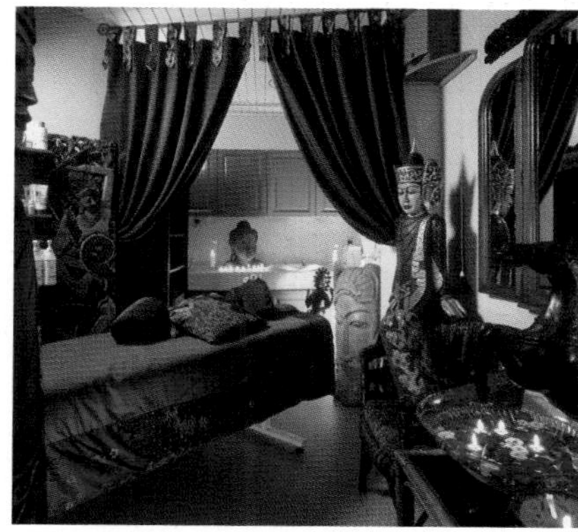

It is important to provide a relaxing environment for your clients

Market research is again a useful tool for collecting the information you require to establish what your potential clients will need. Once you have an established clientele it is easier to collect information as you may already be aware of their requirements, you can question them about their needs, or ask them to fill in questionnaires to collate specific information.

Finding premises

The location of your business is important to ensure that clients will not have to travel too far, will be able to find it easily, be close to public transport and be able to park easily when travelling by car.

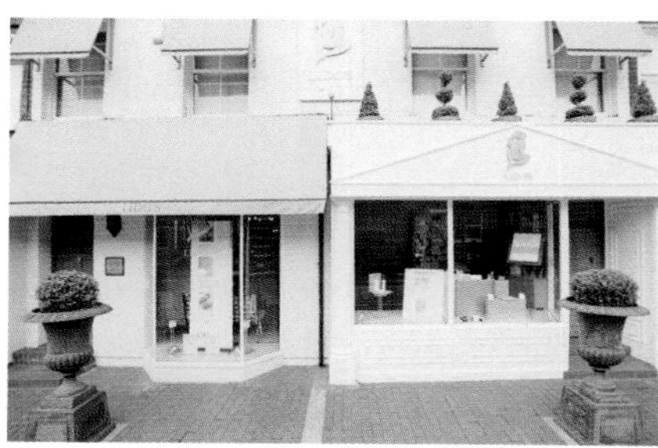

The location of your business is crucial to its success

Your premises should be in the right area and at the right price, and centrally situated in a well-populated area. If it is close to other businesses which have a brisk trade you can benefit from passing trade, e.g. post offices, banks, building societies or chemist shops. Being situated near other businesses such as a hairdressing or beauty salon, or near a medical health centre could also bring in new clients.

The more central the position in a town, the more expensive the cost of buying, renting or leasing premises. The advantage for a reflexologist is the space required is quite small; one or two treatment rooms, a toilet and small reception area is all that is required for a small business. Ensure that the fixtures and fittings are adequate. These may include lighting, heating, electricity and water supplies, telephone and sanitary facilities. If it is necessary to install some or all of these facilities it may add considerably to start-up costs.

One important consideration, to be taken into account, is the expansion of the business as it grows. If you intend to employ staff or take on other therapies, it is best to plan for this initially and buy or lease somewhere of a suitable size, as it may prove costly to constantly move to larger premises as you grow.

Once you have found the right premises there are three options: to rent, lease or to buy.

Renting

A short-term rental agreement is an option for a new business as the financial outlay will not be so great whilst establishing the business; however, the shorter the term of agreement the higher the rental cost. Opting for a long-term agreement will lower the rent but it will commit you to your agreement for several years. A good way to start, as so little room is required, is to find a room to rent within another business or with a health care professional. You have the advantage of sharing costs, gaining clients from an already established clientele, the use of the available resources, such as telephone, computer, fax machine etc. and possibly the services of a receptionist. It is important before signing any agreement to make sure there are no clauses making you liable for the upkeep of the property, unless you have agreed a reasonable rent to reflect this.

Leasing

This is when the business buys the leasehold rights to the premises for a period of time, maybe 25 or 50 years, and then pays an annual ground rent.

The main advantage is that existing capital will be available for the business, rather than being tied up in buying a property with high mortgage repayments that could be a burden, and you have a capital asset for balance sheet purposes with less expenditure than when buying. When negotiating the lease it may be advisable to go for as short a lease as possible with the option to renew the lease for a longer period of time when you feel sure the business will be a success.

The main disadvantage is that over a long period of time the lease will cost as much, if not more, than buying a property. You must also seek permission from the landlord before carrying out any alterations. When the lease expires you have the right to agree new terms but the landlord may refuse if you have not been a good tenant or if they require the premises for their own occupation.

It is advisable to seek the advice of a solicitor before signing a lease and always check the following:

- Can the premises can be used for the purpose you require?
- Will you be able to make any alterations that you need for your business?
- Who is responsible for the repair and maintenance of the premises?
- What is the length of the lease?
- Is subletting part of the premises permitted?
- How often is the rent reviewed?

The Landlord and Tenant Act 1954

The purpose of this Act is to give the tenant some security in remaining in the premises after the lease has expired and to be compensated for improvements which have added to the value of business premises. The landlord has to give six months notice if the lease is to be terminated. This will give the tenant the opportunity to apply to the court to have the lease renewed. The court may refuse the application if the landlord can show the following:

- The rent is in arrears.
- The property has been allowed to fall into disrepair.
- The landlord has found alternative premises for the tenant.
- The premises are to be demolished or reconstructed.
- The landlord needs the premises for his/her own occupation.

Buying

A small business may buy freehold premises along with the business in them. Normally when purchasing a business property you will have to provide 20–25% of the total purchase price and then arrange a commercial mortgage, which may be difficult to obtain for a new business.

The advantages are: it is a good long-term investment, particularly if a good property is bought at the right price and then sold at a profit some years later; you will have no rent to pay and tax relief can be claimed on interest payments and capital allowance claimed against the purchase price.

The disadvantages are: finding the high deposit required, tying up available finance in the property, which could be used to invest in the business itself, and the cost of maintaining and improving the property yourself.

It is essential to seek professional help and advice when buying a freehold property and check that there are no undeclared mortgages or charges existing against the premises. It is also advisable to check that there are no proposed building plans or changes to the area which may adversely affect your business.

Business from home

The final option is using a room in your own home for your business. You may wish to consider converting an integral garage or changing part of your home into a small treatment room. If you consider the latter then you must obtain planning permission to change from domestic use to business use. You will generally not require planning permission if you do not alter the structure of your home and the room you use is still primarily for domestic use, but always check with your local planning authority if in doubt.

If you build a structure to accommodate your business then you will require building regulations approval and an inspector will regularly check that foundations are sufficient and that the builder is complying with the approved details of the building plan.

Finding equipment and product suppliers

Transport may be required if you intend to set up a mobile business. You may already own a vehicle but is it suitable for carrying all your equipment and is it reliable? It must be in good working order so that it doesn't let you down. Consider the size you need, how many miles you will be travelling and if you are intending to buy a new or second-hand vehicle. When lifting equipment in and out of your car it is important to have a model which allows you to do so with ease and to prevent strain or injury. It will be a major cost so it is important to research all options carefully – seek advice if necessary and make sure it creates the right image for your business.

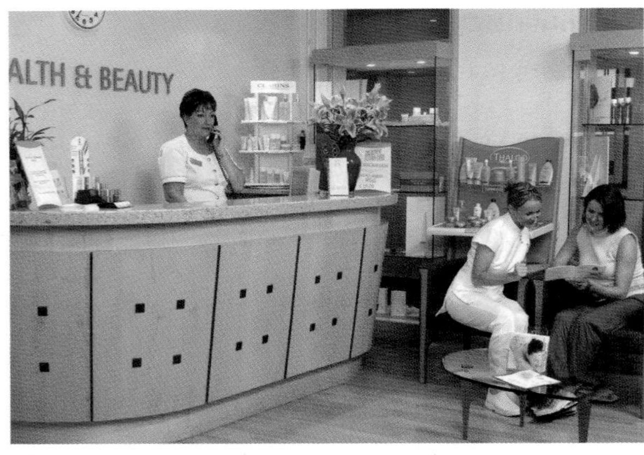

Make a list of the equipment you will need for the reception area

Make a list of the equipment and products you will need, as well as essential requirements for the administration of the business, such as computer, chairs, table, reception desk, display materials, refreshment making facilities, appointment book, record cards, filing systems and health and safety equipment. Divide this list into what you already have and the necessary or desirable items you have to get, as the cost of equipment must be considered. You must, therefore, research your potential suppliers carefully.

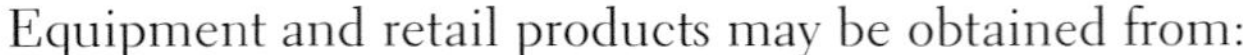

Equipment and retail products may be obtained from:

- the manufacturer directly
- through a company agent or representative
- from a wholesaler
- from a retail outlet.

Wholesalers are a link between the manufacturer and your business. They will buy in bulk and sell smaller quantities to you. The advantages of using a wholesaler are:

- They may be local and can deliver quickly, allowing you to keep a low level of stock in the business with the knowledge that it can be replaced as soon as you require new stock.
- They will offer a wide range of products and equipment providing you with choice.
- They will carry stock from a variety of companies.
- They provide a more personal service and you can establish a professional relationship which is mutually beneficial. They will provide you with up-to-date information about products and market trends.

Manufacturers will provide their product more cheaply but may insist that you place large orders, which a small business may not be able to afford. Buying directly from a retail outlet is expensive but may be necessary if you only require small items or need to replace something very quickly. Once you are an established business you can obtain discounts on many items from wholesale warehouses providing a large range of products suitable for most businesses.

To find a supplier you may look in the local edition of Yellow Pages or the Thomson Directory, or in the advertising section of a professional magazine such as *International Therapist*, *Health and Beauty Salon* or *Professional Beauty*. If you belong to a professional society or association they will be able to offer you assistance and advice, as will your tutor at the establishment or college where you completed your training. A useful source of information will be other professionals; personal recommendation is always good, as you know the products or equipment have already been tried and tested.

Whatever your choice, the considerations are:

- quality products at a reasonable price
- quick efficient service and delivery
- acceptable payment terms to ease your cash flow
- a mutually beneficial professional relationship.

Establishing legal requirements

There are many Acts of Parliament, European Directives and local bylaws that may affect the small business. As we continue to become more closely involved with European law, there appears to be a rapid increase in legislation particularly in the area of health and safety, which has been discussed in detail in Chapter 24.

- The **Town and Country Planning Acts 1971** give responsibility to the local authority in the approval and control of new developments and the approval of change in use of premises. They also have to monitor the appropriate use of 'listed buildings'. The local authority will also undertake the inspection and approval of building work which changes the structure of a building, to comply with building regulations and ensure it is safe.
- The **Local Government Miscellaneous Act 1982** gives the local authority power to grant a license to provide certain services such as epilation, ear piercing, massage and tattooing; they then visit the establishments to ensure that strict hygiene methods are in use. As local councils vary, it is wise to check with your local authority if you think your business may be offering a service or treatment that applies.
- When you have chosen a name for your business you must ensure that it conforms to the rules laid down by the **Companies Name Act 1985** and the **Business Names Act 1985**. The main purpose of these Acts is to enable anyone dealing with a business to know the owner's name and address. The owner of the business must disclose his/her surname as a sole trader and all partners in a partnership, the full corporate name if it is a limited company, and in each case the address. The information must appear on all stationery if trading under a name other than the surname or corporate name.
- If you intend to play background music in the reception area or the treatment room, which will be heard by members of the public (a public performance), you may need to obtain a license. The **Copyright Designs and Patents Act** provides protection for composers, whose music is played for public performance. A license may be obtained from Phonographic Performance Ltd which, together with the Performing Right Society, collects license payments for distribution in the form of royalties to performers and record companies who are members of those bodies.

Obtaining specialist advice

There are many training courses available which will help anyone starting a new business.

Local authorities

Many local authorities, supported by private industry, central and local government, provide training courses in starting and running your own business. The aim of these agencies is to promote economic growth and employment opportunities in local communities. They will provide advice on matters ranging from raising finance and finding premises to marketing and planning the business. They will also have a list of specialists in all areas relating to business — solicitors, accountants, book-keepers, bank managers and insurance companies – to help with starting up a new venture.

Government

The Department of Trade and Industry publishes 'A Guide to Help for Small Businesses' which contains details of government and other schemes specifically to help small businesses. This may be ordered from the DTI Publications orderline – tel: 0870 150 2500.

Business Link

For any advice relating to practical or financial help in setting up a new business, contact Business Link. There may be a small charge or an initial free review and then a subsidised consultancy charge.

To contact your local Business Link operator, call 0845 600 9006.

The bank

Your bank manager will provide advice about business accounts, loans and possibly financial support. He will also know of other professionals who may be able to provide you with assistance in specialist areas. The bank will also be able to provide you with brochures and booklets about starting your own business.

Estate agent

You may need to seek the advice of an estate agent who specialises in commercial property to help you buy or lease premises which will be suitable for your business. This may save you time, as they will know what is currently available, the local developments and any local planning restrictions. They may also be able to provide advice on the best location for your type of business.

Accountant

As a self-employed small business owner it is advisable to employ an accountant. He or she will help you present your case when trying to raise finance. Once the business is established, the accountant will set up an efficient accounting system, explain the tax laws and provide you with invaluable advice about the wide range of expenses that may be deducted from your tax liability, thus reducing your overall tax bill. The fee they charge for this service is also tax deductible!

Solicitor

A commercial solicitor will be able to offer you legal advice on planning, contracts, finance, employment law and consumer protection.

Insurance broker

An insurance broker will be able to find you the best insurance policies for you requirements. Under the Financial Services Act they are required to give you the best impartial advice and not recommend a particular company if it is not appropriate. A free booklet entitled 'Insurance Advice for Small Businesses' is available from the Association of British Insurers tel: 0207 600 3333.

Your business insurance may also be obtained from a professional body such as:

The Federation of Holistic Therapists
3rd Floor, Eastleigh House
Upper Market Street
Eastleigh
Hampshire
SO50 9FD
Tel: 0238 048 8900
www.fht.org.uk

They are experts in the particular fields of holistic and beauty therapy and will be able to provide appropriate cover.

Your insurance broker will advise you of all the required insurance and explain in detail why you may need it, if you so wish; however, you may consider some of the following types of insurance for your particular needs:

- Buildings insurance.
- Building contents to include fixtures, fittings and equipment.
- Motor vehicle insurance.
- Insurance for retail and consumable stock.
- Employers' liability.
- Public liability.
- Product liability.
- Professional indemnity.
- Health insurance.
- Key person insurance.
- Life assurance.

Methods of obtaining finance

If your business proposal is a sound one, with evidence that it will succeed, and your business plan is well presented, you will find that financial support will be forthcoming.

Your own capital

You may have capital of your own that you wish to invest in a business, for example, a lottery win, redundancy or an inheritance. If this is the case, you must ensure that your business is a viable proposition before investing all you have. Producing a business plan and seeking professional advice is just as important for you, as when borrowing money from other sources.

The bank

Your bank may be your first port of call when obtaining finance. If you have been a loyal customer for many years they will be familiar with your accounts and if you have shown that you are reliable and you can provide security then your bank manager may look favourably on your application. Most banks have a business adviser who will help you plan sensibly and help create a successful business and prevent problems occurring.

A partnership

A partnership may be a good idea if you have a colleague, friend or family member who has the necessary skills and the same enthusiasm and motivation as you, and can contribute financially to the business. This will ease your financial burden and as they say 'two heads are better than one'. You may choose a silent partner who will provide financial backing but leave the day-to-day running of the business to you. However many partners you have it is important to have a legal agreement drawn up by a solicitor which will set out all the financial details. These will include details of all parties, the purpose of the loan, the sum of money borrowed, the date of repayment and if there is any interest payable on the loan.

The Prince's Trust

The Prince's Trust is the UK's leading youth charity and will provide grants to people aged between 18 and 30 who wish to start their own business and find it difficult to obtain finance elsewhere. Eligible applicants need to have a good business idea and the determination to turn it into reality.

The Trust's business programme offers a test marketing grant, in addition to low interest loans with beneficial repayment terms.

The Trust also offers an 'aftercare' programme to help new businesses survive during the first three years of trading, in the form of self-help guides, seminars, free advice lines and a business mentor who will provide advice and support in regular meetings during the first three years. You can contact the Trust on:

Freephone: 0800 842 842

Web site: www.princes-trust.org.uk.

Private investors

A private investor may be someone who is looking to invest money in a viable business venture. They may have no knowledge of your business or be interested in the day-to-day running of it; their main concern is the profit they will make on their investment. They are referred to as 'business angels' who tend to be prepared to invest between £10,000 and £250,000. The National Business Angels Network (NBAN) is a non-profit making organisation with government support which brings together business angels across the UK. For more detailed information contact them at:

Tel: 0207 329 4141

Web site: www.nationalbusangels.co.uk.

26 The business plan

The importance of a business plan

It is important for anyone hoping to start a business to produce a comprehensive business plan as this provides a concise document which details the business you wish to establish and the expectations you have for its continuing growth and success. This will then help you decide on the viability of your ideas and give you something to measure the progress you are making once established, as well as allowing you to maintain the course you have set by following the plan and achieving your objectives.

For anyone wishing to raise funds when starting a new business or for expanding an already established business, a thorough and impressive business plan will be essential in convincing potential backers that they should invest their money with you. If a business plan is well written and presented it will show that you have a professional and business-like approach, and it also shows the effort you are making and your determination to succeed.

Setting objectives

Your objectives are the goals you wish to achieve in your business. Your main or primary objectives are often known as your 'mission statement' and will state the purpose of your business and the market it will cater for.

MISSION STATEMENT

I/We will provide a professional holistic service of high quality specialising in Reflexology, Aromatherapy and Stress Management, working in conjunction with medical and alternative therapy practitioners in the North West of England to promote balance in health and vitality.

Once you have stated your primary objectives you must then decide how you will achieve them, what you will require to finance your plans, put them into operation, market the business and monitor the outcomes. This will necessitate defining objectives in much more detail, forming the body of your business plan.

There are many standard formats available from banks or other financial institutions that you may use when writing your business plan; however, to be successful a great deal of thought and preparation needs to go into a good business plan. When raising finance it may be essential to use the format laid down by the institution that you wish to borrow money from, as they will have certain requirements. In some circumstances the standard format may not be quite the right approach for your business, therefore use it as a guide only, using those parts of it which are most appropriate to your business.

Content of a business plan

Details about your business and yourself

- The name and type of business – reflexology clinic, health and beauty salon, mobile holistic therapist, alternative therapist, stress management consultant.

- The services you will be offering – reflexology, aromatherapy, stress management, body massage.
- Why you have chosen this business – your experience in your chosen field, your qualifications and continuing professional development.
- Your legal status – sole trader, partnership, limited company.
- Any previous business experience or courses you may have attended to provide you with skills for running your own business.

These details will serve as a simple but informative introduction to the business plan, providing a brief overview for the reader.

The location

Explain where you will be based. This may be in your own home, in a room you have converted or an extension to provide you with a separate treatment area. You may decide to offer mobile services and visit clients in their own homes or work within another practice, either medical, beauty or complementary, renting a room from another professional. You may even have bought or are leasing your own premises. Whatever the location you need to provide details of the catchment area from which you will be obtaining clients.

The market

To have a successful business and to convince backers of your future success, it is important to demonstrate that there is a market for the services you offer. There are certain points to consider and record in your plan:

- Where is your market and how large is it?
- Does it have the potential for growth?
- Identify the potential clients.
- Identify your competitors, the prices they charge and assess their strengths and weaknesses.

Operating the business

The information required here would include, premises, transport, equipment and suppliers, services and staff.

Premises

For existing premises you should provide details of location, size and type of premises, and if there are any plans for expansion you should give details of future development or change. If the premises are leasehold, state the term of the lease, what period is outstanding and if there is an option to renew, the present rent, when it is paid and date of next review. It is also important to establish who is responsible for the repair and upkeep of the premises. If you are liable you will need to know the extent of this liability. Is it just general painting, decorating and repairs or will you be responsible for the roof, foundations or load bearing walls? This could prove costly!

Transport

A mobile business will rely heavily on the means of transport you choose and, as it will be an expensive outlay, it must be reliable and appropriate for your requirements. State the reasons why you need a particular vehicle, for example an estate car with five doors will be ideal when lifting equipment in and out and will have the capacity to allow you room to store items safely without causing damage in transit.

Equipment and suppliers

State how much equipment will be needed, the cost, the name of supplier and what the alternatives are if they fail to supply. Retail and consumable suppliers may be separate from equipment suppliers. It is important to shop around and find a reliable company who will deliver promptly, offer quality products and not expect you to invest huge sums of money on an initial order.

Services

This will provide details of the services you offer, emphasising anything that is different or special about the various treatments and why it will be successful. List the prices for the treatments and a breakdown of how the cost was established. State whether you are researching new areas or learning new skills which may be added to your treatment list in the near future.

Selling retail products is an important service to the client and essential in maximising profit, therefore detail the lines you have chosen, explain their relevance to your business, the selling price and original cost.

Staffing

As a sole trader you will need to provide a curriculum vitae detailing your personal information, qualifications, professional memberships, career history and any other activities and interests which may be relevant. List all the skills you have which are relevant and all experience you have had which will contribute to the success of the business. Most people sell themselves short when listing previous experience, for example if you have worked in a retail environment you will have been involved in handling cash, customer care, stock control and marketing, all skills relevant to a reflexology practice. In addition you should provide a personal profile to include a description of yourself, your ambitions, reasons and motivation for your proposed business, and your long-term objectives.

In the case of a partnership, details will be required of all concerned and an outline of the roles and responsibilities of all those involved.

If you are employing staff you must provide details to include their name, address, qualifications, relevant work experience and their position in the business. There may be other skills you will require to help establish and operate the business within the next year, state what they are and the staff you will be hoping to employ. You may wish to employ a cleaner, a receptionist, a trainee, book-keeper, other therapists or even a business manager.

Estimate the cost of employing staff and buying in the required skills. These costs should include your own salary and other partners in the business; this could be cost per month or annually.

Financial details

This provides the information required by a bank manager or investor when you wish to borrow money. There is a risk involved when lending money; therefore it is important to show what assets you have available, as insurance against anything going wrong. These may include:

- capital you have available
- other sources of funds – savings, stocks and shares, redundancy money, inheritance, a loan from a member of the family or even lottery winnings!

- another investor
- enterprise fund (help given by the government to encourage small businesses)
- local enterprise agencies which are a partnership between industry and local central government. They will provide advice or recommend experts to help with financial matters as well as marketing, finding premises and planning
- The Prince's Trust, which helps young people aged between 18 and 30 to set up and run their own business.

You must state how much you wish to borrow, for how long and how you propose to pay it back. You will be required to supply a budget and cash flow forecast for 12 months. This will demonstrate your ability to repay the loan after all your business expenses have been met. It analyses your expenditure and receipts for that period.

Expenditure

Expenditure may include such things as:

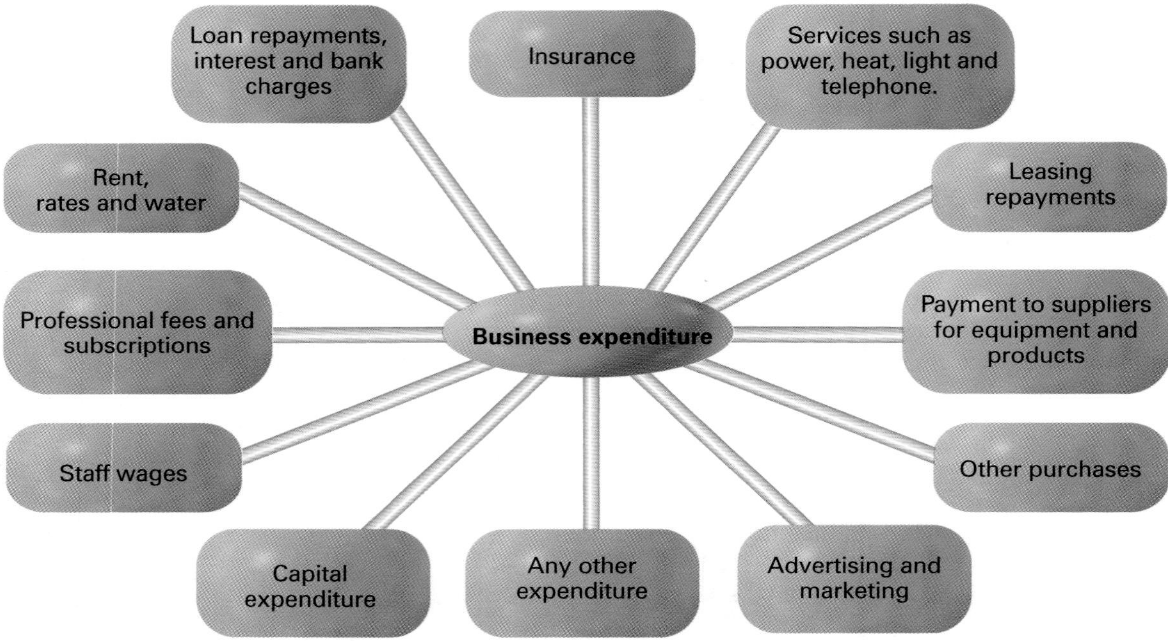

Figure 26.1 *Business expenditure*

Receipts

Receipts or money coming into the business will include:

- the capital you have invested
- loans received initially and at a later date
- cash from treatments, services and retail sales
- other sources of income such as rent from other therapists sharing your premises.

The cash flow forecast is based on assumptions which form a vital part of the financial forecast. It is important therefore to be realistic as it will be evident when your need for cash is greatest and what your funding requirements may be.

- Planning the success of the business
- Recruiting staff
- Marketing the business
- Establishing a retail line

Opening a **Business**

27 Planning the success of the business

The operational plan

Once you have established your business, to ensure its success it is important to put into effect an operational plan. Good planning ensures a smooth running business, providing excellent service and making the best use of the resources available for the benefit of the client. Successful plans will provide adequate detail, be put into operation with ease and achieve the desired result.

Resources

Establish what resources are available to you to achieve the objectives you have set. Resources will include:

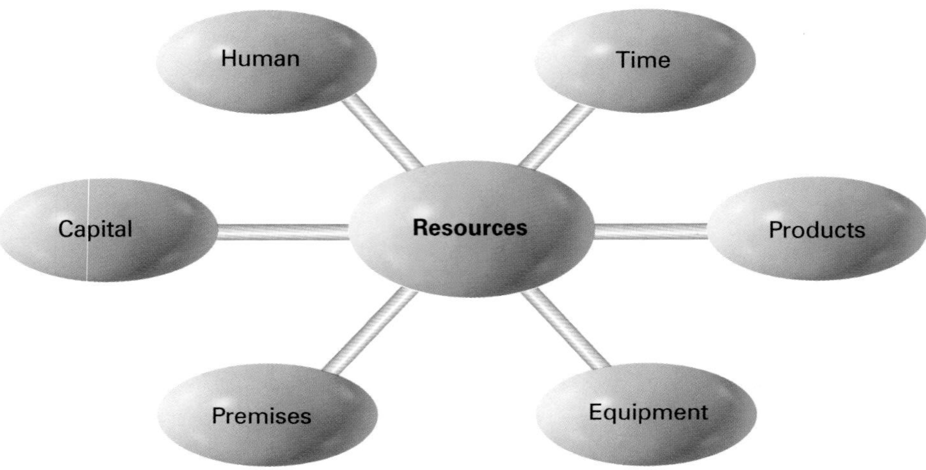

Figure 27.1 *The resources needed to operate a business*

- **Human:** The employees or personnel in the business; you will need to employ the appropriate number with the best qualifications to ensure the highest standards.
- **Capital:** The money invested to set up in business or for expanding an existing business.
- **Premises:** The place from which you will work together with fixtures and fittings; must be well maintained.
- **Equipment:** This will be used to provide the service, must be up to date and of good quality.
- **Products:** These are required for treatment and retail must be appropriate to your clients' needs.
- **Time:** A valuable resource must be used effectively, therefore planning and delegation are important so time is not wasted.

Knowing the resources you have available will help you in the planning process. You need to consider planning a budget, setting a price for the treatments you offer and the retail products you will be selling, advertising and promoting the business, employing the required members of staff, implementing your objectives, monitoring the outcome and making changes if required.

Budget

A budget is a plan based on the objectives of the business. It will show what money is required and how it will be raised. It may be set for a twelve-month period but, if necessary, it can be for as little as one month. A flexible budget is sometimes required to change as a business changes; for example, if there is a sudden increase in demand for treatment, this will result in much higher sales levels, therefore the sales budget may have to be altered. Budgets are usually based on results previously achieved and estimates of future sales, which then determine the budget period and sales targets.

Sales budget

The sales budget contains monthly sales estimates of how many treatments and products will be sold.

Production budget

The production budget shows what the required labour hours will be, the consumables required and the equipment needed to provide the services.

You must ensure that the income from sales covers the production costs and provides a healthy profit.

Price

The price you charge will depend to some extent on the demand for your service and the degree of competition you face.

Whatever the competition, when deciding on a price you must take into consideration your **fixed costs**, those which have to be paid whether you are carrying out treatments or not, rent, rates, electricity, telephone, wages, advertising, insurance etc. Add these to your **variable costs**, the cost of carrying out the treatments and the **profit** you wish to make.

Fixed cost + Variable cost + Profit = Treatment price

There is no standard or ideal way of setting a price for your services as individual business circumstances and costs can vary greatly. There are, however, certain considerations.

The market

Look at your market. It is important to set a price in relation to the clientele you hope to attract. If you are providing a treatment which is unique or better than your competitors, then you can probably charge a higher price. However, if a product is priced too high and the consumer thinks it is poor value for money, then you risk lower sales.

Skimming

Paying a high price appeals to some clients with high incomes or those who like to buy the most expensive products or treatments and be seen to be doing so. This is known as **price skimming** – i.e. you are aiming at the cream at the top end of the market.

Low prices

You may be able to reduce your price to below your competitors if you have very small overheads, for example, a reflexologist working with elderly people in a nursing home. Your overheads will be minimal – your time, your portable treatment chair and a few sundry items – which will allow you to maintain a lower price. All your clients are in one place, you are using their heat, light, electricity, water, etc., therefore you may still have a good profit margin whilst maintaining a lower treatment price to suit your clientele. However, low prices may also generate low sales, with some consumers suspecting that the quality is inferior because of the lower price.

Pricing strategies

Penetration pricing

Penetration pricing may be used to gain a foothold in the market by pricing your treatments and products lower than your competitors, thus gaining business that hopefully you will maintain when the price eventually rises. The drawback to this strategy is that some consumers may think that the service you offer is inferior.

Customer value pricing

This involves charging the price you know the consumer is prepared to pay. When there is prestige attached to the product you may be able to command a higher price.

Price discrimination

Price discrimination is providing a treatment at different prices. This could be time-based, offering lower prices at quiet times to encourage sales, or market-based, discounting prices for particular consumers, for example senior citizens or students.

Competition-based pricing

This is a method based solely on the price charged by your competitors and may be used if there is fierce competition. In this case you must try and develop a strong brand identity, to differentiate your business from the others, allowing you to alter your price with confidence.

Market skimming

This may be used when you have little or no competition but there is a demand for your service. You can charge a high price for a limited period of time. The aim of this strategy is to make as much profit as possible before the competitors join the market.

E'SPA

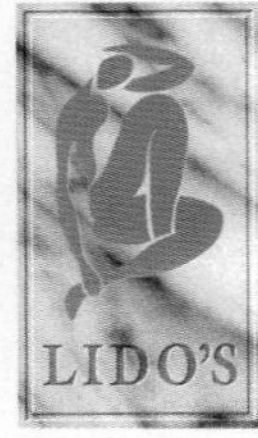

British ▪ Lifestyle concept ▪ Anti-stressing ▪ Organically sourced ▪ Spa treatments ▪ Holistic beauty ▪ Aromatherapy ▪ Cleansing mineral muds ▪ Revitalising seaweeds ▪ 'E' for education

Advanced Concept Treatments			
E'SPA Concept Facial To Lift & Firm	**£60**	£50	1½hrs
Blissfull Face, Back, Scalp Treatment With Hot Stone Therapy	**£60**	£50	1¾hrs
Total Holistic Bodycare With Hot Stone Therapy	**£60**	£50	1¾hrs
Holistic Foot & Nail Treatment With Hot Stones	**£30**	£25	1 hr
Holistic Hand & Nail Treatment With Hot Stones	**£30**	£25	1 hr
ESPA Envelopments			
De-tox Algea Wrap	**£46**	£40	1¼hrs
Purifying Herbal Linen Wrap	**£28**	£23	½hr
Ayurvedic 'Oshadi' Envelopment Warms • Nourishes • Relives Aching Muscles	**£46**	£40	1¼hrs
Warm Marine Mud Envelopment	**£46**	£40	1¼hrs
ESPA Lifestyle Treatments			
Balancing Aromatherapy Facial	**£34**	£30	1 hr
Soothing Eye Treatment	**£22**	£19	½ hr
Cleansing Back Aromatherapy	**£28**	£24	¾ hr
Body Polish	**£22**	£19	½ hr
Hip & Thigh Treatment	**£35**	£30	1 hr
Course of eight	**£260**	£225	
Pre-natal Treatment Essential before or after child birth.	**£50**	£45	1½hrs

Samples of prices from Lido's

Monitoring the business

It is vital to monitor the business to ensure you are achieving your objectives. If you are not then plans may be altered accordingly. This can be done by keeping records of all aspects of the business and should include:

- **Personnel records** – details of all staff, initial application, interview notes, terms and conditions of employment, training given, personal details and appraisal notes.
- **Wages records** – details to include name and address, national insurance number, PAYE reference, pension details and any deductions that have been authorised.

- **Stock records** – details of all incoming stock, regular stock checks, copies of orders and invoices, and stock sold or used for treatments. An inventory of the resources in the business should be made and altered as and when circumstances change.
- **Financial records** – including double entry book-keeping system showing income and expenditure, petty cash book, invoices, bank statements and receipt books.
- **Health and safety records** – to show who is responsible for health and safety, what training has been given and when, and details of any regular safety checks required by law.
- **Client records** – essential for the smooth running of the business, must be kept up to date and in compliance with the Data Protection Act.

Client feedback

It is important to gain feedback from the client to find out exactly what they want, how they feel about the treatment, and the products and the service they receive. It will ensure you are fulfilling their needs, identifying problems which may occur, improving service and monitoring the level of satisfaction.

Feedback is obtained informally each time you speak to the client and you may be aware of any problems and be able to deal with them immediately. More formal methods are used when the feedback is required to help you make business decisions such as taking on new therapies in addition to reflexology, relocating, expanding or changing the way the business operates.

Making a profit

It is the main objective of any business to make a profit, and if this is not happening plans will have to be put into effect to improve the situation. There are several ways to increase your profit: cut costs, increase your range of treatments, increase prices and sell more.

- Costs may be cut by looking for new suppliers who will offer you special deals to save money, but don't cut down on quality.
- Use staff more effectively by using some part-time and ensuring that the maximum number are available at the busy times and the minimum number required at the quiet times.
- Change your working hours to suit your clientele, to ensure all staff are busy and using their time effectively.
- Increase your treatment range if there is a demand. Use market research to establish the need first but make sure you can do this without additional costs that may be difficult for you to recoup.
- Increasing prices may be risky as you could lose some clients; however, the increase in profits may more than compensate for the loss of clients.
- Selling more may be achieved by training staff in sales techniques, providing commission on sales as a staff incentive, and making sure a variety of selling aids are available.

Effective selling

The most effective selling method is the professional recommendation. Once you have established a good client/therapist relationship, the client will always ask for your advice as they rely on your expert opinion. As long as you always sell treatments and products which will benefit the client, they will come back for more.

Learning to recognise buying signals will help. Retail and treatment sales are not always made as a direct response to a client request. There are comments made, questions asked, or actions from the client that may indicate the possibility of making a sale. An experienced therapist will learn to recognise the signals when they occur.

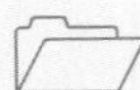

CASE STUDY – BUYING SIGNALS

During treatment, a client tells you she is finding it difficult to sleep, has digestive problems and is looking for information about special diets. She then comments on the lovely music playing in the background.

It is important to sympathise with a client such as the one above, but don't ignore these 'buying signals', which are also pleas for help. For example, you could:

- show her your essential oil burners and choice of relaxing oils to help her sleep
- explain that a course of reflexology will help balance her digestive system
- tell her the dietary advice is contained in a special book you have on offer at the moment
- explain that she can buy a CD or cassette of relaxing music to play at home.

By offering her all these products, you are *helping the client* to satisfy her needs and *increasing turnover*, in the knowledge that it is beneficial to the client and she hasn't purchased your recommendations from other shops.

Cash flow

It is important to maintain a healthy cash flow to ensure there is always money available, allowing you to make the changes you feel will benefit the business. Poor cash flow may be caused by stockpiling, when your stock is surplus to requirements and tying up cash, overspending, overborrowing, reduced turnover caused by seasonal changes, an increase in competition or a reduction in client numbers. By monitoring the business closely you can prevent problems occurring or deal with them as soon as they become apparent.

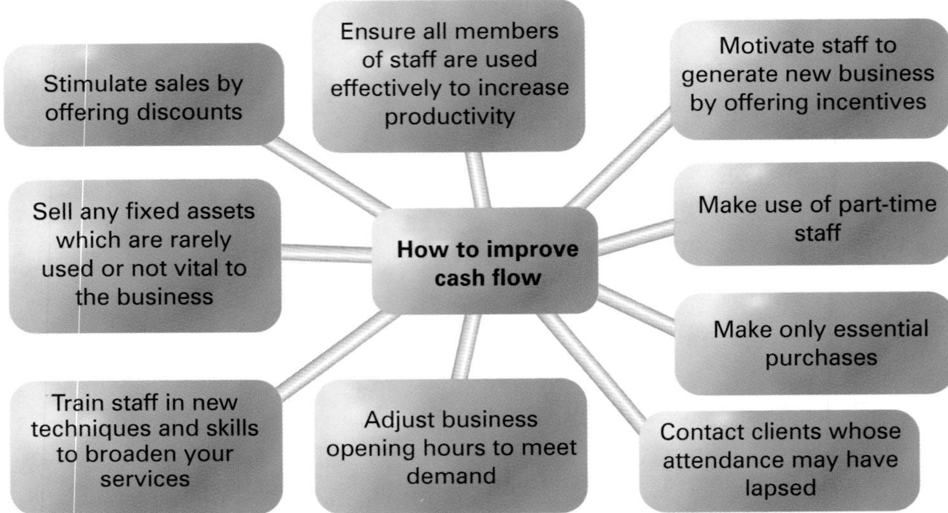

Figure 27.2 There are several ways that a business's cash flow can be improved

Time management

Time is a resource which is often neglected. Poor time management can greatly reduce productivity. Good planning is essential to using time effectively.

There are so many jobs you have to do to operate a successful business that it can be easy to neglect certain aspects of the work. It is important therefore to sit down and analyse the time being spent on each area of responsibility. Good time management will ensure that you are working effectively and contributing to the financial success of the business. It will also serve as a good example to the other staff and, by applying the same principles themselves, they can make their time more effective. Start by making a list of each job that must be done, for example:

- Practical application of treatments
- Stock control
- Planning
- Paperwork/book-keeping
- Appraisal
- Training staff
- Business meetings
- Promotional work
- Interviewing

Rearrange the list in order of importance and the approximate time you devote each week to that task. Make sure you are spending enough time on the more important tasks and reduce the time spent on less important activities. Delegate tasks that you feel others can do and eliminate anything which is not essential. Make a chart of jobs that have to be done daily, weekly and at longer intervals. These may be recorded in a diary on a calendar or business planner.

Finally, work out a daily routine for yourself and other members of staff – less time will be wasted when everyone knows what is expected of them.

Daily routine

Start of the day

- Check the appointment book.
- Deal with staff-related problems such as absence or lateness.
- Check reception and all treatment rooms are well prepared.
- Check stock details.
- Answer any telephone messages.
- Deal with immediate problems.
- Provide treatments.

End of the day

- Check everyone has completed their delegated tasks for the day.
- Consider problems that have arisen during the day.
- Consider action required to deal with the problems.
- Consider jobs which have to be done the following day and work out an approximate timetable.
- Anticipate potential problems and make arrangements to cope with them.

28 Recruiting staff

When starting up your business it may be your intention to employ other reflexologists, other therapists, or you may need the help of a receptionist or book-keeper. Your business plans may include expanding your business over time by increasing the number of people working for you. When looking for staff, it is important to make sure that the right person for the job is chosen first time because hiring the wrong staff and then having to re-advertise will be disruptive and costly to the business.

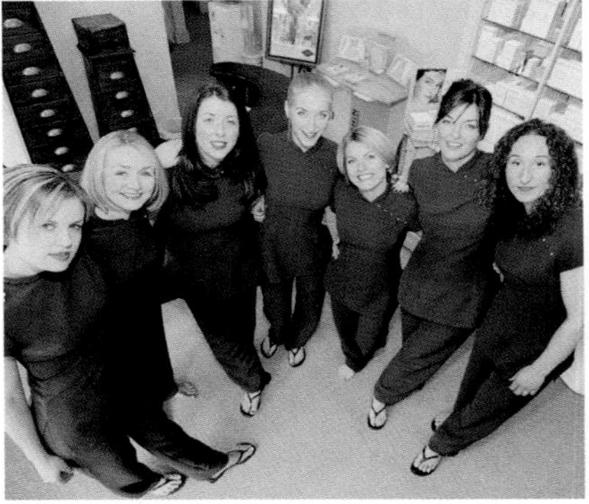

Recruiting the best staff is an important part of making your business succeed

Objectives of recruitment

The objective of recruitment is to attract the best people for the job and then to choose the most suitable for your business. Reflexology provides a personal service and the staff employed must have the right qualifications, appearance, manner and approach to their work. The client–therapist relationship once established can be an enduring one, as a good therapist soon gains the confidence of the client and will therefore generate a great deal of business. When advertising for staff, ensure advertisements comply with the anti discrimination legislation, the Sex Discrimination Act 1975, the Race Relations Act 1976 and the Equal Pay Act 1970.

Part-time staff

When a business is new, the financial commitment of permanent, full-time members of staff may be too big a burden or the work available may not be sufficient for a full-time member of staff. Some employees do not wish to work full-time due to other commitments. Rather than lose a competent member of staff it may be necessary to offer them part-time hours.

Commission

Working on commission only can be an incentive for the reflexologist to increase sales, or it could be a combined basic wage plus commission on achieving set targets.

Procedures

Job description and person specification

Whether you are employing permanent, part time or occasional staff you will need to draw up the following:

- A **job description**, which provides details of the job title, a brief description of the role, specific tasks and responsibilities. This will provide information to the prospective employee, help to identify the requirements for each job, and form the basis of job evaluation for payment of wages.
- A **person specification**, which shows a profile of the person required to do the job and establishes the criteria for selecting the new employee. It should include qualifications, practical and additional skills required, personal attributes required, general fitness and health, and personal interests.

Terms and conditions of employment

You must give these to every employee within two months of starting work .They usually include:

- Name of employer and employee
- Date employment started
- Job title
- Main duties and other responsibilities
- Hours of work
- Rates of pay and how they are calculated, including commission and overtime
- When payment is to be made
- How payment is to be made
- Holidays and holiday pay
- Sickness pay
- Pension schemes
- Period of notice for employee and employer
- Workplace rules and regulations
- Any special terms of employment
- Grievance and disciplinary procedures

Interviewing

If the prospective employee is a reflexologist then it is advisable to ask them to provide you with a treatment, as this will show you first hand how good their practical and communication skills are.

Plan the interview so that it is well organised and relaxed; the candidate will be put at ease and be more open in discussion. Make sure there are no interruptions and allow adequate time for questions and testing practical skills. It is advisable to make notes of the candidates' responses to review later, and also consider the impression they have made on you. Are they what you are looking for and will they fit in with other staff members? Check each candidate against your person specification and finally check references before notifying the successful candidate.

Appraisal

To maintain quality of service it will be necessary to carry out appraisal on a regular basis. This is an evaluation of each member of staff in terms of their job performance or skills. It must be fair and accurate allowing you to assess:

- standards of job performance
- strengths and weaknesses
- training and development needs
- possibilities for promotion
- change in current salary and/or responsibilities.

It also provides motivation and helps in the formulation of business plans. Informal appraisal occurs on a day-to-day basis in the workplace, however a formal appraisal is planned, and uses a standard set of criteria. Use an appropriate appraisal form to record details of appraisal interview or observation of practical skills. Discuss the outcome of appraisal with the employee as soon as possible and agree on a plan of action which is agreeable to both parties. This may include further training, promotion, job improvement or an increase in salary. To be successful the appraisal must be fair and accurate.

29 Marketing the business

The market for your business may be defined as a group of existing clients and potential clients (consumers) who will use your services and products. A very important function in any business is to increase turnover and profits. Marketing is an ongoing process or business philosophy, which helps to provide what the client needs and wants and allows a business to be prepared to respond to change. Marketing, therefore, is essential, particularly in a business which is so highly customer orientated.

Marketing your business

To market your business you need to:

- assess clients' needs and wants
- monitor changes in the market place
- anticipate future trends
- promote the business.

Marketing activities will include carrying out market research, creating the right image, advertising the business, selling and promotions. To achieve your marketing objectives a business must consider the **marketing mix**, which is:

- Product
- Price
- Promotion
- Place

To meet the needs of the consumer you must have the right **product** at the right **price**, make it available in the right **place** and inform consumers through **promotion**.

Your products are the treatments you offer and the retail lines you have established. The price you will have set for treatments and retail products will be based on your overheads, the competition and the area in which you are working. The place will be either your own premises, within another organisation, working from home or a mobile service, covering a specified area. The final part of the marketing mix is 'promotion', which is vitally important to help maintain the market share you already have and increase it further by attracting new business. Clients will buy the product which provides the greatest benefit to them; therefore when promoting your business you must emphasise what the end result will be in having a particular treatment or buying a particular product.

Promotion

Promotion is a form of indirect advertising, which provides incentives to stimulate sales and is used for the following reasons:

- to draw the client's attention to a new business, treatment or product
- to stimulate sales
- to encourage bookings in off-peak times
- to increase turnover.

Types of promotion

- Introducing a new treatment at a special introductory price for a limited period.
- Booking a course of treatments at a discount.
- Providing a free gift with purchase.
- Including a discount voucher in a newspaper advertisement or article.

- Introduce a friend and receive a free treatment.
- Open evenings with demonstrations and refreshments.
- Birthday cards with treatment vouchers sent to existing clients.

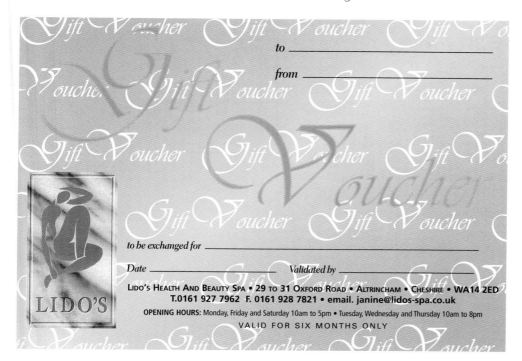

A Lido's gift voucher

The first promotion you may have is the launch of the business. This can be an enjoyable social occasion for your clients. Contact all the relevant people and send invitations to as many prospective clients as possible. Friends and relatives should also be invited as they are potential clients and they may know at least one other person who may be interested. If you provide refreshments and have a special opening offer, you will persuade more people to attend and hopefully establish some new clients. Make sure that all those people involved in the business are on hand to discuss any issues, provide information and book appointments.

Advertising

All businesses will benefit to some extent from advertising at some time.

The aims of advertising are to inform potential clients about the nature and availability of treatments and products, and to persuade them to buy these treatments and products.

Informative advertising

Here is an example of advertising that informs people of a product or service.

The Complementary Therapy Clinic
Hardwicke Crescent Sheffield SH5 10A

will be offering
***Shiatsu** massage and **Reiki** healing*
on
Thursday and Saturday 10.00 – 15.00
from
Monday 10th April 2002

Appointments now being taken Tel: 202 4275

Persuasive advertising

Here is an example of advertising to persuade people to buy a product or service.

> *The Complementary Therapy Clinic*
> *Hardwicke Crescent Sheffield SH5 10A*
>
> *Reflexology is a gentle balancing treatment, which will help to increase energy levels, ease aches and pains, reduce levels of stress, relax the body and calm the mind.*
>
> *For one day only we are offering a free treatment to the first five people to present this advertisement at our reception.*

Advertising is successful when it achieves an increase in sales or in the number of clients.

There are many types of advertising and it is important to select the best method for your business, so that the money spent is used to the best advantage. The method you choose will depend upon the budget you have for advertising, the market you are aiming at and the medium you choose.

Some options are:

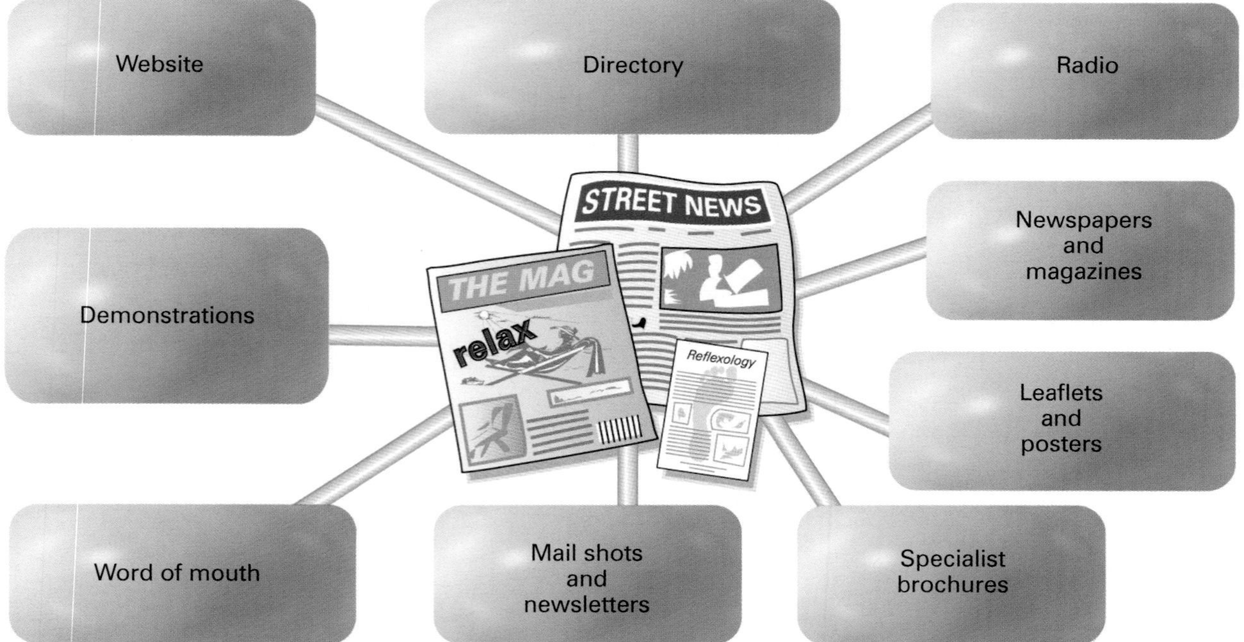

***Figure** 29.1 There are various mediums that can be used for advertising a business*

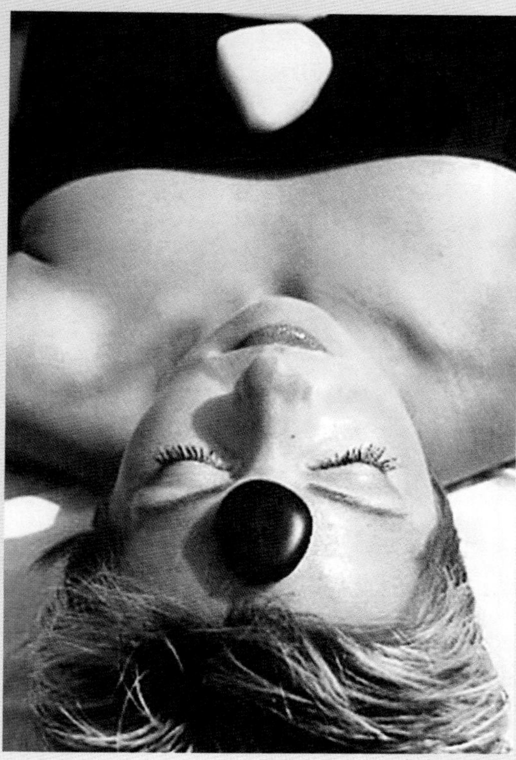
"Getting stoned never felt so good"

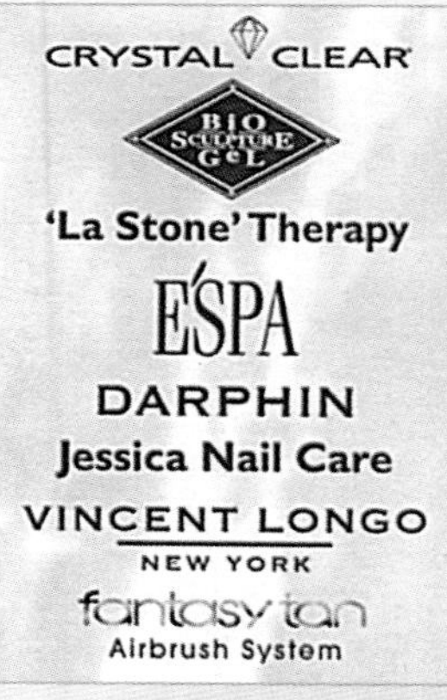
CRYSTAL CLEAR
BIO SCULPTURE GEL
'La Stone' Therapy
ESPA
DARPHIN
Jessica Nail Care
VINCENT LONGO
NEW YORK
fantasy tan
Airbrush System

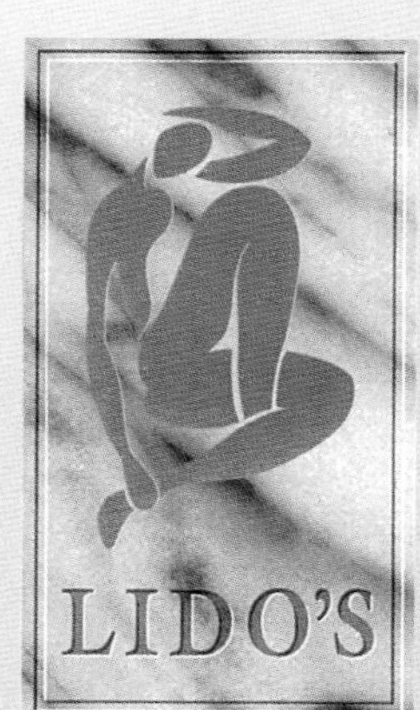
LIDO'S
29 TO 31 OXFORD ROAD
ALTRINCHAM CHESHIRE
WA14 2ED
T. 0161 927 7962
F. 0161 928 7821
email. janine@lidos-spa.co.uk
www.lidos-spa.co.uk
2001 British Beauty Award Winners

A Lido's advertisement

Newspapers

Many areas have free newspapers delivered to everybody in each particular area. Therefore the paper will probably reach more of the market than an advertisement placed in a paper which is bought only by a small percentage of the population in that area. Features contributed by experts are gratefully received by the publishers of free newspapers, so contact the editor and offer to write articles or an advice column related to your business. This will then provide you with valuable free advertising. If your budget allows, use a professional to design an advert for you as this will catch the reader's eye. A good advertisement should draw attention to the services or products you are selling, be easily understood and convince the reader of the benefits, creating the desire to try the treatments or buy the products!

An interesting story about you or your business, particularly if accompanied by an unusual photo, may be deemed by an editor to be worthy of including in their publication. This type of free advertising is often worth far more than an expensive written advertisement.

Radio

This is an expensive advertising medium, but sometimes helpful in reaching a niche market. Take the opportunity of providing advisory services on phone in programmes or take part in discussions when an expert is required.

Magazines

Specialist magazines will allow you to reach your target audience; however, there will be many similar advertisements, so yours will need to stand out from the others.

Specialist brochures

These will be helpful in reaching a target audience, for example, hotel brochures, if you are providing mobile services, or a company's in-house brochure for large businesses.

Leaflets and posters

Leaflets are useful to give to existing clients as they may be passed on to potential new clients. You also have ready-made details of the business to pass on to people requesting information, which they may then read at leisure. You can use them to send out in mail shots, hand post through letterboxes or give out at exhibitions and demonstrations. You may also leave them with other businesses, at medical centres or chiropodists, and in return you could do the same for them.

Posters are effective if placed in a position where they will be read, in a salon or clinic, or in a busy local shop with a considerable amount of passing trade. It is a cheap form of advertising, therefore good value for money even if you only achieve a small response.

Mail shots

Start to record the names and addresses of any enquirers and clients who are interested and compile a mailing list of people to contact with information, special offers or new treatments. A regular newsletter for clients will keep them informed and is a gentle reminder if they have not attended for a while.

NEW PRODUCT LAUNCH

Darphin hair care

All those fans out there of Darphin's must have skin care, can now indulge in their fantastic new hair care products which are based on plant extract and essential oils!

Our favourites are the CREAM MASK with shea butter priced at £24.00 for 200ml. Great for transforming frizzy curls into glamourous twirls. And also the REGENERATING AROMA CARE OIL with essential oils of grapefruit, to re-oxygenate the scalp and improve body. Priced at £24.00

Winter Chill Out!!!

Sea Salt Body Scrub
Aromatic Steam
Indian Head Massage

PRICE £30.00!!! 1hr 15mins BOOK NOW!!!

OFFER RUNNING FROM 1st DECEMBER – 28th FEBRUARY

We have a tester stand in reception for you to have a play with.
We know you will **love** everything!!!

FORTHCOMING EVENTS...

DECEMBER Saturday 1st - CHRISTMAS OPEN DAY

JOIN THE LIDO'S TEAM FOR A DAY OF FUN WITH LOTS OF FREE GIVEAWAYS AND HELP IN CHOOSING THOSE SPECIAL GIFTS.

LADIES: on arrival you will be greeted with a glass of champagne and chocolates to enjoy. You will be escorted to a private area where you can view all our Christmas gifts in a calm environment with advice given if needed.
Once your gifts have been chosen our Jessica Nail Specialist will treat you to a FREE nail varnish application, so you can relax while your presents are being wrapped.
On departure you will receive a FREE COPY of a ladies magazine.!!!

GENTLEMAN: On arrival you will be greeted with a chilled beer and mince pies to enjoy.
Once we have helped you choose your gifts you will receive a FREE scalp massage to help you get over the shock!!! On departure you will also receive a FREE COPY of a leading mens magazine.

The event will take place all day from 10.00am to 5.00pm. Please bring along a friend, no appointment is necessary but it will be on a first come first served basis.

JANUARY Thursday 24th - LUNCH AT JUNIPER'S

GUEST SPEAKER: JANE SCRIVNER - AUTHOR OF THE DE-TOX.

Make a date to join us in the new year when we will be holding a special lunch with speakers from Espa and the author of the must have de-tox book, Jane Scrivner. Advice on spa treatments that really do work and special offers on detox kits will be available.
Tickets are £35.00. To include 3 course lunch with coffee and Complimentary gift bag.

Book now through Lido's reception 0161 927 2962

NEW TREATMENT LAUNCH

Lido's will now be offering CRYSTAL CLEAR FIRMING FACE LIFTS, from the 20th November.
This new treatment will be suitable for anyone who needs to smooth out age lines and brighten up their complexion in just under 45 minutes!!! Consisting of gentle exfoliation, stimulation of oxygen and elastin cells and finishing with a moulding firming face mask this is going to be THE facial just before a special night out!!!

45 MINUTES	£45.00	MEMBERS PRICE	£40.00
COURSE OF 8	£340.00	MEMBERS PRICE	£300.00

Christmas shopping doesn't have to be so stressful any more. Just pop in to Lido's!!!

Autumn colour make-up

Bored, Bored and just Bored with your face make up then check out these two new arrivals. Rumour has it that Madonna stocked up on the lip due pencil when it was launched in London, so see what all the fuss is about.

Trio eye shadow £20.00 Due Lip pencil £13.00

Electrolysis gets the Golden Touch

Having recently completed an update course our 2 therapists Gemma and Melanie came away with new techniques that can reduce redness, and improve results with less discomfort for the client. One of these techniques include using 24 ct gold needles!!!

Why Gold???

1. It's the best conductor for the current allowing the therapist to reduce discomfort by using a lower level with the same results!
2. Gold is very smooth so there is less trauma to the skin so less redness is present!!!
3. Gold has less chance of causing an allergic reaction!!

Due to these new techniques and upgrading our equipment to give you a better result it is necessary to review our prices.

As from the 20th November prices will be:

15 minutes	£15.00	*members*	*£11.00*
30 minutes	£28.00	*members*	*£25.00*

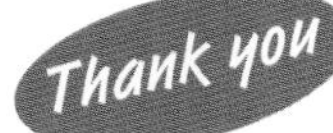

A Lido's newsletter informing people of their products and services

Word of mouth

This is the most valuable form of advertising as it is free, and once you have established a reputation for quality, professionalism and good client care, your clients will not hesitate in recommending you to others.

Demonstrations

This is an ideal way to bring your business to the notice of the public in general. It is an interesting way to educate the public about holistic therapies, coping with stress and the benefits of reflexology. For a successful demonstration:

- find out the type of audience and the general age group that will attend
- be sure of the numbers attending so that you can provide everybody with the necessary samples, advertising literature and information leaflets
- have a basic format to follow and time the demonstration well – not too long or the audience may lose interest
- prepare a set of cards with key points to ensure everything of importance is covered
- use interesting anecdotes and case histories to add interest and reinforce the benefits of reflexology
- know your subject well and prepare answers to questions that you think may arise or are most commonly asked
- involve the audience whenever possible, in particular encourage them to ask questions and use them as demonstration models
- know the retail prices of treatments and products and the advantage they have over your competitors
- practise the demonstration in advance if it is your first.

Directory

Entering your name, address and telephone number in a directory, such as Yellow Pages, is a useful form of advertising. Many people who are looking for a service may automatically refer to a directory. It is important therefore when choosing a name for the business to consider choosing one which begins with one of the first letters in the alphabet.

Internet website

The newest form of advertising allows you to reach a large audience.

The business image

The image the business portrays will be an important part of marketing as it provides an instant visual picture to prospective clients. Image may be expressed in terms of:

- the location of the business
- the external appearance of the establishment
- the name and logo
- the interior décor
- the staff uniform or clothes
- the prices charged.

- the treatments offered and products sold
- the ambience or atmosphere created
- the stationery, price lists, gift vouchers and business cards.

The right image for a reflexology business would be one of quiet calm and reassurance. There are some that are clinical and professional and, in some cases, the décor has been minimalist or with an eastern influence. The image will also be influenced by the location, particularly if it is part of another business or practice.

The reception area will provide the client with the first impression of the business once inside, so it should be attractive, relaxing and inviting.

For continuing success you must regularly identify, review and analyse your clients' needs and respond quickly to change.

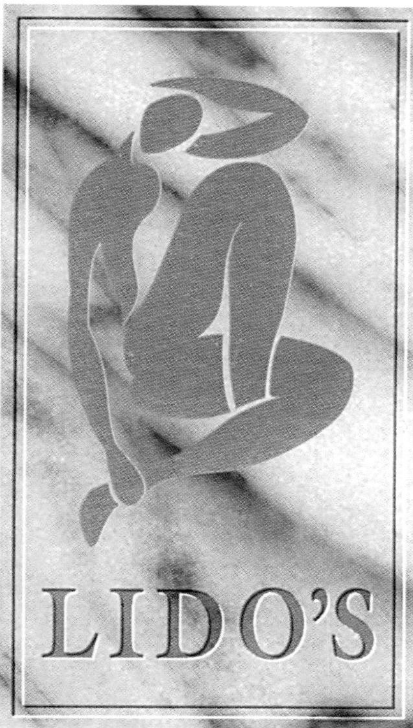

The Lido's business logo

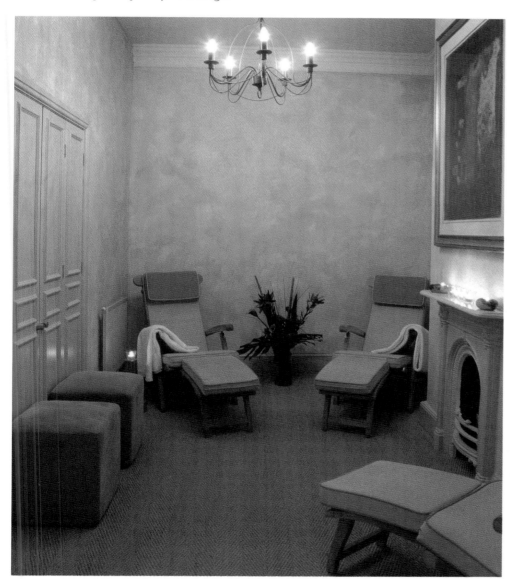

The rest area at Lido's

30 Establishing a retail line

Selling products

Selling retail products to clients is essential for business growth and should account for at least 40% of turnover. While performing treatments, there is a limit to the profit made as there are set prices for treatments and a specific time allocated. You do, however, have a captive audience and every opportunity to sell your clients products and materials for their benefit. There are many things that may benefit your clients and they may include:

- foot care products and implements to improve skin condition
- holistic books relating to topics of interest such as self-help, aromatherapy, diet and nutrition etc.
- reflexology charts and diagrams
- music CDs and cassettes
- candles
- essential oils and burners
- gifts
- herbal teas.

Product knowledge

Once you have found your suppliers it is important to gain product knowledge, be able to provide up to date, accurate information and explain the features and benefits of products that will inspire confidence in the client. The features are a description of the product and the benefits are what the features will achieve for the client (the reasons to buy). Advertising literature in the form of leaflets and brochures should be available for the clients to read. Place them in reception or use them as a visual aid when selling.

The following is an example of the features and benefits of a special foot cream used as a moisturiser and exfoliant.

Features	Benefits
A rich cream	Moisturises and softens dry flaking skin, helps to reduce hard skin on the feet
Contains lavender essential oil	Soothing and antiseptic, beneficial for treating aches and pains, eczema and athlete's foot, and has a lovely fragrance
Contains glycolic acid, a naturally occurring fruit acid	Gently exfoliates, preventing a build up of hard skin, corns and calluses
Has a pump dispenser	Easy to use, economical as it prevents waste
Comes in three sizes	Choice of size and price – small size ideal for carrying in a handbag; the large sizes are more economical

Product display

Retail products need to be visible so the client can look, sample them and become familiar with what is available.

- The reception area is an ideal location as the client can browse when entering and before leaving.
- An eye-catching window display attracts passing trade but must be changed regularly and kept clean to maintain interest.
- Posters, props, materials and products can be used to create the image you wish to portray. What you use will depend on the space you have and if the back opens directly into the reception or treatment area.
- Most manufacturers and suppliers provide display stands, which show products to their best advantage.

To be effective a display should:

- be well balanced
- use lines to draw the eye in to the focal point
- reflect an image or theme
- use the correct props and materials to complement the product
- be colourful
- achieve the desired effect
- be clean
- be safe and secure.

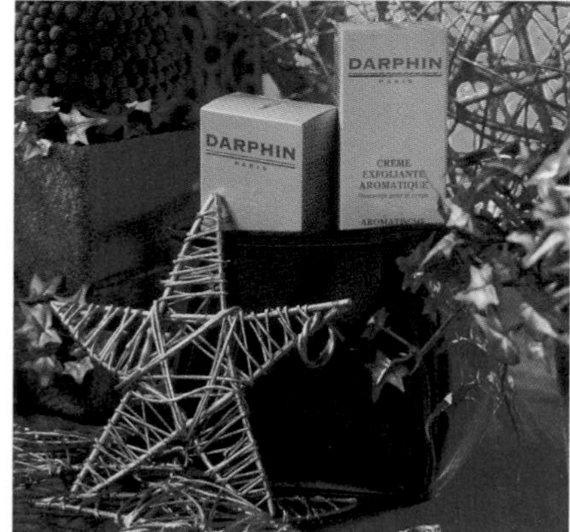

A display stand of products

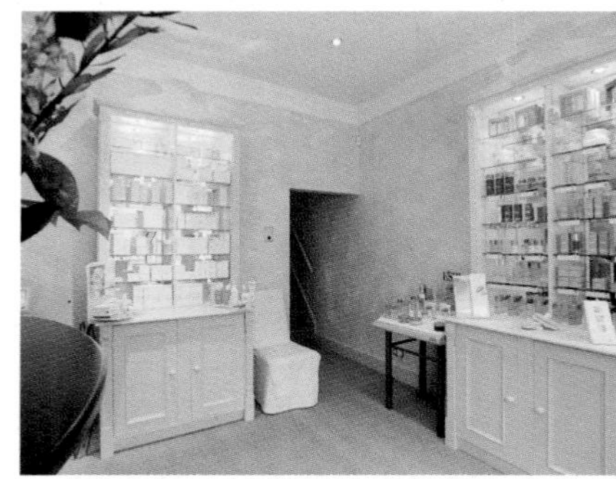
A shelf/cabinet display of products

The individual work area or treatment room could have a small display of relevant products. If the reception is left unattended it would be advisable to store retail products in a glass-fronted cabinet which can be locked, but the goods are on permanent display. Using a cabinet also ensures that the goods remain in mint condition and do not become dusty and dirty.

The price for retail products is often determined by the manufacturer or supplier. Some are inflexible in their approach to setting a retail price for a product but others are happy to help with discounts and special offers. This needs to be discussed with companies before you make any decisions.

Selling skills

It is important that each member of staff has training in sales techniques, as selling does not come easily to everybody. These skills include:

- recognising opportunities to sell
- offering the client advice when asked
- explaining the features and benefits of products and treatments
- offering literature about the products and treatments
- displaying products in an attractive way
- enthusiasm and good treatment and product knowledge
- only recommending treatments and products that are suitable for the client
- knowing when and how to close a sale.

The key to successful selling is to be honest with clients and ensure that the products you are selling to them are appropriate, will be effective and good value for money.

Stock control

Controlling stock is important, as there can be a large amount of capital invested in it. Strict records must be kept to ensure stock does not run out and overstocking does not occur, tying up large amounts of capital, and leading to stock deteriorating with age. The main person responsible for stock control will order, receive and check stock, keep records and carry out regular checks.

Stock should be stored somewhere safe, for example a room or cupboard with adjustable, washable shelving. Liquids should be stored in plastic bottles if possible to prevent breakage, and large or heavy items should be stored on the lower shelves. The most frequently used stock should be placed at eye level to prevent unnecessary bending or stretching. New stock must always be placed behind existing stock to ensure it is used in the correct order.

Case
Studies

Case studies

Each of the case studies that follows includes a brief personal profile of the client, their main concerns and how often they attended for treatment. Details of visual assessment and the main reflexes (MR) and associated reflexes (AR) which are of most benefit to the client have been listed. The lifestyle changes that were discussed and the treatment outcomes have also been noted. A complete reflexology treatment was carried out at each session with special attention to the main reflexes and associated reflexes at each visit, depending upon the feedback from the client after each session.

These are followed by two additional case studies (Client 4 and Client 5) that students can attempt to complete from the information provided.

Client 1

The client is twenty years of age, lives at home with her parents and suffers with **eczema** on the face, hands, elbows and behind the knees. Her doctor has prescribed a steroid cream, which she is unhappy about using, as it will thin the skin. She cannot eat strawberries as they cause her **skin to itch**, or be exposed to horses and dogs, as this makes her **eyes water** and become **swollen**. There is a family history of asthma, eczema, hay fever and metal allergies. She has **painful periods** and finds it **difficult to lose weight** as she favours fast foods, fizzy drinks and sweets.

Regularity of reflexology treatment

One each week for six weeks.

Visual assessment

A yellow colour in the lung and intestinal areas with hard skin on the ball of the foot in the thyroid area.

Reflexes

Condition	MR	AR
Eczema	Face, hands, and elbow and knee joints	Pituitary gland, to help balance hormones Adrenals, to help counteract itching Lymphatics, kidneys and the intestines, to help detoxify Solar plexus, to calm and relax
Allergy	Eyes and sinuses, to help with the congestion in the area Head and the respiratory system	Adrenal glands for the anti-inflammatory effect Upper lymphatics and large intestine to detoxify
Painful periods	Ovaries, fallopian tubes and uterus	Pituitary, to help balance hormones Adrenals, to help in balancing fluid Lumbar spine and pelvic area, to help minimise pain Solar plexus, to induce relaxation
Weight	Thyroid and parathyroids, liver and digestive system, to aid metabolism	Kidneys and lymphatic system for elimination.

Lifestyle advice

Avoid the irritants which cause the eczema and allergic responses and use oil of evening primrose oil on the eczema. Try to eat more fresh fruit, vegetables, salads and cut down on fatty fast foods and sweet sugary drinks, and replace with water. Suggest supplementing her diet with a beneficial drink containing natural bacteria to balance the digestive system.

Treatment outcomes

This client was able to discontinue using the steroid creams as after two sessions the eczema had cleared on the face and was less evident in the other areas. The itching had subsided and a concerted effort had been made to improve the diet, although little weight was lost she had increased energy levels. There was a noticeable improvement in the colour of the feet.

Client 2

The client is seventeen years of age, outwardly very fit and healthy but has a serious kidney complaint, **glomerular nephritis**, which was triggered by a severe throat infection when he was twelve. The condition was treated with oral steroids over a period of eighteen months, but it resulted in **damage to the kidneys** and there have been two much less severe re-occurrences in the last two years, both triggered by **throat infections**.

He has a **sporting injury** to his right **shoulder** caused when it was **dislocated** in a rugby tackle. This prevents a full range of movement and is painful when knocked. He has recently had ultrasound and sports massage to relieve the symptoms and is on a waiting list to have an operation to repair the damage and restore normal movement in the joint. He lives at home but has a busy social life and does not eat at normal meal times, often snacking rather than eating well balanced meals. He finds it difficult to sleep and equally difficult to get up in the morning. This is a problem as he has recently started his first full time job.

Regularity of treatment

Weekly sessions for six weeks.

Visual assessment

Grey pallor over the kidney reflex and puffiness in the bladder and ureter.

Reflexes

Condition	MR	AR
Nephritis	Urinary system and circulatory system, to maintain optimum functioning of the urinary system	Lumbar spine and lymphatic system, to maintain elimination
Throat infections	Throat, eyes, ears and sinuses	Lymphatic system and kidneys, helps elimination and boosts the immune system Adrenals, to reduce inflammation and cervical spine
Dislocated shoulder	Shoulder joint and cervical spine, to aid mobility and ease pain	Kidneys, adrenals and lymphatics, to improve elimination and reduce inflammation

Lifestyle advice

Try to balance social and work life more and improve eating habits by having regular meals to include more fresh fruit, vegetables and fibre.

Treatment outcomes

General feeling of well-being, slightly easier movement in the shoulder joint after three weeks and less pain in the area.

He has decided to have a treatment every four weeks to maintain balance in his immune and urinary systems, as his goal in the long term is to prevent a recurrence of the glomerular nephritis.

Client 3

This client is 41 years old, single and a dedicated career woman, working long hours in a **stressful** environment, managing large numbers of people, in a job which requires exceptional communication skills, tact and diplomacy. She has suffered from **endometriosis** for nearly fifteen years, which now causes severe pain for at least two weeks out of every month. She also had **one ovary removed** after the formation of a blood cyst fourteen years ago. Bowel movements are erratic and she has lower back pain and spasmodic abdominal pain.

She feels **tired and run down** and has recently suffered an **outbreak of spots** on her face. She has had skin care treatments but they have not cleared. Her periods have become very painful and heavy and are lasting for up to two weeks at a time, and the last one was four weeks. Her diet is mainly organic vegetarian food as she is following a special diet which has been recommended to reduce the painful symptoms of her endometriosis. She has limited free time for relaxation but occasionally does aerobic exercise and weight training to improve her fitness level.

Regularity of treatment

Can only attend once a week due to work commitments. Treatments were booked for a period of eight weeks.

Visual assessment

Swelling in the reproductive area, sluggish and yellow in colour in the intestine area with tightness in the region of the coccyx.

Reflexes

Condition	MR	AR
Stress	Solar plexus, to induce relaxation	Brain, pituitary, lungs, diaphragm, adrenals
Endometriosis	Reproductive and endocrine systems	Large and small intestines
Tiredness	Pituitary, pineal, adrenal glands	Kidneys and large intestines
Blemished skin	Endocrine system	Liver, kidneys and large intestine, for detoxifying Adrenal glands, for anti-inflammatory effects

Lifestyle advice

To cut out dairy products and replace with soya to ease endometriosis. Take up a relaxing form of exercise such as yoga. Speak to GP about the recurring spots on her face and the problems she has with her menstrual cycle. Use essential oils to revitalise such as bergamot, camomile to aid digestion and abdominal spasms, and palmarosa for relaxation.

Treatment outcomes

After the first treatment she suffered with headaches and nausea. By the third treatment she was feeling less stressed and much more relaxed, so increased her treatments to twice a week for two weeks. Her GP sent her for a scan, which revealed a cyst on her remaining ovary and arranged an appointment to see her gynaecologist to discuss further treatment for the cyst and the endometriosis. The spots on her face had disappeared after six treatments and she felt 're-energised' as the pain in her ovary had subsided. Recommended maintenance treatments to provide longer lasting effects.

Additional case studies

Read the following case studies and decide how often the client should attend for treatment, which are the main reflexes to work, the associated reflexes, which will support them and any changes in lifestyle you can suggest.

Client 4

The client is a retired teacher, aged 76. She has **osteoporosis** and **arthritis of the spine**. The arthritis was a result of damage sustained during her teaching years, when a child inadvertently moved a low chair as she was sitting down and she fell heavily, jarring her spine. Four years ago she underwent surgery to remove her gall bladder. She suffers with **high blood pressure**, which can be erratic even though she is taking medication to control the condition. She lives alone, eats a well balanced diet, drinks approximately eight cups of tea a day and occasionally enjoys a glass of wine with her meal. She has recently complained of recurring bouts of **cystitis** and she complains of being constantly tired and has **difficulty sleeping** through the night, often waking three or four times after retiring to bed, often to go to the toilet. She has dry flaky skin on her feet with cracks around the heels. Both feet were pale in colour, lacking energy and quite frail. There was hard skin present in the lung area and the bladder area was hot, red and puffy.

Client 5

The client is a full-time hairdresser in her mid-thirties. She is married with two young children and her occupation requires her to be on her feet for most of the working day. She **smokes** 10–15 cigarettes a day and has a couple of glasses of alcohol with her evening meal. Her mother recently died from **bowel cancer** and several other close relatives have suffered with this condition. She has suffered with **asthma** since the birth of her second child three years ago and has recently developed late onset **acne**, which flares up and becomes very sensitive at certain times. For many years she has suffered from **constipation** and **irritable bowel syndrome**, trying all forms of diet and medication with little success. She is trying to lose weight and is following a low carbohydrate diet and takes antioxidant vitamin supplements daily. Due to her busy lifestyle she is unable to take much exercise; she does, however, attend a yoga class one night a week.

Her main concerns are the high incidence of bowel cancer in her immediate family, the condition of her skin and her difficulty in losing weight. Most recently she has been suffering from **premenstrual tension** and the doctor has prescribed hormone tablets to help this condition. She has hard skin in the ball of the foot and it is yellow in colour over the lung area.

For each case study or case history completed for your portfolio of evidence you will need:

- A detailed personal profile of the client.
- A detailed consultation record (see Chapter 2).
- Details of the visual assessment (see Chapter 7).
- A record of findings during treatment.
- Immediate feedback from the client.
- To write up notes and decide on a plan of action.
- Feedback prior to next session, and on the basis of this information indicate any changes from original action plan.
- Colour photographs of the client's feet.

Appendices

Code of practice

Any organisation or professional association will have a code of practice which sets down rules of conduct for their members to follow.

A professional reflexologist who works to high standards and acknowledges the importance of good client care will follow their own industry's code of practice and abide by any rules laid down by the organisation that they are a member of.

The reflexologist should:

- Be proficient in the practice of reflexology for the benefit of the client, working in a competent manner and within the limits of the training received.
- Ensure the comfort and welfare of the client at all times.
- Develop a professional client–therapist relationship and ensure client confidentiality, except where disclosure is required by law.
- Provide accurate details of price of treatments.
- Respect all the religious, spiritual, political and social views of the client.
- Refuse to give a reflexology treatment when it is not appropriate, in a professional and courteous manner.
- Report infectious disease to the appropriate authority and advise clients to seek medical advice when necessary.
- Co-operate with medical practitioners, health care professionals and other complementary therapists.
- Maintain accurate and up-to-date client records.
- Constantly update the skills required and continue their professional development in all areas. This may include practical skills, business and communication skills or updating knowledge of health matters.
- Provide insurance against public liability and malpractice.
- Adhere to the local bylaws in relation to the business.

The reflexologist should *not*:

- Prescribe, diagnose, or make claims to cure.
- Mislead the client in any way.
- Discredit fellow reflexologists or attract business unfairly or in an unprofessional manner.
- Use advertisements for the business that do not follow the British Code of Advertising Practice.

Membership of an association is helpful in maintaining professional links with others in the same industry. It allows practitioners to share information and good practise as well as discussing relevant issues at regular meetings. It also provides the opportunity for associations from different countries to maintain a world-wide link for the benefit of all members.

Addresses of professional associations and organisations

Europe

Association of Reflexologists
27 Old Gloucester Street
London WC1N 3XX
Tel. 08705 673320
www.aor.org.uk

British Reflexology Association
Monks Orchard
Whitbourne
Worcester WR6 5RB
Tel. 01886 821207
www.britreflex.co.uk

Federation of Holistic Therapists
3rd Floor
Eastleigh House
Upper Market Street
Eastleigh
Hampshire
SO50 9FD
Tel. 023 8048 8900
www.fht.org.uk

Holistic Association of Reflexologists
The Holistic Healing Centre
92 Sheering Road
Old Harlow
Essex CM17 OJW
Tel. 01279 429060
www.footreflexology.com

Institute of Complementary Medicine
PO Box 194
London
SE16 7QZ
Tel. 0207 237 5165
www.icmedicine.co.uk

International Institute of Reflexology (UK)
255 Turleigh
Bradford on Avon
Wiltshire
BA15 2HG
Tel. 01225 865899
www.reflexology-uk.co.uk

Irish Reflexologists' Institute
3 Blackglen Court
Lambs Cross
Sandyford
Dublin
Ireland

Scottish Institute of Reflexology
6/1 Minto Place
Hawick
Roxburghshire
TD9 9JL
Tel. 01450 373125

Society of Reflexologists
39 Prestbury Road
Cheltenham
Gloucester
GL52 2PT
Tel. 01242 512601

International

International Council of Reflexologists
PO Box 30513
Richmond Hill
Ontario L4COC7
Canada
www.icr-reflexology.org/

International Institute of Reflexology
5650 First Avenue North
PO Box 12642
St Petersburg
Florida 33733-2642
USA

Reflexology Association of America
4012 S. Rainbow Boulevard
Box K585
Las Vegas
Nevada 89103-2059
USA

Reflexology Association of Australia
National Enquiries
PO Box 366
Cammeray NSW 2062
New South Wales
Australia
www.reflexology.org.au/

Reflexology Association of Canada
#201-17930 105 Avenue
Edmonton
Alberta T5S 2H5
Canada
www.reflexologycanada.ca

South African Reflexology Society
PO Box 1780
New Germany 3620
South Africa
www.sareflexology.org.za

Assessment guidance for the VTCT Diploma in Reflexology

To achieve this diploma you will be assessed over a period of time with the assessor using different methods of assessment.

Assessment will consist of:

Observation of practical skills to ensure that the treatment performed is fully competent, can be adapted to suit each individual client and is repeatable, thus complying with current professional standards. Students will initially practise their skills on other members of their group and will then carry out treatments on individual clients in a realistic working environment. Over a period of time the student will be expected to treat a range of clients, having different objectives and achieving different outcomes.

Oral questioning to assess understanding. Questions will be asked after practical observation rather than during the treatment, to allow the student to complete the treatment without disturbance. These questions may include current health and safety legislation, hygiene, preventing cross infection, the correct appearance of a professional reflexologist and contraindications. You may also be asked about treatment objectives and the importance of consultation with your client when formulating a treatment plan. Questions will also be asked about reflex areas and their location, your conclusions after assessing individual clients and aftercare advice, and any issue which may have been highlighted during treatment.

Written assessments to ensure the student has the underpinning knowledge required to support the performance of practical skills. These assessments are devised by each individual training centre and may be divided into specific subject areas such as anatomy and physiology, consultation, treatment practice and aftercare advice, and locating reflex points and areas.

Written assignments and research projects may be set to assist the student in developing specific skills, collating useful information or improving knowledge. These may include market research for a new business, putting together a business plan, improving and expanding an existing business or explaining the necessary steps in operating a successful business.

Portfolio of evidence

The student, with the help of the assessor, will develop a portfolio of evidence to show competence. This will include records of practical competence with supporting consultation records, treatment plans, aftercare advice and feedback from clients and tutors. Results of written assessments and written assignments will also be included and any case studies completed during the course undertaken. This evidence will then be approved by an internal verifier from the training establishment and by an external verifier from VTCT.

The responsibilities of the first aid representative

To assess a situation when it arises, identify the problem and take immediate and appropriate action. This may include removing the person from a dangerous position, calling for medical assistance and arranging transport to the doctor or hospital if the condition so requires, dealing with a minor problem when it occurs or providing reassurance to the injured/ill person whilst waiting for medical help to arrive. When dealing with a problem it is important to be prepared, have the essential first aid equipment and materials available and ensure any open cuts on your own hands are well covered with waterproof dressings. Always wash your hands before and after touching the injured person to prevent cross infection and, if necessary, wear waterproof disposable gloves.

It is inevitable that, even in the safest environment, accidents may occur which will require attention from the qualified member of staff. These may include:

Problem	Treatment
Minor burns and scalds caused by dry or wet heat	Cool the area by immersing in or running under cold water. Cover with a sterile dressing. Remove rings, watches or constricting clothing before swelling occur. Cover with a sterile non-fluffy dressing. Do NOT use adhesive dressings, apply lotions or cream or pierce blisters.
Chemical burns that may be caused by undiluted chemicals	Flush with lots of cold water, remove any clothing which may have chemicals on it and cover the area with a sterile dressing. Arrange transport to hospital as soon as possible.
Chemicals in the eye	Must be washed out with a large amount of cold water, preferably sterile water, from an eye irrigator. Cover the eye lightly with a sterile pad and remove to hospital as soon as possible.
Asthmatic attack	Reassure and calm the person, sit them up in a comfortable position, leaning forward slightly, resting on a table or back of a chair. Allow them to take their medication if it is available. Seek medical advice in severe cases.
Cuts or wounds	For a minor cut, clean around the wound with warm water and mild antiseptic, apply slight pressure over a pad of sterile gauze and any bleeding should stop.
Fainting	If feeling faint, sit the person down, leaning slightly forward with their head between the knees, supporting them and advising them to take deep breaths. If unconscious, lie them down with legs slightly raised to stimulate blood flow to the brain or place in the recovery position if there is difficulty in breathing, to maintain an open airway.

N.B. Never provide drinks. If necessary, moisten the lips with a little water as anything ingested may prevent or delay the subsequent administration of anaesthetic.

There are certain conditions which may require immediate medical treatment and it is important to recognise the symptoms.

Heart attack

Sudden crushing pain in the chest which may spread to the arms, sudden dizziness, ashen skin with blue lips, profuse sweating and breathlessness. The pulse may be fast but weak and sometimes irregular, and the person may become unconscious.

Angina pectoris

The symptoms are a pain in the chest often spreading down the left shoulder to the arm. The skin may look ashen and the lips may be blue, and shortness of breath may occur accompanied by a general weakness.

Stroke

This may begin with a sudden severe headache and the person may become disorientated, confused and anxious. There may be a full, pounding pulse and the person may become giddy or unconscious. In more severe cases there may be paralysis of the mouth, weakness of the limbs, unequal pupil dilation and loss of bladder and/or bowel control.

When someone has suffered with shock, reassure and comfort them, and cover them with a blanket to keep warm.

Hand Reflexology

There is some evidence from old Chinese writing that a type of pressure therapy and exercises involving wringing the hands were used to benefit the body. In more recent years Dr William Fitzgerald worked the reflex points on the hands and only later on the feet.

What is hand reflexology?

Hand reflexology works in the same way as foot reflexology. You will use the same techniques as the foot when working the reflex points on the hand, and provide a full treatment covering all the systems.

It may be used when the reflexologist is unable to treat the feet. This might be, for example, when a client has a contraindication, severe damage to the foot or amputation. It may also be used for self-reflexology treatment, as hands are more accessible than the feet. Giving hand reflexology is also more flexible in terms of place of treatment; it can be carried out at any place or any time (within reason!).

Applying pressure to specific reflex points may help to relieve stress or tension and to treat specific ailments in between treatments. The effects are the same as foot reflexology but the area treated is smaller and the reflex points are more condensed.

Client care

Client care and consideration is just as important with hand reflexology as foot reflexology. Make sure your client is warm and comfortable with the hand and arm well supported so he or she can be completely relaxed whilst receiving the treatment.

Anatomy of the hand and wrist

Bones

The wrist consists of eight irregularly shaped bones called the carpal bones, which are roughly arranged in two rows of four. These bones are scaphoid, lunate, triquetral, pisiform, trapezium, trapezoid, capitate and hamate. There are five metacarpals, the long bones of the palm of the hand, and fourteen phalanges, the bones that make up the fingers, three in each finger and two in the thumb.

Muscles

The muscles that move the wrist and hand are located on the forearms. The anterior muscles are flexors and the posterior muscles are extensors, and each group is divided into superficial and deep muscles. Each muscle has a tendon, which attaches to the wrist or continues into the hand and fingers helping to produce movement. The main muscles of the hand are the thenar and hypothenar eminences and they are situated on the palmar surface of the hand.

Nail disorders

Recognising some nail disorders and knowing their possible cause can help the reflexologist to determine when physical or emotional problems may be present. Some common disorders include the following:

White spots or leuconychia is a common condition of the nails and may be caused by injury to the base of the nail causing a tiny air pocket to form between the nail bed and the nail plate.

Horizontal and vertical lines are superficial ridges in the nail plate caused by uneven growth and may be the result of illness. They may also appear if there is a general lack of fats in the diet as the nails become very dry and dehydrated.

Ridges or deep furrows in the nail plate may be caused by a nutritional disorder, injury to the matrix, or illness. Sometimes a nervous habit of constantly rubbing the cuticle produces friction in the area of the matrix (the area of mitosis or cell reproduction) and causes a deep ridge to form, which will continue up the nail plate until it reaches the free edge.

Blue nails are a characteristic of poor circulation and in some cases may be attributed to a heart disorder.

Koilonychia is a condition that causes the nail plate to grow in a spoon shape and appear concave. It is caused by an accumulation of horny cells at the sides of the nail plate, under the nail wall, or an abnormal growth stemming from the matrix. The causes are an inherited abnormality, a side effect of a certain type of anaemia, or an over-active thyroid.

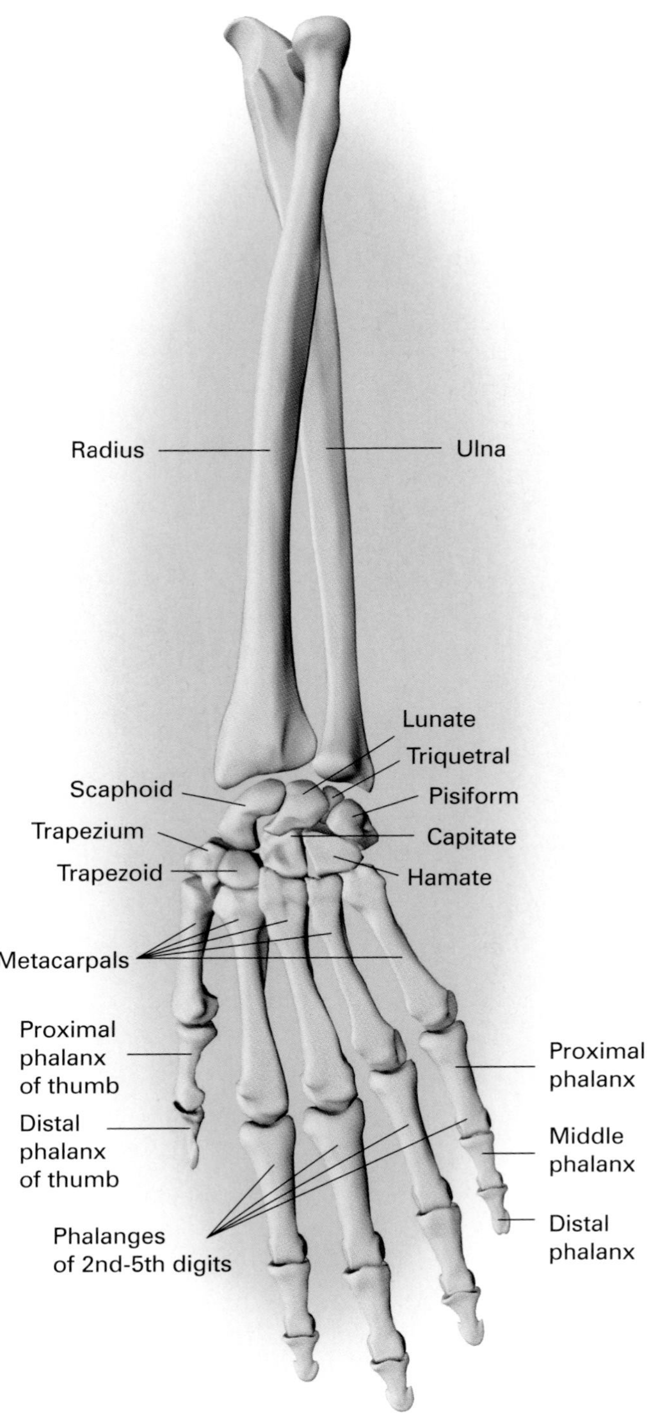

The bones of the wrist and hand

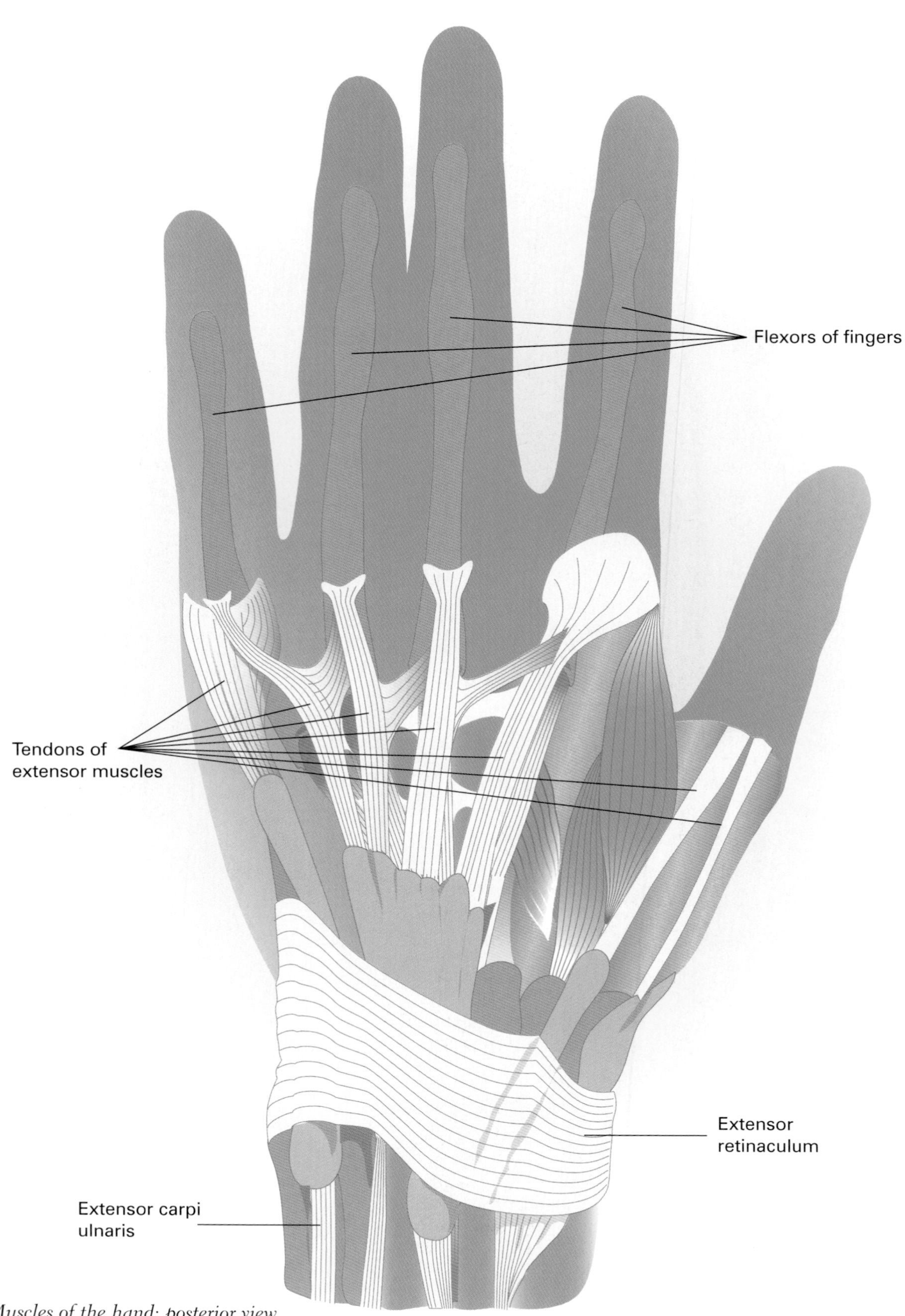

Muscles of the hand: posterior view

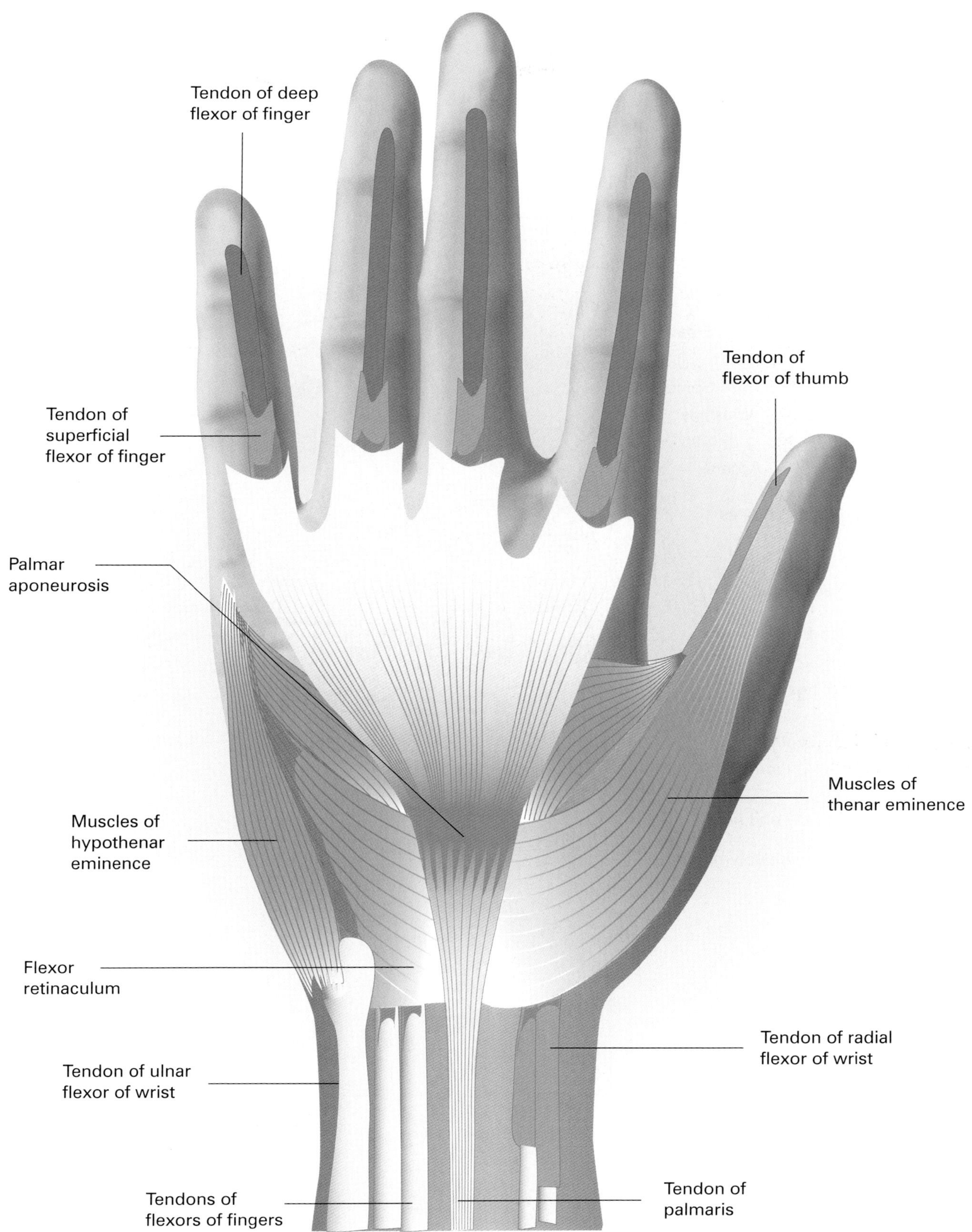
Tendon of deep flexor of finger
Tendon of flexor of thumb
Tendon of superficial flexor of finger
Palmar aponeurosis
Muscles of thenar eminence
Muscles of hypothenar eminence
Flexor retinaculum
Tendon of radial flexor of wrist
Tendon of ulnar flexor of wrist
Tendons of flexors of fingers
Tendon of palmaris

Muscles of the hand: anterior view

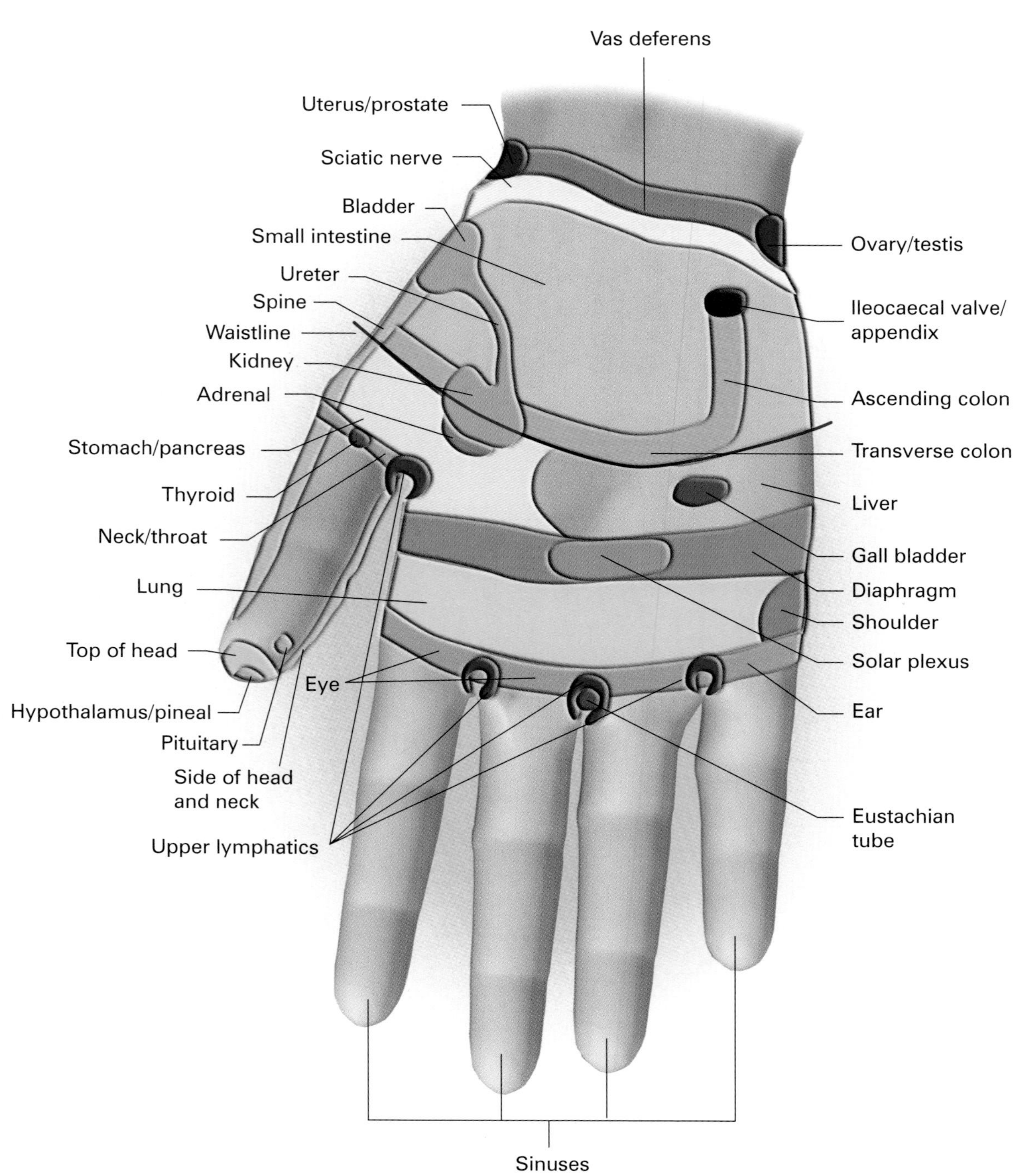
Vas deferens
Uterus/prostate
Sciatic nerve
Bladder
Small intestine
Ureter
Spine
Waistline
Kidney
Adrenal
Stomach/pancreas
Thyroid
Neck/throat
Lung
Top of head
Hypothalamus/pineal
Pituitary
Side of head and neck
Upper lymphatics
Eye
Ovary/testis
Ileocaecal valve/ appendix
Ascending colon
Transverse colon
Liver
Gall bladder
Diaphragm
Shoulder
Solar plexus
Ear
Eustachian tube
Sinuses

Reflex areas on the palm of the rught hand

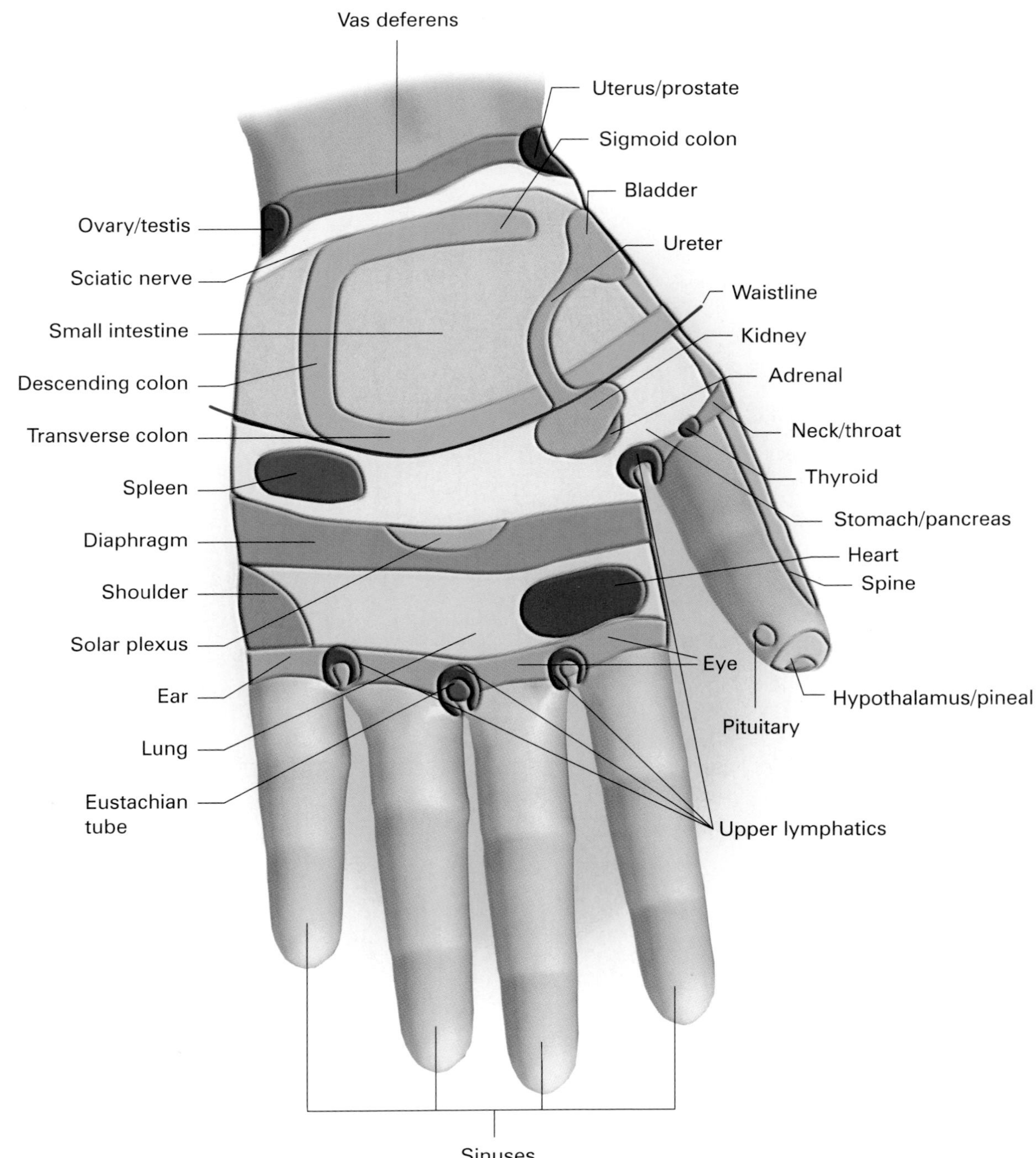

Reflex areas on the palm of the left hand

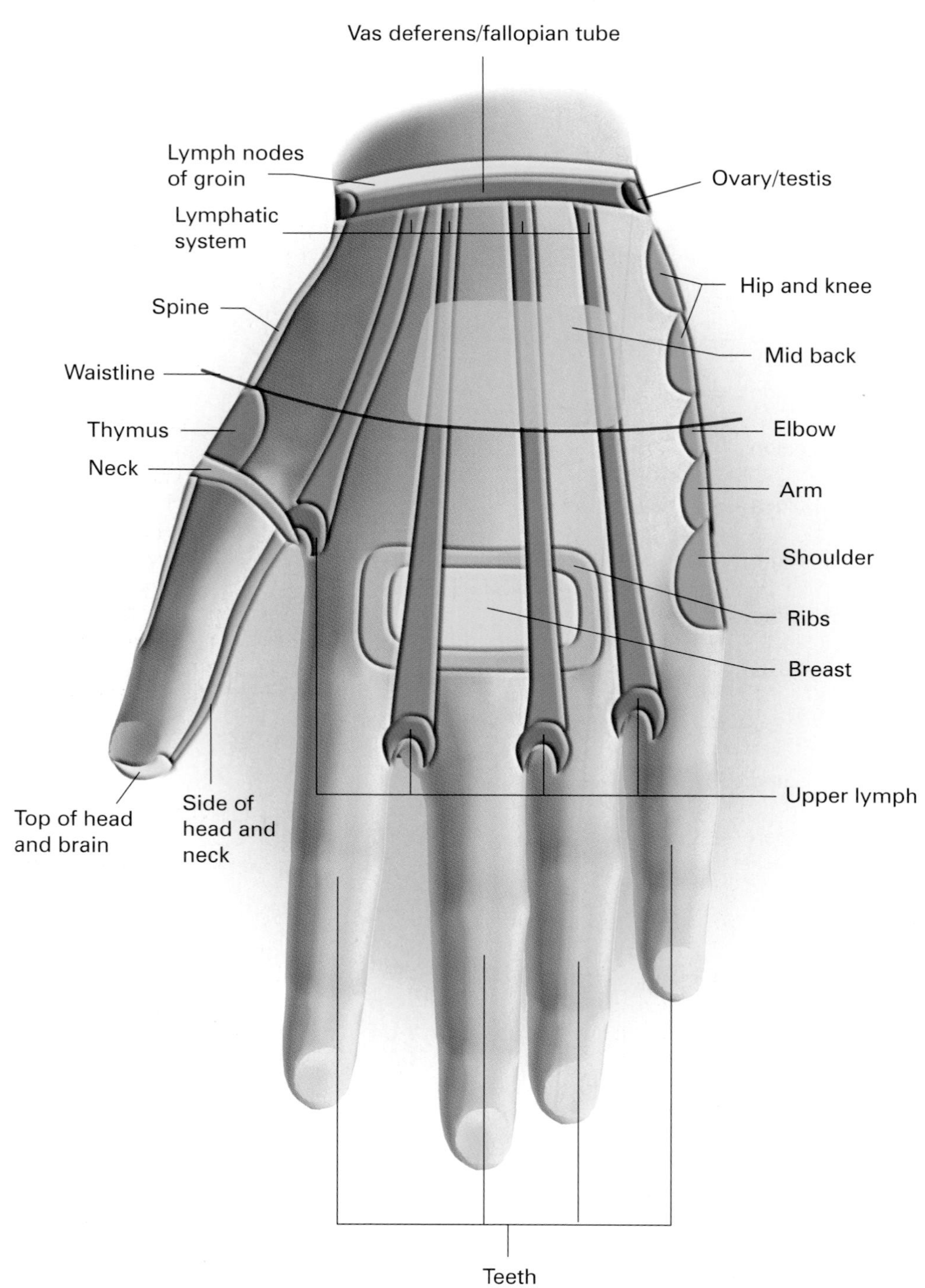

Reflex areas on the back of the hand

Index

S

T

U

V

W

Y

Z